Carcinogens and Anticarcinogens in the Human Diet

A Comparison of Naturally Occurring and Synthetic Substances

Committee on Comparative Toxicity of
Naturally Occurring Carcinogens
Board on Environmental Studies and Toxicology
Commission on Life Sciences
National Research Council

NATIONAL ACADEMY PRESS
Washington, D.C.   1996

NATIONAL ACADEMY PRESS   2101 Constitution Ave., N.W.   Washington, D.C. 20418

NOTICE: The project that is the subject of this report was approved by the Governing Board of the National Research Council, whose members are drawn from the councils of the National Academy of Sciences, the National Academy of Engineering, and the Institute of Medicine. The members of the committee responsible for the report were chosen for their special competences and with regard for appropriate balance.

This report has been reviewed by a group other than the authors according to procedures approved by a Report Review Committee consisting of members of the National Academy of Sciences, the National Academy of Engineering, and the Institute of Medicine.

The National Academy of Sciences is a private, nonprofit, self-perpetuating society of distinguished scholars engaged in scientific and engineering research, dedicated to the furtherance of science and technology and to their use for the general welfare. Upon the authority of the charter granted to it by the Congress in 1863, the Academy has a mandate that requires it to advise the federal government on scientific and technical matters. Dr. Bruce Alberts is president of the National Academy of Sciences.

The National Academy of Engineering was established in 1964, under the charter of the National Academy of Sciences, as a parallel organization of outstanding engineers. It is autonomous in its administration and in the selection of its members, sharing with the National Academy of Sciences the responsibility for advising the federal government. The National Academy of Engineering also sponsors engineering programs aimed at meeting national needs, encourages education and research, and recognizes the superior achievements of engineers. Dr. Harold Liebowitz is president of the National Academy of Engineering.

The Institute of Medicine was established in 1970 by the National Academy of Sciences to secure the services of eminent members of appropriate professions in the examination of policy matters pertaining to the health of the public. The Institute acts under the responsibility given to the National Academy of Sciences by its congressional charter to be an adviser to the federal government and, upon its own initiative, to identify issues of medical care, research, and education. Dr. Kenneth I. Shine is president of the Institute of Medicine.

The National Research Council was organized by the National Academy of Sciences in 1916 to associate the broad community of science and technology with the Academy's purposes of furthering knowledge and advising the federal government. Functioning in accordance with general policies determined by the Academy, the Council has become the principal operating agency of both the National Academy of Sciences and the National Academy of Engineering in providing services to the government, the public, and the scientific and engineering communities. The Council is administered jointly by both Academies and the Institute of Medicine. Dr. Bruce Alberts and Dr. Harold Liebowitz are chairman and vice chairman, respectively, of the National Research Council.

The project was supported by the National Institute for Environmental Health Sciences, U.S. Environmental Protection Agency, the National Cancer Institute, and the U.S. Food and Drug Administration under contract no. NO1-ES-25355, and by the American Industrial Health Council and Nabisco Foods.

Library of Congress Catalog Card No. 95-73149
International Standard Book No. 0-309-05391-9

Additional copies of this report are available from the National Academy Press, Box 285, Washington, DC 20055.

Printed in the United States of America

First Printing, February 1996
Second Printing, October 1996

COMMITTEE ON COMPARATIVE TOXICITY OF NATURALLY OCCURRING CARCINOGENS

RONALD W. ESTABROOK *(Chair)*, Southwestern Medical Center, University of Texas, Dallas, Tex.

DIANE BIRT, University of Nebraska Medical Center, Omaha, Neb.

GARY P. CARLSON, Purdue University, West Lafayette, Ind.

SAMUEL M. COHEN, University of Nebraska Medical Center, Omaha, Neb.

ERIC E. CONN, University of California, Davis, Calif.

NORMAN R. FARNSWORTH, College of Pharmacy, University of Illinois at Chicago, Chicago, Ill.

DAVID W. GAYLOR, U.S. Food and Drug Administration, Jefferson, Ark.

RICHARD L. HALL, Baltimore, Md.

JOHN HIGGINSON, Bethesda, Md.

ERNEST HODGSON, North Carolina State University, Raleigh, N.C.

LAURENCE N. KOLONEL, Cancer Research Center, University of Hawaii, Honolulu, Hawaii

DANIEL KREWSKI, Health Canada, Ottawa, Ontario, Canada

CHARLENE A. MCQUEEN, University of Arizona, College of Pharmacy, Tucson, Ariz.

MICHAEL W. PARIZA, University of Wisconsin - Madison, Madison, Wisc.

JANARDAN K. REDDY, Northwestern University Medical School, Chicago, Ill.

I. GLENN SIPES, University of Arizona, College of Pharmacy, Tucson, Ariz.

Staff

JAMES J. REISA, Director

DAVID J. POLICANSKY, Associate Director and Program Director for Natural Resources and Applied Ecology

CAROL A. MACZKA, Program Director for Toxicology and Risk Assessment

LEE R. PAULSON, Program Director for Information Systems and Statistics

RAYMOND A. WASSEL, Program Director for Environmental Sciences and Engineering

OTHER RECENT REPORTS OF THE
BOARD ON ENVIRONMENTAL STUDIES AND TOXICOLOGY

Copies of these reports may be ordered from the National Academy Press: (800) 624-6242 or (202) 334-3313

Preface

Numerous reports, including some from the National Research Council, have examined the relationship of diet to cancer. It is generally accepted that diet is a contributing factor to the onset or progression of some types of cancer and that a prudent selection of foods, including fruits and vegetables, and avoidance or decreased consumption of other foods might influence the risk to an individual of contracting cancer. But can specific chemicals in our diet be identified as causative agents (carcinogens) or protective agents (anticarcinogens) for cancer? Some naturally occurring chemicals that are part of our diet have been shown in animal models to cause cancer—and therefore might also serve as potential cancer-causative agents in humans. Almost daily, the news media report on the presence of one chemical or another that is claimed to be carcinogenic. Many of these are naturally occurring chemicals. The public is bombarded with reports that raise fear and apprehension.

To make a rational estimate of the risk associated with the diet one must know the level of exposure as well as the carcinogenic potency of a suspected chemical. That basic principle of toxicology is sometimes offset by the belief (often associated with the Delany amendment) that the presence of a potentially hazardous chemical at even minuscule concentrations is dangerous. In addition, the credibility of such a conclusion often depends on the validity of the test used to identify a specific chemical as a carcinogen. Many of the data used in this report are based on studies using the rodent bioassay, where tests are carried out at high exposure levels. The ability to relate results obtained using rodent bioassays to the risk for humans—who are exposed to low levels of a chemical in a complex mixture, such as the diet—is a weakness that puts into question how the results of such evaluations are applied.

This committee has labored diligently and long as it studied, debated, reargued, and wrote the different facets of what some might consider a complex problem that is unsolvable.

As we submit this report we recognize that some readers will look for the identification of a single causative agent to remove from the diet. Others will seek evidence of a panacea—a chemical that will shield them against the causative agents of cancer. Both groups will be disappointed. As the report indicates, we need to know much more than we know today before we can speak with greater certainty about the role of chemicals in the diet as contributors to the burden of cancer in the human population. Such information will come only by continued research, new hypotheses, and a clearer understanding of human biology.

The ability to complete a report of this complexity requires a dedicated staff. We are indebted to efforts and technical expertise of J. David Sandler, project director; Linda V. Leonard, senior project assistant; Carol A. Maczka, program director; Gail Charnley and Richard Thomas (program directors during the early stages of the project); and James J. Reisa, director of the Board on Environmental Studies and Toxicology.

Many distinguished scientists met with the committee and shared their ideas, findings, and interpretations, including: Richard Adamson (National Cancer Institute), Bruce Ames (University of California), Victor Feron (Toxicology and Nutrition Institute, the Netherlands), Adam Finkel (Resources for the Future), Ronald Hart (National Center for Toxicological Research), Donald Hughes (American Industrial Health Council), Richard Jackson (California Department of Health Services), David

Longfellow (National Cancer Institute), Richard Merrill (University of Virginia), Hugh McKinnon (Environmental Protection Agency), Gerard Mulder (Center for Bio-Pharmaceutical Sciences, Sylvius Laboratories, the Netherlands), David Rall, Robert Scheuplein (Food and Drug Administration), Sidney Siegel (National Library of Medicine), and Lee Wattenberg (University of Minnesota). Some of these individuals' affiliations have changed since they provided input to the committee. Our sincere thanks to them for providing guideposts that served to mark the path of progress as the committee deliberated specific issues.

Each member of this committee deserves praise and congratulations for his or her wisdom, dedication, perception, and friendship. Although many sessions were exhausting, the high level of interest of each member made this exercise a rewarding and productive experience. Thanks to each and everyone of you for all your good work.

Ronald W. Estabrook
Chairman

Contents

Executive Summary

From earliest times people have been aware that some plants are poisonous and should be avoided as food. Other plants contain chemicals that have medicinal, stimulatory, hallucinatory, or narcotic effects. The Romans were among the first to enact laws that, over time, have been developed to protect the public from food adulteration, contamination, false labeling, spoilage, and the harmful effects of chemicals added to foods and beverages.

In the past 50 years, great strides have been made in understanding nutrition and the role it plays in human health. This same period has seen vast improvements in the safety and diversity of the diet in the United States, with technological advances in preservation and shipment of foods, and the ability to identify and reduce various food hazards. U.S. laws regulate the safety of the food we eat and the water we drink. Federal agencies, such as the Food and Drug Administration, Department of Agriculture, and Environmental Protection Agency, as well as many state and local agencies, are charged with interpreting and enforcing these laws. As a result, the food supply in the United States is widely recognized as safe, economical, and of high quality, variety, and abundance.

Despite these efforts, concerns remain that some dietary components may contribute to the burden of cancer in humans. For example, the use of pesticides continues to be watched closely, because of indirect exposures of the general public through trace amounts in the food supply (as well as direct exposures of agricultural workers). Yet, by controlling insect vectors, pesticides have

1

profoundly decreased the spread of human diseases, and pesticide usage has increased agricultural yields.

Plants have evolved chemicals that serve as defensive agents against predators. These chemicals may be present in the diet in amounts exceeding the residues of synthetic pesticides used to enhance agricultural productivity. Ames et al. contend that the percentage of naturally occurring chemicals testing positive for carcinogenicity in rodent bioassays does not differ significantly from the percentage of synthetic chemicals testing positive, and that these proportions are likely to hold for untested agents, leading to their conclusion that the cancer risk from natural chemicals in the diet might be greater than that from synthetics. There are, after all, many more naturally occurring chemicals than synthetic. In fact, although the number of naturally occurring compounds in the human diet is certainly far greater than synthetic compounds, the implications concerning health risks—particularly impact on cancer in humans—remain controversial. In addition, it should be noted that synthetic chemicals are highly regulated while natural chemicals are not. This report addresses several elements of this controversy, including the relevance of animal bioassays (including those using the maximum tolerated dose) for identifying human dietary carcinogens, the adequacy and availability of human exposure data, and the complexity of the human diet.

Since the 1930s, scientists have recognized that the occurrence of certain cancers may be related to substances in the diet or to patterns of food consumption. They have also recognized that some chemical constituents of food—either initially present in the food, formed during preparation (especially cooking), or added for preservation or presentation—are capable of inducing tumors in high-dose rodent tests. Many of the early studies on chemicals that cause cancer were carried out to determine what levels of exposure to specific chemicals, such as polycyclic aromatic hydrocarbons (PAHs) and certain food colors, such as butter yellow (N,N-dimethyl-4-amino-azobenzene), resulted in the formation of cancers in the liver and gastrointestinal tract of rodents. Later it was recognized that a number of naturally occurring chemicals present in some foods, such as mycotoxins (chemicals produced by fungi that often contaminate grains and nuts) and plant alkaloids, could also cause cancer in experimental animals. These findings have stimulated research to better understand the health consequences of naturally occurring chemicals found in our diet.

Doll and Peto, in their 1981 review, concluded that 10% to 70% of human cancer mortality in the U.S. is attributable to the diet, with the most likely figure being about 35%. Epidemiologic studies linking the aforementioned mycotoxins to human liver cancer provide convincing evidence that some constituents of foods can cause cancer. Less firmly established, however, is the contribution to human cancer of other naturally occurring chemicals present at low levels in the food we eat. In addition, the diet is a source of calories derived from fats, carbohydrates, and proteins. Calories and macronutrients (principally fat and oxidation products of fatty acids) in excess of body needs serve as an important risk factor that can contribute to the processes of tumor formation and growth. The observations of Doll and Peto are based on statistical and epidemiologic data which many regard as inconclusive. It is important to note that diet also plays a role in protecting against cancer, since diets rich in fruits and vegetables have been associated with reduced rates of cancer. Although dietary factors are certainly involved in carcinogenesis, the percent of cancer attributable to diet has remained uncertain.

THE CHARGE TO THE COMMITTEE

This report was prepared by the Committee on Comparative Toxicity of Naturally Occurring Carcinogens, which was convened in 1993 by the National Research Council upon the recommendation of its Board on Environmental Studies and Toxicology. The committee was charged to "examine the occurrence, toxicologic data, mechanisms of action, and potential role of natural carcinogens in the causation of cancer (in humans), including relative risk comparisons with synthetic carcinogens and a consideration of anticarcinogens." In addition, the committee was charged to assess "the impact of these materials (natural carcinogens) on initiation, promotion, and progression of tumors." Further, the committee was charged to "focus on the toxicologic information available for natural substances" and to "develop a strategy for selecting additional natural substances for toxicological testing."

In this report, the "initiation, promotion, and progression" stages of carcinogenesis were considered from a mechanistic point of view. However, most of the available carcinogenicity data on the compounds that were reviewed do not provide precise information on the specific stage or stages of the multistage process of carcinogenesis at which these compounds act. Since the terms initiator, promoter, and progressor are especially difficult to apply to specific agents, particularly as they pertain to human carcinogenesis, the committee chose primarily to discuss agents as being genotoxic or nongenotoxic. The committee viewed its charge to address toxicologic issues as limited to cancer.

For this report, the committee adopted the definition of a carcinogen proposed by the International Agency for Research on Cancer (IARC). IARC defines a carcinogen as any agent, the exposure to which increases the incidence of malignant neoplasia. It is recognized that many factors can influence the process of tumor formation and that the application of this definition does not always identify the influence of high dose levels of chemicals used in rodent testing, nor does it identify the uncertainties in extrapolating results from these rodent bioassays to much lower exposure/dose in humans. In this report, the term "exposure" means the amount of a synthetic or naturally occurring agent (including contaminants) ingested from the diet.

The number of naturally occurring chemicals present in the

food supply—or generated during the processes of growing, harvesting, storage, and preparation—is enormous, probably exceeding one million different chemicals. Actions of these chemicals in the complex mixture of our diet may be additive, synergistic, or inhibitory to one another. The observed level of a specific naturally occurring chemical in a food may vary greatly, because, in addition to actual variability, which often is great, such levels can be determined by analysis of the intact plant, analysis of the processed food as consumed, or determined as the form absorbed, distributed, and metabolized in the body for presentation at a target molecule. Further, the concentrations of such chemicals in plant and animal tissues used for food are highly variable, depending on the specific variety of the crop studied, the season of year tested, the geographic location and conditions of growth, the type of harvesting and storage used, etc. Intestinal microflora should also be recognized as important contributors to the availability of chemicals that might be carcinogens.

This report provides a perspective on the importance of chemicals in the diet, in terms of the magnitude of potential cancer risk from naturally occurring chemicals compared with that from synthetic chemical constituents. Also addressed are the protective effects of some chemicals (anticarcinogens) in the diet, which may reduce the risk associated with exposure to cancer-producing agents.

Conclusions

Several broad perspectives emerged from the committee's deliberations. First, the committee concluded that based upon existing exposure data, the great majority of individual naturally occurring and synthetic chemicals in the diet appears to be present at levels below which any significant adverse biologic effect is likely, and so low that they are unlikely to pose an appreciable cancer risk.

Much human experience suggests that the potential effects of dietary carcinogens are more likely to be realized when the specific foods in which they occur form too large a part of the diet. The varied and balanced diet needed for good nutrition also provides significant protection from natural toxicants. Increasing dietary fruit and vegetable intake may actually protect against cancer. The NRC report *Diet and Health* concluded that macronutrients and excess calories are likely the greatest contributors to dietary cancer risk in the United States.

Second, the committee concluded that natural components of the diet may prove to be of greater concern than synthetic components with respect to cancer risk, although additional evidence is required before definitive conclusions can be drawn. Existing concentration and exposure data and current cancer risk assessment methods are insufficient to definitively address the aggregate roles of naturally occurring and/or synthetic dietary chemicals in human cancer causation and prevention. Much of the information on the carcinogenic potential of these substances derives from animal bioassays conducted at high doses (up to the maximum tolerated dose, or MTD), which is difficult to translate directly to humans because these tests do not mimic human exposure conditions, i.e., we are exposed to an enormous complex of chemicals, many at exceedingly low quantities, in our diet. Furthermore, the committee concluded upon analyzing existing dietary exposure databases, that exposure data are either inadequate due to analytical or collection deficiencies, or simply nonexistent. In addition, through regulation, synthetic chemicals identified as carcinogens have largely been removed from or prevented from entering the human diet.

Third, the committee concluded that it is difficult to assess human cancer risk from individual natural or synthetic compounds in our diet because the diet is a complex mixture, and interactions between the components are largely unknown.

The committee's major conclusions are presented in detail below. They address the complexity and variability of the human diet, cancer risk from the diet, mechanisms and properties of synthetic vs. naturally occurring carcinogens, the role of anticarcinogens, and models for identifying dietary carcinogens and anticarcinogens.

Complexity of the Diet

• The human diet is a highly complex and variable mixture of naturally occurring and synthetic chemicals. Of these, the naturally occurring far exceed the synthetic in both number and quantity. The naturally occurring chemicals include macronutrients (fat, carbohydrate, and protein), micronutrients (vitamins and trace metals), and non-nutrient constituents. Only a small number of specific carcinogens and anticarcinogens in the human diet have been identified (e.g., aflatoxin). However, it seems unlikely that important carcinogens are yet to be identified. In part, this may reflect the limited number of studies performed.

• Human epidemiologic data indicate that diet contributes to a significant portion of cancer, but the precise components of diet responsible for increased cancer risk are generally not well understood.

Carcinogenicity and Anticarcinogenicity

• Current epidemiologic evidence suggests the importance of protective factors in the diet, such as those present in fruits and vegetables.

• Current evidence suggests that the contribution of excess macronutrients and excess calories to cancer causation in the United States outweighs that of individual food microchemicals, both natural and synthetic. This is not necessarily the case in other parts of the world.

• Epidemiologic data indicate that alcoholic beverages consumed in excess are associated with increased risk for specific types of cancer.

• Given the greater abundance of naturally occurring substances in the diet, the total exposure to naturally occurring carcinogens (in addition to excess calories and fat) exceeds the exposure to synthetic carcinogens. Regarding dietary exposure, the committee reviewed data, including those generated by the Department of Agriculture and the Department of Health and Human Services through the Nationwide Food Consumption Surveys, the National Health and Nutrition Examination Surveys, and other related data bases. However, data are insufficient to determine whether the dietary cancer risks from naturally occurring substances exceeds that for synthetic substances (e.g., these databases do not include concentration data on many of the potential carcinogenic constituents found in foods). Indeed, at the present, quantitative statements cannot be made about cancer risks for humans from specific dietary chemicals, either naturally occurring or synthetic.

• Current regulatory practices have applied far greater stringency to the regulation of synthetic chemicals in the diet than to naturally occurring chemicals. The committee reviewed data and findings of IARC, the National Toxicology Program (NTP), and in the general literature to ascertain the status of carcinogenicity testing of naturally occurring versus synthetic chemicals. Only a very small fraction of naturally occurring chemicals has been tested for carcinogenicity. Naturally occurring dietary chemicals known to be potent carcinogens in rodents include agents derived through food preparation, such as certain heterocyclic amines generated during cooking, and the nitrosamines and other agents acquired during food preservation and storage, such as aflatoxins and some other fungal toxins.

• The human diet also contains anticarcinogens that can reduce cancer risk. For example, the committee evaluated relevant literature on antioxidant micronutrients, including vitamins A, C,

E, folic acid, and selenium, and their suggested contributions to cancer prevention. Human diets that have a high content of fruits and vegetables are associated with a reduced risk of cancer, but the specific constituents responsible for this protective effect and their mechanisms of action are not known with certainty. The vitamin and mineral content of fruits and vegetables might be important factors in this relationship. In addition, fruits and vegetables are dietary sources of many non-nutritive constituents, such as isoflavonoids, isothiocyanates and other sulfur-containing compounds, some of which have inhibited the carcinogenic process in experimental animal studies. Foods high in fiber content are associated with a decreased risk of colon cancer in humans, but it is not yet clear that fiber per se is the component responsible for this protective effect.

• Carcinogens and anticarcinogens present in the diet can interact in a variety of ways that are not fully understood. This makes it difficult to predict overall dietary risks based on an assessment of the risks from individual components due to uncertainties associated with rodent-to-human extrapolation and high-dose to low-dose extrapolation. It is likely that there is also considerable interindividual variation in susceptibility to specific chemicals or mixtures due to either inherited or acquired factors.

Synthetic Versus Naturally Occurring Carcinogens

• Overall, the basic mechanisms involved in the entire process of carcinogenesis—from exposure of the organism to expression of tumors—are qualitatively similar, if not identical, for synthetic and naturally occurring carcinogens. The committee concluded that there is no notable mechanistic difference(s) between synthetic and naturally occurring carcinogens. To assess relative potency, the committee compiled and analyzed data on over 200 carcinogens— 65 of which were naturally occurring. The data set included agents identified by IARC as having sufficient evidence of carcinogenicity in humans or animals, or by the NTP as known or reasonably anticipated to be human carcinogens. Based in part on this limited sample, the committee concluded that there is no clear difference between the potency of known naturally occurring and synthetic carcinogens that may be present in the human diet. Of the selected agents tested, both types of chemicals have similar mechanisms of action, similar positivity rates in rodent bioassay tests for carcinogenicity, and encompass similar ranges of carcinogenic potencies. Consequently, both naturally occurring and synthetic chemicals can be evaluated by the same epidemiologic or experimental methods and procedures.

• Although there are differences between specific groups of synthetic and naturally occurring chemicals with respect to properties such as lipophilicity, degree of conjugation, resistance to metabolism, and persistence in the body and environment, it is unlikely that information on these properties alone will enable predictions to be made of the degree of carcinogenicity of a naturally occurring or synthetic chemical in the diet. Both categories of chemicals—naturally occurring and synthetic—are large and diverse. Predictions based on chemical or physical properties are problematic, due in part to the likely overlap of values between the categories.

Models for Identifying
Carcinogens and Anticarcinogens

• The committee evaluated current methods for assessing carcinogenicity and concluded that current strategies for identifying and evaluating potential carcinogens and anticarcinogens are essentially the same. The methods can be grouped into epidemiologic studies, in vivo experimental animal models, and in vitro systems. The committee recognized the value and limitations of each approach for identifying dietary carcinogens and anticarcinogens.

• In its assessment of traditional epidemiologic approaches to identifying dietary carcinogens and anticarcinogens, the committee concluded that these can be beneficially expanded by incorporating into research designs more biochemical, immunologic, and molecular assays that use human tissues and biologic fluids. Furthermore, incorporating the identification of biologic markers into these approaches may provide early indicators of human carcinogenicity—long before the development of tumors.

• The committee analyzed the applicability of rodent bioassays—specifically the long-term bioassays conducted by the National Toxicology Program—for identifying dietary carcinogens and anticarcinogens. The committee concluded that, despite their limitations, rodent models (involving high-dose exposures) have served as useful screening tests for identifying chemicals as potential human carcinogens and anticarcinogens. Concerns about the use of data generated from these models for predicting the potential carcinogenicity and anticarcinogenicity of chemicals in food arise from the fact that they do not mimic human exposure conditions, i.e., we are exposed to an enormous complex of chemicals, many at exceedingly low quantities, in our diet.

RECOMMENDATIONS

Numerous and extensive gaps in the current knowledge base were apparent as the committee endeavored to examine the risk of human cancer from naturally occurring versus synthetic components of the diet. These gaps are so large—and resources are so limited—that careful prioritization of further research efforts is essential. The following recommendations emphasize the need for expanded epidemiologic studies, more human exposure data, improved and enhanced testing methods, more detailed data on dietary components, and further mechanistic studies, if these gaps are to be filled. These research endeavors may prove inadequate, however, when the complexity and variability of diets and food composition, as well as human behavior, are considered.

Epidemiologic Studies and Human Exposure

• *Improved methods are needed to enable the incorporation of relevant cellular and molecular markers of exposure, susceptibility, and preneoplastic effects (DNA damage, etc.) into epidemiologic studies.*

While existing markers are useful, additional molecular markers of exposure and susceptibility need to be developed, and their relevance and predictivity to the carcinogenic process need to be evaluated. These markers should then be incorporated into epidemiologic studies. In particular, methods are needed to identify high- and low-risk populations. Biologic markers for both genotoxic and nongenotoxic agents need to be developed and validated.

• *Additional data on the concentrations of naturally occurring and synthetic chemicals in foods and human exposures to them are needed.*

To determine exposures to specific dietary chemicals, it is necessary to know the concentration of a specific chemical in individual food commodities, as well as the patterns of consumption of those food commodities. At present, the concentrations are known for relatively few chemicals. In addition, more information is needed on the factors that modify these concentrations.

Current methods for assessing food consumption based on personal recall or food diaries have limitations; they may entail a substantial degree of error and lack of reproducibility. Furthermore, the sample sizes of existing food consumption surveys are limited, particularly when subpopulations such as infants and children or the elderly are considered. To minimize the resources needed to acquire these data, consideration should be given to building on other large population-based studies, such as the Women's Health Initiative Study currently supported by the National Institutes of Health.

Testing

• *Improved bioassay screening methods are needed to test for carcinogens and anticarcinogens in our diet.*

The rodent bioassay currently used in screening chemicals for potential carcinogenicity or anticarcinogenicity has major problems and uncertainties, especially in providing quantitative estimates of dietary cancer risk to humans or the magnitude of protection by anticarcinogens. These uncertainties relate to the variability of the composition and caloric content of the human diet and the bioassay's inability to mimic this range of variability. In addition, human exposures to individual naturally occurring or synthetic chemicals are far lower than experimental test conditions. (The committee recognized that of the NTP bioassays netting positive results, only 6% were from test levels exclusively at the maximum tolerated dose.) Uncertainties also result from variation in responses among species. The factors causing these and other uncertainties should be further evaluated and minimized wherever possible. New methods are needed for assessing complex mixtures such as those present in food. Because some chemicals may produce or prevent cancer in animals by mechanisms not relevant to humans, or do so only at high doses, information on the mechanisms of action of chemical carcinogens and anticarcinogens is crucial to improving the science of human risk assessment.

• *Further testing of naturally occurring chemicals in the food supply for carcinogenic and anticarcinogenic potential should be conducted on a prioritized basis.*

At present, only a limited number of naturally occurring substances present in the human diet have been subjected to testing for carcinogenic and anticarcinogenic potential. Selected additional substances should be subjected to appropriate testing in order to develop a more comprehensive database on which to base comparisons of the potential cancer risks or protective effects of naturally occurring and synthetic chemicals in the diet. Because resources for toxicological testing are limited and because there is a vast number of naturally occurring dietary chemicals, further testing of appropriately selected naturally occurring food chemicals requires the establishment of selection criteria. For potential carcinogens, priority should be assigned to those suspected naturally occurring nonnutritive chemicals that occur at relatively high concentrations in commonly consumed foods, and/or those whose consumption is associated with diets or life styles known to be deleterious. Research should be conducted only when there is substantial evidence that an important problem exists and when there is a reasonable expectation of a meaningful result. Unless a suspected carcinogen or anticarcinogen occurs at high and measurable levels in a diet, its risk to humans cannot be predicted using present methods (experimental animal studies or human epidemiologic investigations).

Additional criteria should be based on knowledge of known carcinogens and anticarcinogens. For example, naturally occurring chemicals could also be accorded a higher priority for testing if they 1) fall in the same chemical class as known chemical carcinogens or anticarcinogens; 2) contain chemical groups also found in known chemical carcinogens or anticarcinogens; 3) are likely, based on structural comparisons with known chemical carcinogens or anticarcinogens, to form reactive intermediates, in vivo; 4) are known to be mutagenic and/or to bind to DNA; 5) share biologic effects similar to those of known nongenotoxic carcinogens; or 6) are likely, based on structural comparisons with known chemicals, to be unusually stable (i.e., long lasting) in vivo.

High priority for identifying potential anticarcinogens might be considered, in view of the fact that they do offer the possibility of new approaches to cancer control and prevention.

• *To help fill the data gaps on the cancer risk of dietary constituents, improved short-term screening tests for carcinogenic and anticarcinogenic activity should be developed, especially for detecting nongenotoxic effects that are relevant to carcinogenesis.*

Currently available short-term screening tests, usually employing cell-culture systems, often provide useful information, but new methods need to be developed and validated. Emphasis should be placed on developing systems that use human genes, enzymes, cells, or tissues. Because most present short-term tests detect DNA-reactive compounds, new methods are needed for screening chemicals for nongenotoxic end points, such as cell proliferation, hormonal effects, receptor-mediated events and effects on cell-cell interactions, gene expression, differentiation, and apoptosis (programmed cell death). Great promise exists for the use of transgenic mice.

Dietary Factors

• *The risk of cancer from excess calories and fat should be further delineated vis-à-vis naturally occurring and synthetic substances in the diet.*

There is considerable evidence that excessive calorie (energy) intake (i.e., in excess of body needs and including fat) is associated with increased cancer risk for several sites. In rodents, and especially in humans, mammary cancer is associated both with excess calories and with high proportion of calories as fat. The mechanisms responsible for this effect have not been clearly identified. Possible mechanisms that have been implicated include increased cell proliferation, decreased cell death, changes in hormonal status, and alterations in the activity of enzymes which metabolize endogenous and environmental agents, and increased oxidative stress. Further studies are needed to elucidate the precise mechanisms and to better define what is optimal or excess caloric intake. Dietary fat has also been associated with increased risk of some forms of cancer, but it is not clear if this is related to the high caloric contribution of fat, to specific constituents in foods high in saturated fats (such as specific fatty acids or other lipid oxidation products), or heterocyclic amines produced in cooking. These relationships and the underlying mechanisms need further study and clarification.

• *The specific chemicals that provide the protective effects of vegetables and fruits should be identified and their protective mechanisms delineated.*

The consumption of diets rich in fruits and vegetables is associated with reduced incidence of several forms of human cancer. The specific factors accounting for this relationship are not known with certainty and require further investigation. A number of vitamins, minerals and non-nutritive components of fruits and vegetables may contribute to the protective properties of these foods. Further research is needed on the independent and interactive effects of these compounds and on the identification of additional protective components. At present, a sound recommendation for cancer prevention is to increase fruit and vegetable intake. Concerning specific plant derived chemicals, we do not have adequate information to recommend supplementation beyond the recommended daily requirements for particular vitamins or other nutrients.

FUTURE DIRECTIONS

New research approaches and enhanced resources are needed to address the precise roles of both naturally occurring and synthetic dietary chemicals in human cancer causation and prevention. Multidisciplinary efforts in food chemistry, analytical chemistry, toxicology, nutrition, carcinogenesis, biochemistry, molecular biology, and epidemiology are needed. Such understanding would improve our ability to apply, with greater confidence, results of animal studies to the estimation of human risk. Mechanistic understanding will also improve our ability to foresee and interpret the effects of mixtures. As noted earlier, our diets are one of the most complex mixtures to which we are exposed. As an example, epidemiologic studies will become far more informative when they routinely employ improved biologic markers for exposure, individual susceptibility, and early cellular response. (The NRC addressed biologic markers in a recent series of reports.) The use of human tissues in cell systems has been limited by the obvious fact that they are not the entire organism and that there have been many technical difficulties in maintaining them. Improved techniques from biotechnology can permit us to employ human tissues and cell systems with greater confidence in how the results will relate to responses in the living person. Also, greater mechanistic knowledge will support and expand our understanding of structure-activity relationships.

CLOSING REMARKS

At the present time, cancers are the second leading cause of mortality in the United States, resulting in over 500,000 deaths per year. It is agreed that smoking-related lung cancer is a major contributor to this statistic. However, it appears that dietary factors play an important role in the causation of a major fraction of these cancers. Current knowledge indicates that calories in excess of dietary needs, and perhaps fat or certain components of fat, as well as inadequate dietary fruits and vegetables, have the greatest impact. Most naturally occurring minor dietary constituents occur at levels so low that any biologic effect, positive or negative, is unlikely. Nevertheless, a significant number of these chemicals have shown carcinogenic or anticarcinogenic activity in tests. Overall, they have been so inadequately studied that their effect is uncertain. The synthetic chemicals in our diet are far less numerous than the natural and have been more thoroughly studied, monitored, and regulated. Their potential biologic effect is lower.

The subject of this report is, therefore, of major relevance to public-health protection and disease prevention. The assessment by this committee indicates that our current knowledge of the specific naturally occurring chemicals (or mixtures) that are involved in cancer causation or prevention, the mechanisms by which they act, which types of cancer they affect, and the magnitude of these affects, is inadequate. New research approaches at the fundamental and applied levels are urgently required to address this important problem.

Coupled with the requirement for research efforts in these areas is the need to better characterize the chemical composition of our diet and its variations in the American population. Advances in analytic and survey techniques should facilitate this endeavor.

Finally, as advances are made in identifying with certainty specific naturally occurring dietary chemicals that either enhance or inhibit cancer risks in humans, it will be possible to formulate rational dietary guidelines for the American public. It may also be possible to use this information to modify the composition of our food sources through breeding methods, genetic engineering, and other advances in biotechnology, so as to optimize the quality of the diet with respect to cancer prevention. Above all, a major effort will be needed to educate the American public regarding appropriate life-style modifications if we are to achieve these goals.

1

Introduction

Each of us personalizes values of risk whenever we cross the street, fly in an airplane, or learn of possible threats to our health and well-being. Risks associated with the presence of possible cancer-causing agents in the air we breathe, the water we drink, or the food we eat, evoke a large emotional response—often demanding a full evaluation of the source and immediate correction of the situation. The safety of air, water, and food is considered beyond the average citizen's control; it is regulated, monitored, and evaluated by laws and government agencies. However, a steady flow of articles and reports describes the risks associated with exposure to chemicals that may be present in many situations. These reports have saturated the capacity of most people to differentiate the important from the trivial and to discriminate fact from hypothesis.

In the past 50 or 60 years, our knowledge of nutrition and the role it plays in human health has developed enormously. This same period has seen vast improvements in the safety of the U.S. diet, with technological advances in preservation and shipment of foods and with our ability to identify and reduce risks from various food hazards.

The U.S. diet contains both naturally occurring and synthetic substances that are known or suspected to affect cancer risk. Although many substances present in the food supply have been shown to increase cancer risks under certain conditions—usually not the conditions encountered in consuming food—others may, in fact, decrease risk. The level of risk associated with a carcinogenic agent depends on both the potency of the agent and the level of exposure to it. Carcinogenic potency can be estimated, fairly crudely, using clinical and epidemiologic data on humans or toxicologic data derived from animal cancer tests. Potency of chemical carcinogens varies over a wide range. Ames et al. (1987) introduced a useful measure of carcinogenic potency known as the human exposure/rodent potency (HERP) index. The HERP index reflects the ratio of human exposure to carcinogenic potency determined in rodents; the larger the value of the HERP, the closer the level of human exposure to the dose estimated to cause a 50% excess cancer risk in animals (Gold et al. 1992). Over the past decade, Ames and his colleagues have assembled a Carcinogenic Potency Database (CPDB), which now contains information on the potency of over 1,000 chemicals evaluated in animal cancer tests. However, neither toxicokinetic nor mechanistic considerations are included in this assessment.

Exposure to carcinogenic agents present in the diet depends on both food consumption patterns and the concentration of the particular agent in foods consumed. Food-consumption data can be collected by the maintenance of food diaries or by national surveys or questionnaires designed to gauge how often specific foods are consumed or to identify by recall those foods recently consumed. Concentrations of specific, known carcinogenic agents in the food supply can be determined by analytic techniques, such as chemical analyses for pesticide residues present in foods as consumed.

Using data from the CPDB, Ames et al. (1990a) compared the potency of naturally occurring compounds with synthetic (chemical) agents found in food that are capable of causing cancer in animals. They argue that the toxicology of synthetic chemicals is similar to that of natural chemicals, which represent the great majority of chemicals present in the human diet. Ames et al. (1990b) note that plants have evolved bioactive compounds to protect themselves from fungi, insects, and predators. Of 50 such natural "biocides" evaluated in animal cancer tests, about half have demonstrated carcinogenic properties, a number similar to the proportion of synthetic chemicals that test positive. Considering plant biocides as "natural pesticides," Ames concluded that the amount of such naturally occurring compounds in the diet far exceeds that of residues of synthetic pesticides used to enhance agricultural productivity.

Inferences about dietary cancer risks are complicated by the fact that the human diet is a highly complex mixture containing a large number of chemical substances that are mostly natural, but also some that are synthetic. Some chemical substances and mixtures, such as pesticide residues, spices and flavoring agents, and indirect food additives, are usually present only in very low concentrations; other macroingredients such as saturated fats comprise a large percentage of the total diet by weight. Dietary cancer risk assessment thus requires study both of the risks associated with individual microcomponents and macrocomponents of the diet and of the manner in which their effects may be modified when consumed as part of the total diet. One's diet is the result of individual choice and depends on many variables: ethnic custom, economic availability, personal likes and dislikes, fads, etc.

Although risk assessors state that risk estimates are a statistical expression of probability, the lay public often wants to know the meaning of such a risk to the individual. For example, a risk estimate of 1 in 10,000 means that up to one additional death (or case of cancer) from a designated cause, in a population of 10,000 people, may occur in the next 70 years. The controversial concept of *de minimis* is generally recognized to represents one additional death (or case of cancer) from a designated cause, in a city of one million people, expected in the next 70 years. One approach used for translating risks into more personalized terms is to rank them by developing a scale of comparative risks. Is the danger of death from a shooting in Washington, DC, greater than the risk associated with smoking a full pack of cigarettes per day for 40 years? Or is the cancer risk from exposure to a chemical by eating a charbroiled steak greater than the risk of driving from Dallas to Chicago? Some feel that in such a personalized ranking, the statistical probability of risk may be translated into meaningful lay terms. However, individuals perceive risks in different ways, and voluntary risks may be perceived differently from involuntary ones.

Estimates of dietary cancer risks are subject to uncertainty. Specifically, uncertainty exists about the potency of carcinogenic substances, about food consumption patterns, and about the concentration of carcinogenic—as well as anticarcinogenic—constituents in foods. When inferences about human risks are based on laboratory studies using animals, several reasons for uncertainty exist: uncertainty about extrapolations from the high dose levels used in the laboratory to the lower levels of exposure typical of the human diet; about the relative sensitivity of animals and humans to the effects of carcinogenic or anticarcinogenic agents; about the relevance of the animals themselves as suitable surrogates for humans; and the possibility of interindividual variations in susceptibility related to age, body size, and specific inherited or acquired factors. These uncertainties are nearly always addressed by using conservative assumptions or procedures intended to err on the side of overstating the probable risk. Thus, the result is often considered to be a plausible, but a probable upper bound of human risk, accompanied by great uncertainty. In evaluating dietary cancer risks, it is important that this uncertainty be recognized and, if possible, characterized.

Epidemiologic studies suggest that a diet with excess fat and caloric intake levels increases risk for some cancers. Studies with rodents have likewise documented the role of excess calories in sensitivity to chemicals that cause cancer. This is a highly important factor to consider in the United States where—although most people recognize that there is a relationship between diet and health and that a life style including a well-balanced, nutritionally adequate diet can have a positive effect on the quality and duration of life—more than 3 in 10 adult Americans weigh at least 20% in excess of their ideal body weight (Kuczmarski et al. 1994).

Animals maintained on a calorie-restricted diet have shown significant reduction in the rate of onset of tumor formation and adverse toxicity to chemicals recognized to initiate cancer or cell death. The specific relevance to humans of this caloric restriction is, as yet, undetermined. However, the inclusion in the human diet of vegetables and fruits is associated with a decreased risk of cancer. This association may be due to one or more of several causes: the antioxidant or other biological effects of specific vitamins or polyphenols; the protective effect of fiber; the inhibition of those enzymes functioning in the enzymatic conversion of procarcinogenic chemicals to carcinogens; the enhanced synthesis of enzymes (often the conjugating enzymes) that combine with reactive metabolites to form inactive derivatives; the stimulation of enzymes participating in the repair of modified DNA; or other mechanisms yet to be discovered. Other dietary components induce the synthesis of detoxifying enzymes, thereby reducing the formation of toxic oxygen products, such as the superoxide anion, formed by redox reactions of quinones.

This report focuses on the presence of naturally occurring chemicals that might be carcinogenic ("naturally occurring carcinogens") in the diet of the average U.S. citizen and compares the risk from these chemicals with synthetic chemicals that may also be present in the food we eat. Although much of the current concern about the risks of naturally occurring carcinogens is motivated by concern about the potential effects of bioactive natural chemicals, the committee addressed the broader comparison between naturally occurring chemicals that may possess carcinogenic potential and other naturally occurring dietary carcinogens, such as aflatoxin and other mycotoxins.

Naturally occurring agents suspected of carcinogenic activity are frequently normal chemical constituents of foods, or they may be chemicals formed during the processing, cooking, or storage of foods. They range from those chemicals that function as part of the plant's normal physiology (e.g., plant hormones, such as auxins, gibberellins, cytokinins, ethylene, and abscisic acid required for growth and development); or naturally occurring protective chemicals that make up the defense system against diseases or predators (phytoalexins); or color and aroma chemicals (anthocyanins and monoterpenes) that serve as pollinator attractants, repellants, or feeding inhibitors to limit the predation of herbivorous pests; to those chemicals that are formed as breakdown products of naturally occurring chemicals during the preparation of a food (e.g., pyrolysis products of amino acids generated during the charbroiling of meat and fish).

For the chemist, there is no distinction between a naturally occurring chemical and its equivalent counterpart, a manmade (synthetic) chemical. One significant operational difference, however, is that naturally occurring chemicals in the food supply are not subject to the same government regulations as manmade chemicals, a fact that raises questions about their safety and role as a possible threat to the health and well-being of an individual.

In 1938, the U.S. Congress passed the Food, Drug, and Cosmetic Act, which contained food-related provisions, such as tolerances for unavoidable toxic substances, and prohibited the marketing of any food containing such substances. In 1948, the Miller Pesticide Amendment was passed by Congress to streamline procedures for setting safety limits for pesticide residues in raw agricultural commodities. The Food Additive Amendment, which contains the "Delaney Clause," was passed on September 6, 1958. That clause states that no additive (either natural or manmade chemical) is to be permitted in any amount if it has been shown to produce cancer in animal studies or in other appropriate tests. This amendment also provides that an additive may be permitted at not more than the amount necessary to produce the intended effect. The amendment does not apply to all food ingredients, because it excludes substances classified as "generally recognized as safe" (NRC 1984), as well as several other categories of food components. The Color Additive Amendment, enacted in 1960, allowed the Food and Drug Administration (FDA) to regulate the conditions of safe use for color additives in foods, drugs, and cosmetics, and to require manufacturers to perform tests to establish safety. The Food, Drug, and Cosmetic Act and its various amendments are administered by the FDA. These regulations affect approximately 60% of the food produced in the United States. (The remaining 40% is under state regulations, which in many cases are tailored after federal legislation [NRC 1989]). These highly compartmentalized laws are concerned in part with what humans put into food, rather than with what occurs naturally. In addition, at the time each part of the legislation was drafted, many of the questions being asked today—particularly involving quantification—were not (and could not be) envisioned, much less answered. Furthermore, increasingly sensitive, sophisticated technologies have been developed that can detect minuscule amounts of chemicals, unimaginable when these legislative initiatives were enacted, and when "not detectable" meant "safe."

But what of the naturally occurring carcinogens? How many of them are there? What is the burden of exposure for the average person? Is there a difference in the ability of natural and synthetic chemicals to cause or prevent cancer? The report presented here attempts to address these questions.

Plants are the major source of naturally occurring chemicals. Historically, in addition to serving as a major food source, they have served as a source of medicines, potions, amulets, poisons, and panaceas to alleviate pain and cure illnesses, enhance physical and sexual performance, or terminate a rival. A vast history of folk medicine exists based on the cumulative experience of observations and trials through centuries. Even today there remains a constant search for chemicals in plants (phytochemicals) that can serve as therapeutic agents. The plant kingdom is a vast reservoir of chemical variety. It is estimated that millions of chemicals are synthesized by plants as a result of the diversity of products that biochemical processes have produced over millions of years.

Many chemicals present in the growing plant are modified during harvesting, storage, processing, and cooking, making the listing of all the chemicals present in the diet a gargantuan task. Very few of them have been tested to determine if they are carcinogens.

Do naturally occurring and synthetic chemicals, considered as general classes, differ in their chemical and physical properties? Can the principles and techniques used for the evaluation of the carcinogenic and toxic properties of synthetic chemicals be used in the evaluation of naturally occurring chemicals? As examples for comparing the characteristics of naturally occurring and synthetic carcinogens, the committee used peroxisome proliferators, nitrosamines, hydrazines, phenolic antioxidants, methylenedioxyphenyl (benzodioxole) compounds, sodium salts (e.g., saccharin and ascorbate), aromatic amines, and naturally occurring versus synthetic α_{2u}-globulin binding compounds. Each of these was considered as a single chemical species (not present as mixtures), evaluated using the rodent carcinogen bioassay system currently employed to assess the cancer-causing properties of a chemical. The committee considered whether the same principles governing toxicity and carcinogenicity apply to a naturally occurring chemical and a manmade chemical. Unexplored were questions evaluating the importance of so-called "organic foods" and claims that they protect an individual by reducing the level of exposure to a potentially deleterious synthetic chemical in the food supply.

STATEMENT OF TASK AND DELIBERATIONS OF THE COMMITTEE

The Committee on Comparative Toxicity of Naturally Occurring Carcinogens was convened in 1993 by the National Research Council of the National Academy of Sciences on the recommendation of the Board on Environmental Studies and Toxicology. The committee was charged to "examine the occurrence, toxicologic data, mechanisms of action, and potential role of natural carcinogens in the causation of cancer (in humans), including relative risk comparisons with synthetic carcinogens and a consideration of anticarcinogens." In addition, the committee was charged to "include the assessment of the impact of these materials (natural carcinogens) on initiation, promotion, and progression of tumors." It was also charged to "focus on the toxicologic information available for natural substances" and to "develop a strategy for selecting additional natural substances for toxicological testing."

The committee met frequently during its 2 years. A number of distinguished individuals presented their views to the committee, and a public forum was scheduled for the presentation of comments by interested individuals and organizations.

The committee was burdened by the complexity of the issues involved and the paucity of data available for analysis. Extensive discussion of key issues resulted in consensus—based many times on the best professional judgment of the committee members. Readers seeking rigorous scientific evidence on the issues will need to review the many references included in the report. Considerably more research will be required to identify the comparative risks for cancer of naturally occurring chemicals ranked against manmade chemicals. The committee has identified the directions for this research that it considers most promising to resolve scientifically testable hypotheses. Factoring in the elements of life style as contributors to any calculation of risk must be considered as unresolved, except for the oft-repeated admonition to reduce calories as a risk factor for cancer as well as heart disease.

It should be noted that although the committee was charged to assess the impact of naturally occurring carcinogens on initiation, promotion, and progression of tumors, it is difficult to define precisely these stages in most animal model systems and especially in human carcinogenesis. It is particularly difficult to classify chemicals or other agents as initiators, promoters, or progressors. It was decided to use more contemporary and accurate terminology. This report addresses the impact of agents in carcinogenesis in terms of DNA reactivity or DNA and chromosome damage (genotoxicity) and DNA replication and possible other nongenotoxic effects. This subject is covered in detail in Chapter 3 of the report. The committee also viewed its charge to address toxicologic issues as limited to cancer.

DEFINITIONS

For the purpose of this report, the term *diet* refers to the foods and beverages one consumes intentionally and customarily, not as a result of accident or deprivation. The diet will vary depending on age, customs, preferences, and availability of foods. It is not possible to describe a diet that will be common for all humans, not even when restricted to the confines of a single country, particularly not in such a country as the United States, with its population of multiethnic origins. Most significant are differences in the diets of infants and young people (NRC 1994). Diets often include at least low levels of potentially hazardous substances associated with some common foods and beverages. Estimates of exposure to these hazardous substances may be determined from knowledge of the aggregate amount of food consumed—but data permitting the further identification of food consumed by subgroups of the population are largely lacking.

The term *naturally occurring chemicals* comprises those that are constitutive, derived, acquired, pass-through, or added (see Table 1-1). In addition to these naturally occurring chemicals, food often contains a number of synthetic chemicals, although at a far lower level and in less variety. An *additive* is any minor ingredient added to food to produce a specific effect. Direct additives include natural and synthetic noncaloric sweeteners, antioxidants, colorants, flavor ingredients, and preservatives. Indirect additives are those chemicals present in the food because of their use in raw or packaging materials but no longer effective in the food as sold

Table 1-1 Definitions

Term	Definition	Examples
Constitutive naturally occurring substances	Substances synthesized by physiological and biochemical processes present in food organisms themselves	Furano coumarins, isoflavanoids, phytoalexins, cutins, alkaloids
Derived naturally occurring chemicals	Substances formed as a result of the breakdown of constitutive chemicals during stress, storage, processing, and preparation of foods	Polycyclic hydrocarbons, pyrazines, and heterocyclic amines that provide characteristic flavor of roasted and cooked foods—coffee, chocolate, nuts, meats, and browning products that add color and flavor to foods, such as toast and tawny port wine
Acquired naturally occurring chemicals	Substances present by infection or spoilage caused by bacteria or fungi or passively acquired from the environment	Aflatoxin B_1 or botulism toxin, as well as chemicals such as the residues of persistent pesticides no longer used but remaining in the soil
Pass-through naturally occurring chemicals	Materials present in animal products consumed by humans that are derived from food eaten by an animal	Any seafood toxins sometimes present in shellfish, toxol in snakeroot, or aflatoxin, which can appear in cows` milk, or arsenic (a carcinogenic, toxic metal found naturally in seawater and marine microorganisms), assimilated by shrimp from consumed zooplankton

Table 1-1 (continued)

Term	Definition	Examples
Added naturally occurring chemicals	Constitutive or derived naturally occurring substances that are isolated from raw or traditionally processed plant or animal sources then added to the same or other foods	Sucrose, glucose, isolated soy protein used in infant formulas, flavors extracted or distilled from spices, numerous gums and starches (e.g., corn or tapioca starch) that, because of specific functional characteristics, are used in other food

and consumed. Examples are pesticides, solvents, and chemicals derived from packaging.

The definition of *carcinogen* proposed by IARC is used in this report: a carcinogen denotes any agent, exposure to which is capable of increasing the incidence of malignant neoplasia (IARC 1993). The term *exposure* is restricted to mean the amount of a naturally occurring substance ingested orally in the human diet. The substance may be a solid or liquid. The presence of a specific chemical in a food may vary greatly for the reasons discussed in the report. Of greater relevance to safety, however, is the amount of a chemical determined as the form absorbed, distributed, and metabolized in the body for presentation at a target organ.

A *carcinogenic risk factor* is a contributor to the process of tumor formation and growth. For example, the diet is a source of calories (dietary energy, now often expressed as joules) derived from fats, carbohydrates, and proteins. Calories in excess of body needs can serve as an important contributor to cancer (Kritchevsky 1995). Likewise, smoking or alcohol consumption may serve as confounding life-style risk factors when considering the statistics associated with the frequency of occurrence of neoplasia in relation to diet. The committee recognized that the diet consists of a complex mixture of natural and synthetic chemicals and that additive, synergistic, or inhibitory interactions may occur between chemicals, influencing one or several steps in the multistage mechanisms associated with the formation and development of cancers.

Toxicity is defined by the dose at which adverse effects are produced by chemicals. Many chemicals, either natural or manmade, that induce cancer require metabolic activation for conversion from a procarcinogen to a carcinogen. For the purpose of this report, the terms *procarcinogen* and *carcinogen* will be used interchangeably, except where identified.

Other terms used in this report include *anticarcinogens* known to inhibit the formation of cancers or the growth of tumors. (Carcinogens and anticarcinogens are not mutually exclusive, as discussed in detail in Chapter 2.) More than 600 chemicals are claimed to be anticancer agents. These range from natural chemical constituents present in garlic, broccoli, cabbage, and green tea, to manmade antioxidants, such as butylated hydroxyanisole (BHA) and derivatives of retinoic acid. Much about how anticarcinogens act remains to be explained before they can be considered and employed as an effective part of any anticancer strategy.

STRUCTURE OF THE REPORT

The results of the committee's deliberations are found in the chapters that follow. Chapter 2 provides an analysis and assessment of naturally occurring chemicals that may be carcinogenic in the diet, as well as anticarcinogenic chemicals. The chapter discusses exposure, the effects of processing and contamination on the formation of carcinogens, and the effects of macronutrients and micronutrients in carcinogenesis.

Chapter 3 presents an overview of direct and indirect synthetic food additives that might be carcinogenic and provides comparisons with naturally occurring chemicals.

Chapter 4 discusses methods for evaluating potential carcinogens and anticarcinogens, from studies in human populations to rodent bioassays and various short-term tests, and provides criteria for selecting and testing of carcinogens and anticarcinogens.

Chapter 5 addresses the following critical questions:

• Does dietary exposure to naturally occurring carcinogens differ from dietary exposure to synthetic carcinogens?

• Do the potencies of naturally occurring and synthetic carcinogens differ (also addressed in Chapter 3)?

• Does cancer risk due to naturally occurring substances in the diet exceed that due to synthetic substances?

• Do naturally occurring and synthetic substances cause cancer by similar mechanisms (also addressed in Chapter 3)?

• Does diet contribute to an appreciable proportion of human cancer?

• Are there significant interactions between either synthetic or naturally occurring carcinogens and anticarcinogens in the diet?

Chapter 6, the final chapter, provides the committee's conclusions and recommendations for future directions.

REFERENCES

Ames, B.N., R. Magaw, and L.S. Gold. 1987. Ranking possible carcinogenic hazards. Science 236:271-279.

Ames, B.N., M. Profet, and L.S. Gold. 1990a. Nature's chemicals and synthetic chemicals: comparative toxicology. Proc. Natl. Sci. U.S.A. 87:7782-7786.

Ames, B.N., M. Profet, and L.S. Gold. 1990b. Dietary pesticides (99.99% all natural). Proc. Natl. Acad. Sci. U.S.A. 87:7777-7781.

Gold, L.S., T.H. Slone, B.R. Stern, N.B. Manley, and B.N. Ames. 1992. Rodent carcinogens: Setting priorities. Science 258:261-265.

IARC (International Agency for Research on Cancer). 1993. IARC Monographs on the Evaluation of Carcinogenic Risks to Humans.

Some Naturally Occurring Substances: Food Items and Constituents, Heterocyclic Aromatic Amines and Mycotoxins. Volume 56. Lyon, France: IARC.

IOM (Institute of Medicine). 1984. Cancer Today: Origins, Prevention, and Treatment. Washington, D.C.: National Academy Press. 132 p.

Kritchevsky, D. 1995. Fat, calories and cancer. Pp. 155-165 in Dietary REstriction: Implications for the Design and Interpretation of Toxicity and Carcinogenicity Studies. R.W. Hart, D.A. Neumann, and R.T. Robertson, eds. Washington, D.C.: ILSI Press.

Kuczmarski, R.J., K.M. Flegal, S.M. Campbell, and C.L. Johnson. 1994. Increasing prevalence of overweight among US adults: The National Health and Nutrition Examination Surveys, 1960-1991. JAMA 272(3):205-211.

NRC (National Research Council). 1989a. Diet and Health: Implications for Reducing Chronic Disease Risk. Food and Nutrition Board, Committee on Diet and Health. Washington, DC.: National Academy Press.

NRC (National Research Council). 1989b. Drinking Water and Health. Vol. 9. Selected Issues in Risk Assessment. Washington, DC: National Academy Press.

NRC (National Research Council). 1994. Science and Judgment in Risk Assessment. Washington, DC: National Academy Press.

2

Naturally Occurring Carcinogens and Anticarcinogens in the Diet

This chapter addresses two questions: (1) what is the current state of knowledge regarding the presence and availability of carcinogens and anticarcinogens in the human diet? and (2) how much do we know about the dietary factors that modify carcinogenesis?

EXPOSURE TO NATURALLY OCCURRING CHEMICALS

Naturally occurring chemicals present in our food supply can be classified into the following five categories: constitutive naturally occurring substances, derived naturally occurring substances, acquired naturally occurring substances, pass-through naturally occurring substances, and added naturally occurring substances. These are defined in Chapter 1.

Environmental exposures to naturally occurring chemicals occur principally from the food and water we consume (approximately 1-1.5 kg/day of each) and from inspired air (approximately 18 kg/day). While air and water frequently contain at least trace levels of contaminants of human origin, they are seldom a source of naturally occurring substances that raise health concerns, including those about cancer. Among the uncommon exceptions is arsenic. Although it occurs at a few parts per billion (ppb) in most drinking waters, it occurs at the part per million (ppm) level in spring, well, and surface waters in arsenic-rich areas in the United States and in many other countries (Underwood 1973, NRC 1977). Food, however, is overwhelmingly our major source of exposure to naturally occurring chemicals and is therefore the focus of this report.

THE COMPOSITION OF FOODS

Food, of course, is simply what we choose to eat, a choice heavily influenced by availability and culture (Pyke 1968, Jenner 1973, Tannahill 1973, NRC 1975). Although practical experience has taught us to avoid certain plants or animals because eating them results in illness, that experience is limited, largely anecdotal, and incomplete. We usually avoid acute toxicants—those things that make us unpleasantly sick immediately. However, we rarely possess sufficient knowledge about foods that contain naturally occurring toxicants that could cause delayed or chronic effects, including cancer.

In contrast, there are many potentially useful foods we avoid or disregard for reasons of unawareness, aesthetics, religion, culture, or cost. All human diets that sustain life and normal activity must supply at least the minimum quantity of the essential nutrients, including calories. Even given differences in age, body weight, and activity level, the range of those requirements for children and adults is fairly narrow—less than threefold. The range of variation in the foods that supply those nutrients, however, is enormous. Contrast the traditional Eskimo diet, high in animal fat and protein, with the vegetarian diet of the Seventh-Day Adventist or Hindu. Many diets in developing countries are low in animal protein simply because it is too expensive or unavailable. The use of spices and seasonings is often a distinctive cultural mark (Rozin 1973). The foods we choose to eat are merely a fraction of those we could eat. Furthermore, many dietary patterns shift over time, as demonstrated by our current—but recent—broad North American fondness for traditional Italian, Asian, and Latin American foods.

The variety in our modern food supply is due largely to the many different species of plants we consume. There are estimated to be about 250,000 species of flowering plants, and at least 11,000 are used as foods, spices, or flavoring agents (Tanaka 1976), including vegetables, fruits, and nuts. In some cases, different parts of the same plant are used as food, such as celery stalks, celery seeds, and celery essential oil (derived from the seed). The constituents of each plant part, and hence the expected biological activities, may be entirely different.

The Major Components

In biochemistry and nutrition, it is customary to think of food in terms of its major components. Across the entire U.S. food supply (plant, animal, and microbial), these component classes are, in descending order of concentration, water, carbohydrate, fat, protein, the non-nutrients, and the micronutrients, including minerals and vitamins. On average, carbohydrates supply 46% of our calories, fats supply 42%, and proteins supply 12% (Whistler and Daniel 1985). Of these component classes, proteins are the only primary gene products, i.e., the only class of components (other than DNA and the RNAs) produced directly by the operation of the genetic code of the organism. Minerals are absorbed from the environment, including the diet. All the other component classes are secondary gene products, produced in each organism by the action of the primary gene products, the proteins.

Carbohydrates consist of single or polymerized multiple units of simple sugars, such as glucose or fructose. Glucose, by itself, occurs naturally in foods only to a very limited extent; however, it is the most abundant sugar in the world. Combined chemically with other simple sugars in disaccharides such as sucrose and in starch, a polysaccharide composed solely of glucose, it constitutes about three-fourths of total dietary carbohydrates (Whistler and Daniel 1985). In the American diet, sucrose, fructose, and glucose supply more than half of carbohydrate calories and starch the remainder. The overall structure of nearly all dietary carbohydrates is remarkably similar—simple sugars in their ring (hemiacetal pyranose) form, linked together in chains. The large differences in their digestibility and functional characteristics lie in the length of these chains, the degree of branching, and in more subtle aspects of structure.

Lipids are a broad group of naturally occurring compounds that typically are freely soluble in organic solvents and nearly insoluble in water. The glycerol esters of fatty acids (triacyl glycerols, also called triglycerides) form up to 99% of the lipids of plant and animal origin and are customarily called *fats*, or somewhat more precisely, *fats and oils* (Hawk 1965; Anonymous 1970, 1986; Nawar 1985; NRC 1989b). Fats is the more specific term for those that are solid or semisolid at room temperature and are typically of animal origin, e.g., lard and butter. Oils, such as soy, olive, and corn oils, are liquid at room temperature and are usually of plant origin, although these distinctions have exceptions, e.g., whale oil. Those lipids that are not triacyl glycerols are quantitatively minor but of enormous physiological importance. They include cholesterol, the phospholipids in cell membranes, prostaglandins, and a host of other substances of structural and functional significance (Stryer 1975). Although all triacyl glycerols share the same basic structure, the differences in melting point, oxidative stability, nutritional qualities, and other important characteristics depend on structural aspects, such as fatty acid chain length and degree of unsaturation.

The basic structure of all proteins is that of a polypeptide—a polymer of α-aminocarboxylic acids linked by amide bonds. In terminology parallel to that used for the carbohydrates, two amino acids form a dipeptide, and three form a tripeptide. Peptides containing more than three, but fewer than ten amino acids, are often called oligopeptides, and those with ten or more are polypeptides. More than 400 different amino acids occur in nature (Harborne 1993), but only 20 are found in the major food proteins. Of these, nine are essential in human diets. As will be discussed later, proteins serve several diverse and essential purposes in the organisms that produce them. Although all are polypeptides, the number and sequence of the different amino acids, the nature of the chain—linear, branched, or ring, the additional functional groups (e.g., amino or carboxylic acid) on certain amino acids, and the three-dimensional conformation of the entire molecule determine the physiological role of each protein (Cheftel et al. 1985).

Alcohol, a nutrient only in the sense of a source of calories, is discussed in the section on "Identifying Potential Human Dietary Carcinogens."

The Minor Components

Minor components of food include the micronutrients (minerals and vitamins), the enzymes that all organisms produce and use as essential catalysts for their own life processes, and the DNA and RNAs that determine the nature of all constituents. In addition, plants and animals, and therefore foods derived from both, contain an almost unlimited variety of largely non-nutrient organic compounds often termed *natural products* or *secondary metabolites.* In this report, natural products or secondary metabolites are categorized as constitutive naturally occurring chemicals. Although chemically quite distinct, these chemicals are formed by modification of the same building blocks and biosynthetic pathways that produce carbohydrates, fats, and proteins. Examples of these chemicals are volatile oils, waxes, pigments, alkaloids, sterols, flavonoids, toxins, and hormones. Most plants contain one or a few minor constitutive naturally occurring chemicals of toxicologic or pharmacologic interest. This report intentionally focuses on the minority of these chemicals that are known or are suspected to cause, enhance, or inhibit cancer in humans. However, because of inherent low toxicity or low concentration, the vast majority of these naturally occurring chemicals are known or can reasonably be presumed not to pose a toxic threat.

Within the higher plants—excluding animals, fungi, and microorganisms—the enormous complexity arises from variations on only a few major biosynthetic pathways, all of which use as their starting materials compounds derived from carbohydrates produced by photosynthesis. In addition to photosynthesis, the principal pathways are

• The shikimic acid pathway, which produces compounds containing benzene rings and related structures (including the three aromatic amino acids—phenylalanine, tyrosine, and tryptophan and a host of secondary metabolites derived from them—numerous quinones, benzoic acid derivatives, lignin, and many other benzenoid compounds)

• The acetate (polyketide) pathway, which adds two carbon atoms at a time and is responsible for fats, waxes, hydrocarbons, certain phenols, and for portions of the structures of many minor constituents

• The isoprenoid pathway, which combines 5-carbon isoprene units (derived from acetate) and is the source of terpenes (e.g., volatile flavor compounds such as menthol and camphor), plant pigments (e.g., carotenes, including Vitamin A), sterols, and rubber

• Protein synthesis, which combines amino acids to produce the primary gene products, proteins, including enzymes

Still further complexity is found in products such as alkaloids that arise from combinations of these pathways.

Complexity and Variability

The identity of the specific constituents in the minor and major components of food—the qualitative composition—is in large part determined genetically. Environmental factors also affect qualitative composition and influence quantitative composition. Any particular crop is the result of the interplay of genetics and environment. Thus the genetic promise inherent in highly productive and disease-resistant new varieties of rice and wheat—the "green revolution"—cannot be realized without more intensive and better controlled cultural practices, including fertilization and irrigation. For plants, the relevant environmental factors include

- Latitude, which determines hours of daylight
- Climate (long-term temperature and rainfall trends)
- Weather (short-term temperature and rainfall)
- Altitude, which affects temperature independently of latitude, climate, and weather
- Agricultural practices, such as fertilization and irrigation
- Maturity at harvest
- Post-harvest processing
- Soil conditions (e.g., selenium content)
- Storage conditions

For foods of animal origin, the factors are diet, geographic origin, animal husbandry practices, season of harvest or slaughter, and environmental conditions prior to and at harvest or slaughter. All such factors have a major influence on the chemical composition of foods consumed in the diet.

Because of genetic and environmental factors, variation in the quantitative composition of individual foods is often great and can be dramatic. The usual food composition tables provide a useful overall picture, but the average values they contain give little indication of this variation.

Of the major components, water, carbohydrate, and protein vary the least and are typically, though not always, within 20% of the average value. Fat content varies somewhat more, from 50 to 200% of the average value, in foods of both vegetable and animal origin.

This greater variation in fat content reflects genetic and cultural practices, ones that are now changing because of recent appreciation of the role nutrition plays in chronic disease. Trace nutrients, constitutive naturally occurring chemicals, and natural contaminants are subject to much wider variation in foods derived from plants. Table 2-1 presents data representative of these variations in the U.S. diet.

Some foods, e.g., paprika, demonstrate inherently great variability in composition, reflecting variation in plant strain, climate, geographical source, and post-harvest processing. Some constituents, e.g., vitamin C, are highly variable in most of their dietary sources and for the same reasons. When these factors combine, the variability can be extreme: note, for example, the ascorbic acid content of paprika, for which the standard deviation (SD) is nearly equal to the mean. Standard deviations that are large compared with the mean imply that circumstances have combined and led to high production of that particular constituent. In general, variation is greater, i.e., the SD is larger relative to the mean, for

- Plant foods rather than animal foods (animal foods are usually subject to greater genetic control and less environmental influence with the exception of fat content)
- Microconstituents (those present at less than 1%), as opposed to macroconstitutents (those present at more than 1%)
- Plant foods that have a broad genetic base and are produced in many areas (e.g., paprika), as opposed to those that have a narrower genetic base and are produced in a few areas (e.g., California Valencia oranges).

Microconstituents such as selenium vary even more dramatically than those shown in Table 2-1, because of the great variation in the selenium content of soils.

Although the minor constituents account for only small percentages of total composition by weight, they are by far the largest num-

Table 2-1 Partial Quantitative Composition of Individual Foods

| | Mean Standard Deviation[a] | | | | | | | Retinol Equivalents/100g |
| | g/100g | | | mg/100g | | | | |
Food	Carbohydrate[b]	Fat	Protein	Sodium	Ascorbic Acid	Iron	Thiamin	Vitamin A
MEAT, FISH								
Beef, ground, extra lean, raw	†	17/4.6	19/1.2	66/7.6		2/0.29		
Lamb, shoulder, arm, separable lean, choice, raw	†	5.2/0.35	20/1.1	69/19		1.7/0.52	0.12/0.028	
Herring, Pacific, raw	†	14/5.4	16/1.1	74/3.5				
Pork, ham, separable lean, raw	†	5.4/1.4	20/1	55/12		1/0.31	0.88/0.19	
Tuna, Yellowfin, fresh, raw	†					0.73/0.26		
Veal, sirloin, separable lean, raw	†	2.6/0.30	20/2.3	80/14		0.80/0.11	0.08/0.02	
GRAIN								
Wheat, soft, white	75.36/-*	2/0.18	11/1.7			5.4/3.6	0.41/0.056	

43

Table 2-1 Continued

| | Mean Standard Deviation[a] | | | mg/100g | | | | Retinol Equivalents/100g |
| | g/100g | | | | | | | |
Food	Carbohydrate[b]	Fat	Protein	Sodium	Ascorbic Acid	Iron	Thiamin	Vitamin A
FRUITS AND VEGETABLES								
Beans, snap, raw	7.14/-	0.12/0.10	1.8/0.50					670/190
Broccoli, raw	5.24/-	0.35/0.16	3/0.51	27/10	93/8			
Cabbage, raw					32/18			
Cauliflower, raw				30/17	46/22			
Carrots, raw	10.14/-	0.19/0.11	1/0.14					28,000/2,000
Celery, raw	3.65/-	0.14/0.083	0.75/0.17	87/39				
Cherries, sour, red, raw	12.18/-		1/0.21					1,300/330
Mangoes, raw	17/-	0.27/0.27	0.51/0.22				0.058/0.030	3,900/2,300
Melon, cantaloupe, raw	8.4/-	0.28/0.077	0.88/0.35					3,200/670

Oranges, raw, California, navels	12/-		1/0.08	57/8.4			0.087/0.017	180/66
Oranges, raw, California, Valencias	12/-		1.04/0.14	49/8.8			0.087/0.009	230/79
Peppers, sweet, raw	6.4/-	0.19/0.14	0.89/0.080					
Pineapple, raw	12/-	0.43/0.57	0.39/0.049	15/1.8				
Spinach, raw	3.5/-	0.35/0.13	2.9/0.34		2.7/1.7			
Tomatoes, red, ripe, raw	4.6/-	0.33/0.26	0.85/0.14	19/4.4		620/92		
SPICES								
Cinnamon, ground	80/-	3.2/2.03	3.9/0.88		38/15			
Paprika	56/-	13/4.9	15/1.9	71/69	24/12		0.65/0.25	61,000/31,000

†: negligible

*Because protein content often is determined indirectly, this method of obtaining carbohydrate content does not justify calculating standard deviations.

[a]In all columns except the carbohydrate column, the figure before the diagonal is the average for the set of available samples; the figure after the diagonal is the standard deviation (S_1D_1).

[b]Carbohydrate content is calculated, not measured, by subtracting from total calories, calories from fat and protein, and dividing the difference by four (the number of calories/g of carbohydrate). Where significant, adjustments are made for nondigestible crude fiber.

45

ber of individual substances. For example, more than 200 constituents have so far been isolated and identified in orange oil—a simple oil (Maarse and Visscher 1989). Extensive information is available on single classes of such constituents, e.g., alkaloids (Pelletier 1983-1992, Mattocks 1986), terpenoids (Glasby 1982, Connolly and Hill 1991), and flavonoids (Harborne et al. 1975, Harborne 1988). The number of identified constituents of unprocessed food plants is at least 12,200; undoubtedly the actual number is far greater (Farnsworth 1994).

Geography and environment cause a variability in the concentration of these minor non-nutrient constituents, especially the essential oils and alkaloids, at least as great as that of the micronutrients. *Salvia officinalis* (sage) grows luxuriantly in many temperate areas of the world. Sage from the Dalmatian coast has an oil content of about 2.5% and is the industry standard for defining the characteristic flavor of the herb. However, sage grown in the mid-Atlantic states of the United States has an oil content of about 1.0%, and the flavor quality is variable and not as characteristic. We consume members of the red pepper family (*Capsicum annuum* or *C. frutescens*) for their color and flavor, as with paprika, or for color, flavor, and heat (piquancy), as with those used in Tabasco™ sauce. That heat is caused by a family of constituents called capsaicins. The capsaicin content of mild paprika ranges from 0.0002 to 0.0003 percent, that of jalapeño peppers is typically from 0.02 to 0.03 percent, and that of cayenne pepper from 0.2 to 0.3 percent—a thousandfold variation (Hoffman 1994). Ideal environmental conditions for maximum value are often unique to each species or variety and are found only in limited areas. Thus, the spice industry historically is international.

Coevolution, the long-term mechanisms by which environment exerts its effect on composition, is discussed in "The Functional Role of the Components of Food" section. However, short- and long-term events can result in the formation of secondary metabolites, even on plants of identical genetic background. For example, in the wine industry, the highest concentrations and quality of flavor constituents are often coupled with unfavorable growing conditions and low yields. Even without understanding the interrelationship between environment and biosynthetic mechanisms, it seems obvious that the minor secondary metabolites created are the products of general stress on the plant. Such a conclusion differs from but is consistent with the presumption that these metabolites act as agents for combatting specific predators, pests, or pathogens. Biotechnology techniques have been developed to supplement and extend classical breeding methods, and we now have the opportunity to modify the chemical concentrations in plants (see the section at the end of this chapter).

We complicate the variability of food by processing, especially by cooking, the most widely used and probably the oldest form of processing. We enjoy many foods in the raw state, but most foods must be processed, primarily to delay or prevent spoilage and thus avoid the resultant waste and hazard. Cooking, canning, aseptic packaging, pasteurizing, refrigeration and freezing, dehydration, curing, smoking and salting, and the use of chemical preservatives, fermentation and pickling, and irradiation all preserve food. Moreover, many foods, such as soy beans, must be processed to render them digestible. Others, such as cassava (manioc, *Manihot esculenta*), a major starch source in the tropics, contain cyanogenic glycosides and must be rendered safe. Neurological damage from chronic cyanide poisoning due to inadequate processing can still be found in central Africa. Processing is also used to eliminate sometimes unwanted constituents, such as caffeine from coffee or tea, or to introduce, increase, or restore desirable constituents, such as iodine in salt, vitamins A and D in milk, and niacin, iron, thiamine, and riboflavin in enriched flour. We process still other foods to make them more acceptable or convenient. Thus, in addition to genetic modification, processing provides a broad set of options for modifying the concentration of constitutive or added naturally occurring chemicals.

Even the simplest processing of the simplest mixtures results in amazing complexity. A single sugar such as glucose, in water solution at neutral or near-neutral pH and at the temperatures used for cooking or sterilization, produces an array of monomeric and dimeric anhydrides, fragments, and second- and third-order reaction products (Davídek et al. 1990). All of these are derived naturally occurring chemicals. Complex raw materials yield far more complex final products. For example, because of its cultural, economic, and commercial importance, coffee aroma has been studied extensively, and more than 1,000 components have been identified (Clarke and Macrae 1985). More might yet be measured by more sophisticated analytical technology. It might not seem desirable to include the consequences of traditional and widely used processing in a definition of naturally occurring, but we must take them into account. We may modify processing in the interest of acceptability, improved nutrition, or safety, just as we have modified genetic composition and cultural practices, but processing is not dispensable. It is inevitable and we must deal with the consequences.

Compared with the huge number of naturally occurring chemicals in food, those of synthetic origin are much fewer. The total number of chemicals—natural and synthetic—added directly or indirectly to food is approximately 6,000, slightly more than half of which are indirect additives used as packaging components or constituents (Hall 1992). The majority of indirect additives are synthetic (see Chapter 3). Of approximately 3,000 intentionally added to food, the great majority are constitutive naturally occurring chemicals. A few are used in high volume. Examples are the major caloric sweeteners such as sucrose (ordinary sugar) and glucose, isolated soy protein used in infant formulas, flavors extracted or distilled from spices, and numerous gums and starches, such as corn or tapioca starch, isolated from one food and used in other foods because of their functional characteristics. Such separated and transferred substances are naturally occurring but can create different patterns of dietary exposure than would otherwise occur.

Because of cost, many constitutive naturally occurring substances are duplicated synthetically, then added to food. As is true of the naturally occurring chemicals, most of the synthetic additives are at microgram or nanogram levels or lower.

Toxicants and Nontoxicants

It was Paracelsus who first observed that "Everything is poison. There is nothing without poison. Only the dose makes a thing not a poison" (Paracelsus 1564). But to describe everything as poison avoids the practical and vital distinctions we must make in dealing with naturally occurring substances, many of which we consume with far less than conventional margins of safety.

Today, toxicity is defined as the adverse effects produced by chemicals. The nature and extent of the toxic effect depends on the dose of the chemical. For practical reasons, such as those encountered with naturally occurring chemicals, this broad definition must often be reduced to an operational statement. The International Food Biotechnology Council uses a fairly restricted definition (i.e., operational guideline) for toxicant:

The toxic effects that the substance, i.e., the "toxicant," causes in humans, domestic animals or experimental animals either are irreversible (e.g., carcinogenicity, teratogenicity, certain neurotoxicities) or occur with narrow margins of safety, that is, at low multiples (approximately 25 or less) of ordinary exposures (IFBC 1990b).

Using this definition, the report goes on to note that, less than one-tenth of one percent of the total number of food constituents in our current food supply are toxicants. As analytical chemists identify the hundreds of thousands of constituents yet to be found at still lower concentrations, any toxicants to be discovered will have to be potent indeed to be capable of exerting adverse effects at such low concentrations. However, population growth will probably force the use of new or underused food sources, most of them plants (NRC 1975). In many cases, and especially in developing countries, the populations will not have benefited from the experience that has produced our present western diets. Even in the United States, several people die each year from the toxic constituents in teas made of herbs gathered by amateurs. It is useful to keep in mind that throughout history, plant materials have served as a source of poisons and medicines, as well as food.

Naturally occurring toxicants occur in most plants, in many microorganisms, and also in marine plants and animals. They are, however, essentially absent from the major cereal grains and from farm animals. Clearly, cereal grains have been selectively bred for at least 10,000 years—since the Neolithic Age—and the significant toxicants, e.g., phytic acid, have been bred out or reduced by processing. Naturally occurring contaminants such as mycotoxins are, however, quite common. Domestic animals, under the care of their owners, act as biological screens. Their illnesses have often alerted us to the presence of naturally occurring toxicants. Herd managers are careful to exclude known toxicants from feed and forage, although rare exceptions occur. In some of these exceptions, the naturally occurring toxicant does not affect the domestic animal but does affect the consumer of the animal product. Examples of these pass-through toxicants are the several honey toxins (IFBC 1990c), cicutoxin in water hemlock, and toxol in snakeroot which, when it appears in cow's milk, is suspected of causing the "milk sickness" from which Abraham Lincoln's mother died (Crosby 1969). Pass-through toxicants can be a major concern in seafood, particularly in shellfish. The contamination caused by the "red tide" is the most familiar example, but there are many others, several of which have been identified only in the last few years (Dickey 1989, Hall 1989, Iverson 1989). Much human experience with these toxicants suggests that their potential effects are most likely to become real when the specific foods in which they occur form too large a part of the diet, as in times of food shortages. The varied and balanced diet needed for good nutrition also provides, through dilution, significant protection from natural toxicants, as well as wider exposure to a range of potential anticarcinogens.

Of the human dietary constituents in our western food supply that can reasonably be called naturally occurring toxicants, only some are now regarded as carcinogens. In this report, the committee has assembled a representative list of chemicals for which there is at least some evidence of carcinogenicity in animals. The list comprises the naturally occurring chemicals, closely related groups of chemicals (such as the aflatoxins), and crude extracts or distillates, such as that from calamus. The committee then selected five chemicals, representative of various categories, for discussion in more detail. Very few naturally occurring chemicals have been tested for their carcinogenic potential, and still fewer have been tested by the standard methods used to determine xenobiotics (see the section on "Dietary Plants and Cancer"). Additional data, particularly if obtained in bioassays using the maximum tolerated dose (MTD), could well increase this number substantially. However, use of the MTD has inherent problems and limitations; these are discussed in chapters 4 and 5.

In addition to carcinogens that occur in the diet, some can be formed endogenously in humans from naturally occurring chemicals that are not toxic at levels found in the diet. N-nitroso compounds, including nitrosamines (discussed more completely in this chapter under N-nitrosodimethylamine and in Chapter 3), illustrate this class of potential human carcinogens. N-nitroso compounds are suspected of being a causal factor in gastric and other cancers (Mirvish 1983). They can be formed endogenously in the stomach by nitrosation of secondary and tertiary amines and other nitrogen compounds that occur naturally in the diet. This reaction also requires nitrite and an acidic environment. Nitrite exposure results from the oxidation of NO produced as the result of inflammatory responses or from reduction of dietary nitrate, the primary source of which is green vegetables (usually about 90%) and drinking water. The latter is a significant source only if the drinking water nitrate exceeds the EPA limit of 50 mg/L (NRC 1981). Nitrate in vegetables is accompanied by varying amounts of ascorbic acid and polyphenolics, which inhibit the nitrosation reaction. Nitrosamines are also found to a small extent occurring naturally in foods.

It is important to note that the putative naturally occurring carcinogens in our food are not a separate, easily definable class of constituents. They depend on the definitional criteria applied, on what is selected for testing, or on accidental discovery. They are merely a small part of the complexity of food. A critical purpose of this report is to provide a perspective on their importance, in terms of both the range and the size of the threats they present compared with similar threats from the synthetic constituents in our food supply.

The Functional Role of the Components of Food

It is useful to review briefly the functional role of naturally occurring constituents in the organisms from which we derive our food. The utility of the major components of food is well known. Water is the solvent and vehicle in which all the biochemical reactions of living organisms take place. Carbohydrates are energy stores and, particularly as cellulose, structural elements in plant foods. Proteins and their simpler relatives, peptides, appear as enzymes, hormones, and structural components, such as muscle. Fats, oils, and other constituents related to them serve primarily as energy stores but also have important functional utility as cell membrane components. Minerals serve a structural purpose, as in bones and teeth, but often play key metabolic roles as well. Examples are the iron complexed in hemoglobin and in the cytochromes, the magnesium in chlorophyll, the cobalt in vitamin B12, and the essential minerals in the metalloproteins.

The role of the numerous, minor plant constituents in the organisms in which they are found is seldom obvious. However, their roles and the enormous diversity of such natural products can be accounted for by the theory of biochemical coevolution between plants and animals (Fraenkel 1959, Ehrlich and Raven 1964, Feeny 1975, Visser and Minks 1982, Harborne 1993). Simply described, this theory states that a natural product (or group of products), presumably arising from some random mutation, may provide an advantage to the plant by deterring feeding by phytophagous insects, discouraging competitive plants, or by encouraging pollination (and reproduction). If that advantage is significant, further mutations that enhance the plant may confer further advantage and may survive. If the plant is thereby allowed to occupy a new ecological niche, it will flourish there until some mutant form of insect occurs that can feed on the previously protected plant. In this way, plants tend to increase the diversity of plant-eating animals and vice versa.

Consistent with this concept of coevolution, the study of which is often called chemical ecology, are constituents that have a protective role for the plants or animals in which they occur. This is particularly true of the constituents in the component classes called essential (or volatile) oils, the alkaloids, the nonvolatile components of extracts, gums and oleoresins, and the many animal venoms, toxicants, and repellents. Many of these act as pest or predator repellents, pesticides, fungicides, and pathogen inhibitors (ApSimon 1989, Ames et al. 1990, Harborne 1993, Meinwald and Eisner 1995). Some, found particularly in animals, are pheromones—substances released to communicate alarm or sexual availability or to indicate a path to be traveled. Those used as sexual attractants often are unique to the species and are a means of maintaining species isolation. Some constituents appear to be general attractants; others act as competition inhibitors and feeding deterrents. The flowers of many plants that require birds or insects as pollinators use a sweet and often aromatic nectar as an attractant. We find that same nectar attractive in perfumes, as space odorants in and around our homes, and as a food in the much more concentrated form of honey.

Flower nectars are one of the few examples in which the constituent is used by both humans and the source organisms for a closely similar function. More often, as in spices, plants use a constituent in one role, and humans harvest the same constituent for use in another. Repellents present a different situation. We insist that repellents be pleasant, or no worse than innocuous, to us but noxious to the species to be repelled. Such insistence eliminates many obviously effective repellents, skunk essence, for example.

Similarly, and more significantly, the plant antioxidants such as flavone derivatives, isoflavones, catechins, coumarins, phenylpropanoids, polyfunctional organic acids, phosphatides, tocopherols, ascorbic acid, and the carotenes have clear roles in plants (including dietary plants). They act as reducing compounds, as free radical chain interrupters, as quenchers or inhibitors of the formation of singlet oxygen, and as inactivators of pro-oxidant metals (Simic and Karel 1980, Hudson 1990). Although the plant and animal milieux are quite different, the value to us of antioxidants from each is similar.

Lupines are known in the United States as both wild and cultivated flowering plants. In South America, several species of lupine are used both for domestic animal forage and for human food. Use as food requires careful processing to reduce the levels of naturally occurring quinolizidines which, without such processing, have caused illness and death in both humans and domestic animals. Efforts to breed lupines with lower alkaloid contents have met with success, but these "improved" lupines are susceptible to higher levels of mycotoxin contamination.

"Potato poisoning" was a common occurrence in the 19th and early 20th centuries when potatoes often formed a large part of the diet. Such poisoning was caused by the variable presence of a glycoside, solanine. Even recently, a cultivar of Idaho potatoes had to be taken off the market when it was found to contain toxic levels of the neurotoxin solanine (IFBC 1990b).

When a natural product first appears in a species, it is presumably the result of a random mutational event; however, its perpetuation may at first be for reasons more subtle than those discussed above. Harborne (1993) points out that plants of the legume genus *Astragalus* have been able to adapt to high selenium soils because they can sequester selenium analogs in nonprotein amino acids, which are structurally different and therefore not incorporated into protein synthesis. A large number of plants, e.g., the genus *Prunus*, detoxify cyanide by sequestering it in the form of glycosides. Thus, while plants cannot excrete, in the sense of animal physiology, they can sometimes set aside useless or dangerous substances. In such cases, however, the detoxification products also now serve the protective role discussed above. Hölldobler (1995) cites Morgan (1984) in reporting "that the species-specific trail pheromones from the poison glands of myrmicine ants are generally the metabolic byproducts of venom synthesis." Thus, natural products that may originally have been waste products, byproducts, or detoxification products become simply new factors in the process of coevolution. Any or all of these functions may be consistent with the apparent positive correlation of the concentrations of the minor constituents with environmental stress.

Some naturally occurring plant compounds are virtually ubiquitous. Caffeic acid is a metabolic precursor of lignin, a structural polymer found in all land plants. Caffeic acid is also a component of chlorogenic acid, a phenol found widely distributed in fruits and vegetables. D-limonene is particularly characteristic of the orange and other members of the citrus family, but it is also found in more than 75 unrelated species, including allspice, tea, coffee, hops, passion fruit, peppermint, saffron, and vanilla. Alpha- and beta-pinene are major constituents of the oils from the genus *Pinus* but are also widespread throughout the plant kingdom. The widely distributed anthocyanins, one of several classes of flavonoid pigments, are responsible for the colors of flower petals, ripening fruits, and autumn leaves. Other closely related groups of constituents are found almost entirely in one family, as the glucosinolates in the genus *Brassica* (the cabbage family). Still other constituents are uniquely identified with a single species, e.g., cicutoxin in water hemlock or tetrodotoxin in puffer fish. Furthermore, the range of concentrations is as broad as the distribution is diverse. Some instances demonstrate survival value, but others suggest imprecise and slowly evolving systems.

Many plants and nearly all animals, including unicellular ones, have what appears to be a "chemical sense," i.e., they move or grow preferentially in the direction of increasing concentrations of attractive or nutrient substances; they also move away from or do not grow in the direction of or thrive in the presence of increasing concentrations of adverse substances. Thus there is a clear, if general, explanation for the effectiveness and survival value of many constituents. This phenomenon is most apparent in the case of nutrients or, at the opposite extreme, acutely noxious or toxic constituents. It seems reasonable to accept a role for genotoxic constituents if they have the capability of lowering the survival value of subsequent generations of pests or predators. What is far more difficult to imagine, however, is the survival value of a constituent that is an animal or human carcinogen. The typically long induction periods for chemical carcinogenesis could rarely if ever affect the aggressiveness or reproductive effectiveness of a pest or predator. If correct, this then leads to the conclusion that the carcinogenicity—of such concern to us—is merely an incidental aspect of some constituents, functionally unrelated to whatever role they may have in the physiology of the source organism.

This perspective seems further strengthened by the often substantial differences in susceptibility to toxicants, including carcinogens, among different animal species. This report considers elsewhere the difficulties in interspecies comparisons and the problems of comparative risk assessment for carcinogens from different sources and of different potencies. We simply conclude that, as far as we know now, there is a clear survival value for the plant or animal source in many of the naturally occurring toxicants found in food, but no clear rationale for distinctively carcinogenic constituents as promoters of evolutionary fitness. Carcinogenicity appears to be an incidental aspect—one of many forms of toxicity encountered in the naturally occurring constituents of food.

Certainly, non-nutrient components of foods have the potential to be toxic as well as beneficial, as is discussed below for selected nutrients. It is likely that as purified sources of these chemicals become available, individuals may consume excessive amounts and some people will reach toxic doses. The studies demonstrating toxicity of chemicals that have potential beneficial properties, including nutrients, were conducted using higher doses than those to which people consuming normal diets would be exposed.

Dietary Plants and Cancer

The ability of dietary plant extracts and constituents to induce malignant neoplasms in rodents has not been extensively studied, for several reasons. First, if humans have ingested these plants over the millennia without apparent toxicity, there has been no clear-cut rationale for undertaking such studies. Second, the cost of a two-species, two-sex carcinogenicity study, with the subchronic, metabolic, and analytical work typically needed for proper study design and interpretation, can exceed $2 million per chemical tested. This cost is prohibitive without a compelling rationale for such an effort. Third, traditional food plants are in the public domain. They have no owner or sponsor with a proprietary interest that could justify assuming these high costs.

Moreover, a positive result obtained from testing a plant or crude extract would leave unresolved the question of which constituent, or combination of constituents, produced this result. As discussed earlier, plant composition is complex and highly variable. Useful specifications are sometimes difficult and often impossible, and without them, one cannot be sure what one has tested, or that one can reproduce the results. Lastly, the great majority of these constitutive naturally occurring chemicals are present at microgram or nanogram levels or lower. Unless there are data suggesting that further study is indicated, there is a high probability that nearly all these chemicals are present in the diet at levels that pose no toxicological significance (see Chapter 5).

As a consequence of all this, except for chili peppers (*Capsicum frutescens, C. annuum*), calamus (*Acorus calamus*), black pepper (*Piper nigrum*), and bracken fern (*Pteridium aquilinum*), and some edible mushrooms (*Agaricus* species), very few edible plants or their crude extracts have been shown to be carcinogenic in laboratory animals. Certain plants used as herbal remedies contain carcinogenic pyrrolizidine alkaloids (e.g., lasiocarpine), but are not considered as foods and thus are not included in this discussion. In contrast, animal tests provide some evidence of carcinogenicity for a large number of individual plant constituents (see Appendix A). In many cases, these results were obtained only at or near the MTD. In plants or their crude abstracts, carcinogenic constituents typically are highly diluted by the noncarcinogenic components of the plants and their crude extracts, thus making achievement of an MTD impossible. Because of physical and nutritional limitations, one cannot simply feed more of the plant or crude extract to compensate for the dilution, and also because other constituents, although noncarcinogenic, will often be sufficiently toxic to make the MTD unreachable. In addition, research in this area has been hampered by limited availability of purified plant components and by our limited knowledge about potential interactions between compounds within plants and in humans. Furthermore, studies on toxicity have looked at the effects of plant components in animal systems using the highest doses tolerated, while studies looking for protective properties have generally used somewhat lower doses and have often studied the impact of the agent on the toxicity of a potent chemical or biological agent. These crude approaches certainly result in data that are difficult to use for assessing the risk escalation or risk reduction resulting from human exposure to these chemicals.

Nevertheless, the literature shows that although the crude extracts of more than 50 species of flowering plants have been tested orally for carcinogenic activity in rodents, only 27 of them were dietary plants. Of these, positive results were seen in only the four noted above. Based on the criteria set forth in the next section, and on the apparent quality of the data, only three of the dietary plants just mentioned might be considered to be carcinogenic. On the other hand, dietary plants which have been reported to inhibit carcinogenesis number approximately 28, and secondary metabolites from dietary plants number approximately 55 out of 65 tested (Farnsworth 1994).

According to current knowledge, the limited number of biosynthetic pathways in higher plants produces only a small number of constitutive naturally occurring chemicals found to be carcinogenic in animals. None of these is a potent carcinogen, comparable to the aflatoxins or the nitrosamines. However, as we have noted, food also contains naturally occurring substances that have been acquired and derived. Among these are some of the most potent animal carcinogens that have been identified.

NATURALLY OCCURRING CARCINOGENS FORMED DURING PROCESSING OR CONTAMINATION OF FOOD

Mycotoxins

The category of acquired naturally occurring substances includes those known as mycotoxins, resulting from fungal growth on food either in the field or during harvest and storage. Dietary contamination by one or more mycotoxin is common in most parts of the world, and particularly in hot, humid climates, such as those of Southeast Asia and sub-Saharan Africa (Wogan 1992). Exposure to mycotoxins is a chronic concern worldwide, not only because domestic products from these areas may be contaminated, but also because countries in colder climates import foods from areas where mycotoxin contamination of dietary staples is more frequent and severe (IARC 1993). The presence of one mycotoxin in food generally implies cocontamination by others, because a single fungus can generate several mycotoxins, and also because a food can be contaminated simultaneously by several mycotoxin-producing fungi.

Of several toxigenic species of fungi that can contaminate diet and dietary staples, contamination by two species of *Aspergillus,* namely *A. flavus,* and *A. parasiticus,* both known to produce hepatocarcinogenic aflatoxins, appears ubiquitous. *A. flavus* produces aflatoxins B_1 and B_2, whereas *A. parasiticus* produces aflatoxins B_1, B_2, G_1 and G_2 (Pitt et al. 1993). While all four aflatoxins are toxic and believed to be carcinogenic in animals, B_1 is the most prevalent and the most potent. Grains, peanuts, tree nuts, and cottonseed meal are among the foods on which aflatoxin-producing fungi commonly grow. Meat, eggs, milk, and other edible products from animals that consume feed contaminated by aflatoxins are additional sources of potential exposure. The relative amounts of aflatoxin B_1 on crops such as corn or groundnuts (peanuts), or other grains and cereal products, depends not only on the presence of the toxigenic fungi *A. flavus* and *A. parasiticus,* but also on pre- and post-harvest conditions (IARC 1993). Levels of aflatoxin in crops can also vary geographically and over time, with the southeastern US frequently referred to as an area where high levels can occur in corn. If a particular corn crop is stressed, for example, by drought or insect attack, it is susceptible to *A. flavus* growth and hence aflatoxin contamination (U.S. Food and Drug Administration [FDA], Compliance Program Guidance Manual 7106.10). Available data from various parts of the world suggest that the median levels of aflatoxins in corn range from <0.1 to 80 ng/kg, and that in groundnuts (peanuts) the median levels are always below 26 ng/kg (IARC 1993). The dietary exposure resulting from consumption of aflatoxin-contaminated diets, including milk and milk products from animals that have eaten contaminated feed, ranges widely from about 2.7 (U.S.A.) to 2,027 (Southern Guangxi, China) ng/kg bw/day (IARC 1993).

In view of the ubiquity of *Aspergillus* in the environment and the possibility that food staples may be contaminated at various stages of production and processing, it is unlikely we can ever completely eliminate exposure to aflatoxin. Regulations now in effect or proposed for many countries generally impose a maximum limit of 50 μg/kg food of aflatoxin B_1 or the total of all aflatoxins, and many countries impose far lower limits, e.g., 20 ng/kg in the United States. The carcinogenic properties of the aflatoxins have been extensively investigated, and much of these data are reviewed in somewhat greater detail later in this section.

Epidemiologic studies have provided convincing evidence that dietary consumption of aflatoxins has an etiologic role in hepatocarcinogenesis, and the studies indicate a synergy between chronic viral B (also C) hepatitis and aflatoxin exposure (Ross et al. 1992, Qian et al. 1994). In addition, a synergistic interaction between chronic alcohol consumption and aflatoxin exposure appears to play a role in human hepatocarcinogenesis. This causative role of aflatoxins in human hepatocarcinogenesis has recently been further supported by evidence from molecular epidemiology (see section on aflatoxins). There now can be no doubt that elevated exposure to aflatoxins, and especially to B_1, is a major contributor to human liver cancer. Nonetheless, it should be noted that aflatoxin appears to account for a fraction of liver cancer in the United States because of low aflatoxin concentrations in most U.S. foods and low prevalence of hepatitis B virus carrier status (HBsAg+).

Of the other most widely distributed toxigenic fungi, *Fusarium moniliforme* is a ubiquitous contaminant in corn, and it produces toxins such as fumonisins B_1 and B_2 and fusarin C. Exposure to

Fusarium toxins appears to play a role in the pathogenesis of esophageal cancer in humans. There are limited data on the levels of these *Fusarium* toxins in food; thus, it is not possible to estimate reliably the levels of exposure (IARC 1993).

Ochratoxin A, produced predominantly by *Aspergillus ochraceus* and *Penicillium verrucosum*, occurs worldwide in many commodities from grains to coffee beans, and it is implicated in urinary tumorigenesis in humans and rodents. Furthermore, barley, wheat, and pork products all appear to be human dietary sources of ochratoxin A (IARC 1993).

Although less well-studied, T_2 toxin from *Fusarium* and other species (Rodericks and Pohland 1981, Watson 1985, Ueno 1987) and the toxins found in *Penicillium islandicum* Sopp (Ueno 1987) have been reported to be carcinogenic. Beyond these, a large number of toxicants from many species of lower fungi have been reported to cause liver damage in test animals or to be mutagenic in microbiological assays (IFBC 1990) . At least some of these would reasonably be expected to be carcinogenic in animals if adequately tested.

Unfortunately, mycotoxins are ubiquitous. They can and must be minimized, but they cannot be eliminated entirely from our diet.

Pyrolytic Products

As indicated earlier, cooking is the oldest and most widely used method of food processing. Cooking alters the chemical structure of the food to be consumed by pyrolysis, rendering it safe from microbial growth. The chemistry of pyrolysis is extremely complex. The pyrolysis products of graphite, 60-carbon aromatic bucky balls, received much attention in the early 1990's; however, the chemistry of this process is simple when compared to the real world process of cooking food (Kroto et al. 1985). Nonetheless, the processes are similar and the chemistry not very well understood. When foods (or more properly food juices) are subjected to high temperatures, the amino acids, sugars, and other constituents are degraded and recombined to yield a bewildering array of compounds responsible for the aromas and flavors of cooked foods. Many of these compounds (e.g., the pyrazines) constitute the desirable flavor components that we associate with cooking, yet many others, particularly the more complex polycyclic heterocyclic amines, have been shown to be carcinogenic.

In 1977, Sugimura and coworkers demonstrated that the charred part of a grilled sardine was highly mutagenic in *Salmonella typhimurium*. After isolation and characterization, the agents responsible were determined to be a variety of polycyclic heterocyclic amines (PHAs). When further investigated, it was shown that any amino acid, when pyrolyzed, would produce its own characteristic set of pyrolysis products. Analysis of these products indicated that as many as 25 mutagenic PHAs may be isolated (Nagao and Sugimura 1993, Sugimura et al. 1994). For instance, tryptophan yields Trp-P-1 and Trp-P-2 (Tryptophan Pyrolysis 1 and 2, respectively) shown in Figure 2-1.

Pyrolysis of many other amino acids yields structurally similar compounds (see Lys-P-1, Phe-P-1, IQx, in Figure 2-1). It is important to keep in mind that these compounds are isolated from single amino acid reactions, and that the mixture of amino acids and other metabolites produces still other, more complex compounds, for instance IQ, MeIQ, and MeIQx. These compounds are among the most potent mutagens yet discovered.

The mutagenicity of these compounds correlates well with their carcinogenicity. When Trp-P-1 is fed to mice at the dosage of 15 mg/kg/day (0.53 mg/day per mouse) it induces hepatocellular tumors in 42% of the animals. In well-charred beef, Trp-P-1 may be present at a concentration of 106 ng/gm beef. Thus, assuming the average rate of consumption of beef to be 188 gm/day, the average human exposure from this source is 285 ng/kg/day, or 19.95 μg for a 70 kg person (Prival 1985). Similarly, when Trp-P-2 was adminis-

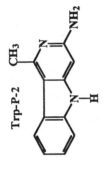

Trp-P-2

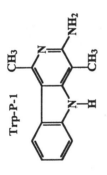

Trp-P-1

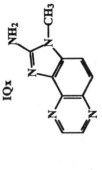

IQx

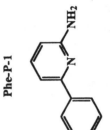

Phe-P-1

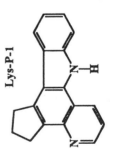

Lys-P-1

Figure 2-1 Pyrolysis Products of Amino Acids

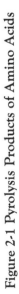

tered for 112 weeks in the diet at 100 ppm to male and female rats, significant increases in the incidences of neoplastic lesions were found in the liver, urinary bladder, and mammary glands in males and in the mammary gland, hematopoietic system, and clitoral gland of females (Takahashi et al. 1993). While these doses are dependent on cooking conditions and their relevance is a matter of dispute, it is clear that there are several orders of magnitude between the human and rodent experimental doses.

The discovery, identification, analysis, and testing of the PHAs provide a useful example of the progress that can be made, although with much cost in time and effort, in dealing with a complex mixture. The problems involved in dealing with mixtures receive further attention in Chapters 4 and 6.

Cooked sugar was also found to be mutagenic and to promote the growth of colonic microadenomas in rats and mice (Corpet et al. 1990).

CURRENT STATE OF KNOWLEDGE
OF HUMAN DIETARY CARCINOGENS

Identifying Potential Human Dietary Carcinogens

Appendix B presents a list of substances evaluated by the International Agency for Research on Cancer (IARC) and U.S. National Toxicology Program (NTP) on the basis of epidemiologic and animal studies and found to pose some specified degree of carcinogenic risk to humans. Those substances are the primary focus of this report. In addition, Appendix A contains a list of other substances that have been tested for carcinogenicity in animals and found to have some positive evidence of it. Most of these are not included in Appendix B. The list in Appendix A provides a more comprehensive summary of the limited carcinogenicity testing done so far on naturally occurring chemicals in the food supply and indicates the wide variability in the apparent quality and solidity of the results.

It is not feasible to discuss in depth each of the substances in either appendix. Instead, the discussion that follows provides some reasonably detailed information on five representative naturally occurring chemicals.

Constitutive Naturally Occurring Carcinogens

Caffeic Acid

Caffeic acid is a constitutive naturally occurring chemical found in higher plants. Of the five chemicals listed in Table 2-2, it is the most widely distributed throughout the plant kingdom, occurring mainly as the three monocaffeoylquinic acid esters, chlorogenic, cryptochlorogenic, and neochlorogenic acid. The chlorogenic acids are apparently hydrolyzed in the stomach to caffeic and quinic acid (Booth et al. 1957, Czok et al. 1974). Caffeic acid also occurs esterified to other hydroxyacids such as malic and tartaric acid and to glucose as a glucoside. It occurs infrequently as a free acid (Herrmann 1989).

The concentration of conjugates of caffeic acid in various fruits and vegetables, expressed in terms of mg/kg fresh weight, has been summarized by IARC (1993). Concentration data summarized by IARC and by Stich (1991) are used in Chapter 5 for making estimates of caffeic acid exposure. Large concentrations of caffeic acid conjugates can be found in apples and lettuce (Herrmann 1989).

There is sufficient evidence in experimental animals for the carcinogenicity of caffeic acid. Administered in the diet, it induced forestomach squamous cell carcinomas in male mice and in male and female rats, and renal tubular cell hyperplasia and adenomas in mice.

Table 2-2   Examples of Carcinogens Naturally Occurring in Normal Human Diets[a]

Substance	Degree of Evidence for Carcinogenicity[b] Human	Degree of Evidence for Carcinogenicity[b] Animal	Overall Evaluation of Carcinogenicity[c]	Nature of Supporting Evidence[e]	Extent of Natural Occurrence in Foods	References[f]
Constitutive Naturally Occurring Carcinogens						
Caffeic Acid	ND	S	2B [56, 1993]	Forestomach tumors in male mice, male and female rats; kidney tumors in female mice, male rats. clastogenic, mutagenic	Occurs widely in plants as esters of hydroxyacids, such as quinic (e.g., chlorogenic and neochlorogenic acid), tartaric, and malic acid; as glucose ester; and as glucosides; released by hydrolysis	68, 28, 21, 58, 63, 75, 26, 34, 25, 60, 36, 40
Urethane	ND	S	2B [7, 1974]	Lung tumors, lymphomas, hepatomas, and melanomas in rats, mice, and hamsters	All fermented and yeast-leavened foods; wines, yogurt, soy sauce 1.0-5.0 ppb; sake, liquors 100-500 ppb; ale, beer, bread ≈1.0 ppb	7, 65, 31, 13, 1, 66, 22, 24, 51, 42

Table 2-2 Continued

Acquired and Pass-Through Naturally Occurring Carcinogens

Substance	Degree of Evidence for Carcinogenicity[b] Human	Degree of Evidence for Carcinogenicity[b] Animal	Overall Evaluation of Carcinogenicity[c]	Nature of Supporting Evidence[e]	Extent of Natural Occurrence in Foods	References[f]
Aflatoxin B$_1$	S	S	1 [56, 1993]	Etiologic role in hepatocarcinogenesis derived from epidemiologic studies involving dietary consumption. Tumors of liver, colon, kidneys in several animal species. Hepatocellular and/or cholangiocellular liver tumors, including carcinomas in rats, hamsters, monkeys. Renal cell tumors, colon tumors in rats. Liver angiosarcomas of gall bladder and pancreas in monkeys. Altered hepatocytes in rats and hamsters. Clastogenic, mutagenic	Most prevalent fungal contaminant found in food. Derived from *fusarium moniliforne*—ubiquitous contaminant in corn. Also found on grains, peanuts, and more rarely, milk	71, 8, 15, 70, 69, 30, 41, 56, 74, 8, 39, 6, 5, 47, 17, 56, 72, 12, 46, 57, 50, 25, 48, 2, 18, 41

Derived Naturally Occurring Carcinogens

PhiP (2-Amino-1-methyl-6-phenyl-imidazo [4,5-b] Pyridine)	I	S	2B [56, 1993]	Lymphomas in male and female mice; intestinal adenocarcinomas in male rats, mammary adenocarcinomas in female rats. Clastogenic, mutagenic	Most abundant heterocyclic amine in cooked food, especially fried ground beef, broiled chicken, fried fish. ≈ 20-70 ng/g	3, 27, 19, 29, 44, 25
N-Nitrosodimethylamine	ND	S	2A [17, 1978][d]	Liver hamangiosarcomas, hepatocellular carcinomas, kidney, lung tumors in mice; kidney and bile duct tumors in rats, hepatocellular carcinoma, bile duct tumors in hamsters, rabbits, and guinea pigs. Clastogenic, mutagenic	Cheese, soybean oil, canned fruit, various meat products, bacon, various cured meats, frankfurters, cooked ham, fish, spices for meat curing, apple brandy, other alcoholic beverages, and beer. Concentrations in foodstuff 0-85 ng/g	38, 52, 74, 4, 59, 64, 65, 62, 11, 16, 14, 35, 49,10, 32, 45, 53, 33, 76, 20, 61, 54, 25, 43

[a] This is not an exhaustive list. Represented chemicals were chosen because they are classified by IARC as carcinogens, represent a range of carcinogenic potencies, and are present in diet for a variety of reasons.
[b] ND, no adequate data; I, inadequate evidence; S, sufficient evidence. For definitions of terms and overall evaluations, see IARC 1993, pp.; 28-29.
[c] Overall evaluation based only on evidence of carcinogenicity in monograph [volume, year].
[d] Other relevant data, as given in monograph [volume, year], influenced the making of the overall evaluation.
[e] Positive results reported in IARC; routes of administration are oral.
[f] Source of data on occurrence as well as carcinogenicity.

References

1   Adenis et al. 1968
2   Aguilar et al. 1994

3   Alink et al. 1988
4   Argus and Hoch-Ligeti 1961, 1968

5   Autrup et al. 1987
6   Bannasch et al. 1985

Table 2-2 Continued

7 Berenblum & Haran-Ghera 1957	31 Klein 1962, 1966	55 Sieber et al. 1979
8 Bulatao-Jayme et al. 1982	32 Kowalewski and Todd 1971	56 Soffritti & McConnell 1988
9 Butler et al. 1969	33 Kuwahara et al. 1972	57 Srivatanakul et al. 1991
10 Clapp and Toya 1970	34 Laranjinha et al. 1992, 1994	58 Stich 1991, 1992
11 Clapp et al. 1968, 1971	35 Le Page and Christie 1969a,b	59 Takayama and Oota 1963, 1965
12 Cusumano 1991	36 Li and Trush 1994	60 Tanaka et al. 1993
13 Della Porta et al. 1963	37 Li et al. 1994	61 Taylor et al. 1974
14 Den Engelse et al. 1969/1970	38 Magee and Barnes 1956, 1959, 1962	62 Terracini et al. 1966, 1967, 1969
15 Epstein et al. 1969	39 Moore et al. 1982	63 Toda et al. 1991
16 Geil et al. 1968	40 Nakayama 1994	64 Tomatis et al. 1964
17 Gil et al. 1988	41 Nishizumi et al. 1977	65 Toth et al. 1961
18 Greenblatt et al. 1994	42 Nomura 1982	66 Toth and Boreisha 1969
19 Gross 1990	43 NTP 1994	67 Toth et al. 1964
20 Hadjiolov and Markow 1973	44 Ochiai et al. 1991	68 Wattenberg et al. 1980
21 Hirose et al. 1988, 1991, 1992	45 Otsuka and Kuwahara 1971	69 Wogan et al. 1971
22 IARC 1974	46 Parkin et al. 1991	70 Wogan 1969, 1974, 1992
23 IARC 1978	47 Peers et al. 1987	71 Wogan and Newberne 1967
24 IARC 1987	48 Qian et al. 1993	72 Yeh et al. 1989
25 IARC 1993	49 Riopelle and Jasmin 1969	73 Zak et al. 1960
26 Inoue et al. 1992	50 Ross et al. 1992	74 Zawirska and Bednarz 1981
27 Isumi et al. 1989	51 Schmähl 1977	75 Zhou and Zheng 1991
28 Ito and Hirose 1987	52 Schmähl and Preussmann 1959	76 Zwicker et al. 1972
29 Ito et al. 1991	53 Shabad and Savluchinskaya 1971	
30 Kalengayi et al. 1975	54 Shinohara et al. 1976	

The relevance to humans of the positive findings in animal studies is uncertain for several reasons: no data are available on the carcinogenicity of caffeic acid in humans; the dose of caffeic acid tested in experimental animals was high; humans do not have a forestomach; and the renal lesions reported in mice and rats were related to toxic lesions. In addition, studying the actions of plant components in isolation can lead to incorrect assumptions about their modes of action and ultimate effects, which represents a specific instance of the general uncertainties about substance interactions. Caffeic acid, which exhibits both carcinogenic and anticarcinogenic activity, appears to be a case in point. In vitro studies indicate that caffeic acid may act either as a pro- or anti oxidant, depending on the experimental conditions. In the presence of free transition metals (e.g., manganese, copper, iron), reactive oxygen species capable of damaging DNA may be formed (Inoue et al. 1992, Li and Trush 1994); however, in their absence, caffeic acid blocks the formation of reactive oxygen species, lipid peroxides, and nitrosamines (Toda et al. 1991; Zhou and Zheng 1991; Stich 1992; Laranjinha et al. 1992, 1994; Li et al. 1994; Nakayama 1994). In vivo studies in which caffeic acid was administered orally in combination with known carcinogens have also yielded seemingly contradictory results with respect to the carcinogenic action of caffeic acid in epithelial tissues. Caffeic acid increased forestomach tumors in rats pretreated with DMBA or MNNG (Hirose et al. 1988, 1991, 1992). However, it inhibited squamous epithelial carcinomas of the rat tongue (Tanaka et al. 1993) and mouse forestomach tumors when administered with benzo[a]pyrene (Wattenberg et al. 1980). The dose range at which caffeic acid has been observed to be protective (500-10,000 ppm) overlaps with the range at which enhancing effects have been seen (5,000-20,000 ppm). A cursory look at the foods in which caffeic acid is present reveals many that are high in fiber, vitamins A, E, C, beta-carotene, and numerous other protective compounds that might significantly affect the fate of caffeic acid in the body.

On the basis of studies in animals, IARC (1993) concludes that caffeic acid is possibly carcinogenic to humans and has classified it as a Group 2B carcinogen.

Urethane (Ethyl Carbamate)

Urethane is a derived naturally occurring chemical found in foods produced or modified by fermentation, including alcoholic beverages, bread, soy sauce, yogurt, and olives (IARC 1974). Urethane is also an artifact resulting from treatment of beverages such as wine, beer, orange juice, and some soft drinks with pyrocarbonate, a fungicide that breaks down in the beverage after treatment (Schmähl 1977).

There is clear evidence for the carcinogenicity of urethane in experimental animals (IARC 1987). Urethane has been shown to be carcinogenic in mice, rats, and hamsters after administration by the oral route, producing lung tumors, lymphomas, hepatomas, and melanomas (Berenblum and Haran-Ghera 1957; Toth et al. 1961; Klein 1962, 1966; Della Porta et al. 1963; Adenis et al. 1968; Toth and Boreisha 1969).

The relevance to humans of animal studies of urethane is not known. No case reports or epidemiologic studies in humans of urethane are available, although clearly alcoholic beverages are carcinogenic to humans. On the basis of animal studies, IARC (1987) concludes that urethane is possibly carcinogenic to humans and has classified it as a Group 2B carcinogen.

Acquired Naturally Occurring Carcinogens: Aflatoxin B₁

As discussed earlier, the aflatoxins are the most ubiquitous of the fungal toxins, and aflatoxin B_1 the most potent and most studied of all. In addition to being an acquired naturally occurring carcino-gen, often found on grains, nuts, and seed meals, it is also a pass-through naturally occurring carcinogen, as it can be found in milk and other edible products from animals that have consumed feed contaminated with aflatoxin.

The carcinogenic properties of aflatoxin B_1 have been extensively investigated, and much information has been generated regarding their metabolic activation and mechanisms of action (Wogan 1992). Aflatoxin B_1 has been identified by IARC (1993) and NTP (1994) as a carcinogen. There is sufficient evidence to indicate the carcino-genicity of aflatoxin in experimental animals (IARC 1993). Admin-istered in the diet, aflatoxin B_1 has been tested for carcinogenicity in many animal species and found to produce tumors primarily of the liver, colon, and kidneys. After oral administration, aflatoxin B_1 caused hepatocellular and/or cholangiocellular liver tumors, including carcinomas, in all species tested (including rats, hamsters, and monkeys) except mice (Wogan and Newberne 1967, 1971; But-ler et al. 1969; Epstein et al. 1969; Wogan 1969, 1974; Kalengayi et al. 1975; Nishizumi et al. 1977; Sieber et al. 1979; Zawirska and Bednarz 1981; Moore et al. 1982; Bannasch et al. 1985; Soffritti and McConnell 1988). In rats, renal cell tumors were also found but a low incidence of tumors at other sites, including the colon (Wogan and Newberne 1967, Butler et al. 1969, Epstein et al. 1969). In monkeys, liver angiosarcomas of the gall bladder and pancreas developed, in addition to hepatocellular and cholangio-cellular carcinomas (Sieber et al. 1979). In rats and hamsters, afla-toxin B_1 administered in the diet induced foci of altered hepato-cytes, the number and size of which was correlated with later devel-opment of hepatocellular adenomas and carcinomas (Wogan and Newberne 1967, Wogan et al. 1971, Kalengayi et al. 1975, Moore et al. 1982, Bannasch et al. 1985, Gil et al. 1988, Soffritti and Mc-Connell 1988).

There is also sufficient evidence to indicate the carcinogenicity of aflatoxin B_1 in humans (IARC 1993). Epidemiologic studies

(Autrup et al. 1987, Peers et al. 1987, Yeh et al. 1989) and several case-control studies (Bulatao-Jayme et al. 1982, Cusumano 1991, Parkin et al. 1991, Srivatanakul et al. 1991) have provided convincing evidence that dietary consumption of aflatoxin B_1 plays an etiologic role in hepatocarcinogenesis. Two correlation studies—one in Swaziland and one in China—indicate a synergy between chronic viral B (also C) hepatitis and aflatoxin exposure (Peers et al. 1987, Ross et al. 1992, Qian et al. 1993). In addition, a synergistic interaction between chronic alcohol consumption and aflatoxin exposure also appears to play a role in human hepatocarcinogenesis. Furthermore, approximately 55% of the hepatocellular carcinomas from people exposed to aflatoxins contain an AGG to AGT mutation at codon 249 of the p53 tumor suppressor gene (Greenblatt et al. 1994), a mutation that is preferentially induced in cultured human hepatocytes exposed to aflatoxin B_1. This fact supports the causative role of aflatoxins in human hepatocarcinogenesis. Less than 4% of liver tumors found in people from developed countries, in which exposure to aflatoxins is relatively low, contain this mutation (Aguilar et al. 1994). Thus, the conventional and molecular epidemiologic studies clearly indicate that aflatoxins are carcinogenic to humans.

On the basis of studies in animals and data in humans, IARC (1993) concludes that aflatoxin B_1 is carcinogenic to humans and has classified it as a Group 1 carcinogen.

Derived Naturally Occurring Carcinogens

PhIP (2-Amino-I-Methyl-6-Phenylimidazo[4,5-b]Pyridine)

In investigations of foods for the presence of multiple polycyclic heterocyclic amines (PHAs), PhIp is usually found to be the most abundant (IARC 1993). PHAs have been isolated from a ordinary human diet cooked simulating household conditions (Alink et al. 1988).

According to IARC (1993), there is sufficient evidence in experimental animals for the carcinogenicity of 2-amino-1-methyl-6-phenylimidazo[4,5-b]pyridine (PhIP). PhIP was tested for carcinogenicity in one experiment in mice and two experiments in rats by oral administration in the diet. It increased the incidence of lymphomas in mice of each sex (Esumi et al. 1989). In rats, it produced adenocarcinomas of the small and large intestine in males and mammary adenocarcinomas in females (Ito et al. 1991, Ochiai et al. 1991). The relevance of these findings to human health is unknown. No data directly relevant to an evaluation of the carcinogenicity to humans of PhIP were available.

On the basis of these studies, IARC (1993) concludes that PhIP is possibly carcinogenic to humans and has classified it as a Group 2B carcinogen.

N-Nitrosodimethylamine

N-nitrosodimethylamine is a derived naturally occurring carcinogen present in a variety of foods, including cheese, soybean oil, canned fruit, various meat products and cured meats, bacon, frankfurters, ham (cooked), fish and fish products, apple brandy, other alcoholic beverages, and beer. Concentrations in these foodstuffs have been measured to be between 0 and 85 ng/kg. Levels of N-nitrosodimethylamine in various foods from several countries, including the United States, have been reported by IARC (1978).

N-nitrosodimethylamine has been identified by IARC (1978) and NTP (1994) as an animal carcinogen. There is sufficient evidence to indicate the carcinogenicity of N-nitrosodimethylamine in several experimental animal species (IARC 1978). When administered orally, it induced liver hemangiosarcomas, hepatocellular carcinomas, and kidney and lung tumors in mice (Takayama and Oota 1963, 1965; Terracini et al. 1966; Toth et al. 1964; Clapp et al. 1968, 1971; Den Engelse et al. 1969, 1970; Clapp and Toya 1970; Otsuka and Kuwahara 1971; Shabad and Savluchinskaya 1971; Zwicker et al. 1972). The chemical also induced kidney and bile duct tumors in rats and hepatocellular carcinomas and bile duct tumors in hamsters, rabbits, and guinea pigs when orally administered (Magee and Barnes 1956, 1959, 1962; Schmähl and Preussmann 1959; Zak et al. 1960; Tomatis et al. 1964; Terracini et al. 1967, 1969; Geil et al. 1968; Le Page and Christie 1969a,b; Riopelle and Jasmin 1969; Kowalewski and Todd 1971; Hadjiolov and Markow 1973; Taylor et al. 1974; Shinohara et al. 1976). N-nitrosodimethylamine is also carcinogenic when it is administered prenatally and in single doses. In several of the studies, dose-response relationships were established.

No case reports or epidemiologic studies are available to evaluate the carcinogenicity of N-nitrosodimethylamine in humans. However, similarities in its metabolism by human and rodent tissues have been demonstrated. Therefore, IARC (1978) concludes that N-nitrosodimethylamine "should be regarded for practical purposes as if it were carcinogenic in humans" and has classified it as a Group 2A carcinogen.

CURRENT STATE OF KNOWLEDGE
OF HUMAN DIETARY ANTICARCINOGENS

Considerable evidence suggests that the consumption of fruits and vegetables is important in the prevention of human cancer (NRC 1989a, Birt and Bresnick 1991, Block et al. 1992, Lelloff et al 1994). Fruits and vegetables are associated with reduced rates of several forms of human cancer, including stomach, lung, breast, and colon. These observations, in addition to other beneficial properties of fruits and vegetables, have encouraged the development of public health campaigns such as the "five-a-day" program designed to increase their intake (NRC 1989a).

A few studies have been conducted in experimental animals on the ability of specific dietary plants to prevent cancer (Birt and Bresnick 1991). Most extensively studied have been members of the cruciferous, allium, and tea families, which were effective in rodents preventing cancers at numerous sites, including esophagus, colon, lung, breast, and skin. There is evidence that some of the inhibition of cancer by fruits and vegetables is due to the essential nutrient vitamins A, C, E, and selenium. There have also been extensive investigations of the particular chemical compounds present in fruits and vegetables, as shown in Appendix C. The results of these investigations suggest that these minor constituents contribute significantly to cancer prevention.

Of particular interest are members of the flavonoid class (apigenin, myricetin, quercetin, robinetin, and rutin), which are widely distributed in foods and which inhibit a range of cancers, such as skin, colon, and lung. Conversely, the most extensively studied flavonoid, quercetin, has also been reported to be a carcinogen under other conditions of feeding (Appendix A). These opposing effects on cancer are not unique to flavonoids. For example, caffeic acid, chlorogenic acid, and eugenol have been observed both to increase and to inhibit the formation of neoplasias. Observations of both positive and negative effects on health have been made for numerous other compounds in foods, such as lectins, phenolic compounds, saponins, and enzyme inhibitors (Thompson 1993). Similarly, synthetic dietary compounds such as butylated hydroxyanisole (BHA) have been found both to induce and to inhibit carcinogenesis in animals (Ito et al. 1989). For example, forestomach cancer was induced by high doses of a number of antioxidants, including BHA. However, these same antioxidants given at low doses, with more potent carcinogens, were effective in inhibiting cancer at a number of sites (Ito et al. 1989). Further studies are needed to define the conditions necessary to achieve inhibition of cancer, avoid undesirable effects, and identify mechanisms of action.

A number of plant phenolics, such as genistein and indole-3 carbinol, have received considerable attention in recent years because of their weak estrogenic activity. Such compounds are called *phytoestrogens*, and it has been hypothesized that these chemicals may block more potent estrogens by binding to estrogen receptors that control gene expression. However, many of the effects of these phenolic compounds do not appear to be related to this binding. It was recently proposed by Safe that some of the potential toxic impact of estrogenic industrial compounds may well be prevented by the large number of phytoestrogens in the diet (Safe, in press).

It is important to note that the results in bioassay testing for carcinogenicity and anticarcinogenicity will probably be skewed by the methods currently used. These methods tend to identify anticarcinogenic properties of chemicals more rapidly than carcinogenic properties, for the following reasons: 1) anticarcinogenicity is typically assayed in the presence of, or following treatment with, a potent carcinogen in a 15-50 week animal bioassay, while to demonstrate potential carcinogenicity, tests require two years with a larger number of animals, and 2) because of the tremendous difference in cost for these two types of studies, it is likely that more chemicals will be studied for their anticarcinogenic effects than for their carcinogenic effects.

There are, moreover, issues of relevance. Compounds are tested for carcinogenicity at high doses to be as certain as possible of detecting weaker effects that would occur rarely and possibly be missed in low dose testing. However, as noted in Chapter 4, high doses introduce problems of extrapolating properly to low human exposures, even when no other factors render the high-dose effects uninterpretable. High-dose exposure to a potent carcinogen, as described above in animal testing for anticarcinogenic effects, is hardly the typical human situation, and the interpretation of such high-dose exposures in anticarcinogenicity studies is open to the same criticisms that apply to high-dose testing for carcinogenicity. It would be more realistic to look for the effects of putative anti-carcinogens on background tumor rates or on rates in animals with genetic predisposition to certain cancers parallel to human genetic patterns, or on animals fed ad libitum vs. calorie-restricted diets. Biological markers, discussed in Chapter 6, may also prove to be of value here.

Many of the compounds listed in Appendix C are reported to have antioxidant properties. However, there are numerous other mechanisms whereby these dietary components may modify carcinogenesis. These include activating detoxification pathways or deactivating toxification pathways, inhibiting cellular proliferation, affecting hormonal modulation, inhibiting interaction of growth factors with their receptors, etc. Equally important, the impact of any single compound on cancer development will almost certainly be the sum of numerous effects of the chemical, rather than a single biological effect. This complexity will inevitably make it difficult to determine mechanisms of dietary prevention of cancer.

The compounds in Appendix C have been assessed individually in experimental animals, or in cell or tissue culture studies. There is no current evidence that these compounds are effective in cancer prevention in humans. Diets rich in plants or in particular types of plants, however, have been associated with reduced rates of some forms of human cancer.

It is important to note that about 70 constitutive naturally occur-ring chemicals from dietary plants are reported to possess both mutagenic and antimutagenic and, in some cases antioxidant prop-erties. Most of these fall under the following classes: flavonoids, phenolic acids, phenylpropanoids, coumarins, depsides, cyclitols, isothiocyanates, catechins, simple phenols, monoterpenes, sesquiterpenes, amino acids, and anthraquinones (Farnsworth 1994).

EFFECT OF DIETARY MACRONUTRIENTS ON CARCINOGENESIS

In this and the following section, we discuss the effects of dietary nutrients (macro- and micro-) separately from non-nutrients, because the data available on these two categories are considerably different. In general, nutrients have been extensively studied and attempts have been made to identify optimal ranges of intakes. Studies on the modulation of cancer by nutrients compare low dietary intakes with optimal and high intakes. Few studies assess nutrient-free diets in cancer modulation because of the known adverse health consequences of consuming deficient diets. In contrast, diets that contain non-nutrient additives have been compared with diets that are free of these agents. Since these components, by definition, are not known to be required, their impact on cancer development has been studied by an approach more typical of toxicology than of nutrition.

Dietary macronutrients include carbohydrates, protein, fats, and alcohol (NRC 1989a). With the exception of alcohol, each class consists of a number of substances that are structurally related.

The dietary substances that ordinarily constitute these classes of macronutrients are generally not carcinogenic. However, carcinogens may be generated when foods containing these substances are cooked excessively, as described in the section on pyrolytic compounds (see previous section on pyrolytic mutagens) (Lijinsky and Ross 1967, Sugimura 1985, Felton et al. 1986). Furthermore, macronutrients may influence the development of cancer by acting as enhancers or, in some cases, inhibitors of carcinogenesis. This section is intended to summarize some of the more important, generally accepted findings concerning the effects of dietary macronutrients on cancer development. This subject was previously reviewed by the Committee on Diet and Health (NRC 1989a).

Calories

Reducing calorie intake results in a reduction in cancer. This phenomenon, known as the *caloric effect*, appears to be the major effect of dietary macronutrients on carcinogenesis in experimental animals.

The caloric effect, discovered early in this century, is one of the most well-documented and generally effective anticarcinogens known for rodents (Pariza and Boutwell 1987). As an example, conducted an experiment in which a group of 50 female BDA mice were fed a mixture of dog chow meal and skimmed milk powder. Supplementation with 1 gm of corn starch in addition to the 2 gm basic feed given to controls increased the spontaneous breast cancer incidence from 0% to 38%. Similar studies conducted in rats reported approximately 20% reduction of lifetime malignant tumor incidence, and many of the tumors observed in the animals whose diets were restricted appeared only when most of the rats fed ad libitum had died. The cancer potency value calculated for the rat study fell between the values derived from the mouse study. These observations suggest that rats and mice might react in a similar manner to excess food and that generalizations to humans may be possible. Haseman and Rao (1992) demonstrated an association in rats between body weight and leukemia, pituitary, and mammary tumors. In male mice an association was also demonstrated between body weight and liver and lung tumors. Hart and Turturro (1994) observed reduced tumor incidences at these sites in calorie-restricted animals. These results are consistent with the finding that excess calorie intake by rodents is associated with higher tumor rates for some tissue sites.

There is considerable epidemiologic evidence that the balance between calorie intake and energy expenditure influences the risk of cancer in humans as well (Kritchevsky 1993, Willett 1994). Nevertheless, independent associations between macronutrients and selected cancers have been found in many epidemiologic studies after controlling for caloric intake (Van't Veer et al. 1990, Willett et al. 1990, Giovannucci et al. 1993b). It appears that the biochemical mechanism of the caloric effect involves changes in hormonal balance (Pariza and Boutwell 1987, Kritchevsky 1993). Specifically, the effect may be mediated by elevated secretion of adrenal hormones such as glucocorticoid hormone and/or dehydroepiandrosterone (Schwartz and Pashko 1994). A considerable body of evidence suggests that glucocorticoids inhibit inflammation, a concomitant of many cytotoxic-regenerative processes associated with enhanced tumorigenesis in some tissues. It is also known that caloric restriction can affect metabolic processes, including enzymes involved in carcinogen activation and inactivation (ILSI 1995). Reduced caloric intake also reduces the rate of cell proliferation or increases the rate of apoptosis (programmed cell death) (Lok et al, 1988, 1990; Grasl-Kraupp et al. 1994; ILSI 1995). Effects on cell proliferation appear to be a particularly significant means of modulating carcinogenesis, including effects on spontaneous tumors in rodents. The effect on apoptosis is particularly prominent in preneoplastic lesions such as hyperplastic nodules in the rat liver (Grasl-Kraupp et al. 1994). A major consequence of inhibiting apoptosis is to increase the number of cells available for replication, in contrast to increasing the rate of proliferation. The resulting effect of either is an increase in the number of DNA replications.

The caloric effect is recognized as markedly influencing the quantitative assessment of carcinogenic potency of chemicals tested by the rodent bioassay (ILSI 1995). Animals fed ad libitum appear to be more responsive when tested in the standard rodent bioassay. In this way, calories play a central role in our evaluation of chemicals and the extrapolation of potency data from rodent studies to humans.

Carbohydrates

The effects of carbohydrates on carcinogenesis have been studied primarily in relation to their contribution to dietary energy. Recent studies have compared the impact of carbohydrate energy on carcinogenesis with that of fat energy on carcinogenesis (see below).

A more extensively studied macronutrient that is often categorized with carbohydrate is fiber, which is not a single substance but rather a collection of many different carbohydrate-containing materials (NRC 1989a). These include cellulose, hemicellulose, pectin, and lignin. Fiber is not degraded by mammalian digestive enzymes but may be partially metabolized by colonic microflora. Some fibers are water-soluble, others insoluble.

The consumption of fiber-rich foods, including those high in pentoses, is associated with decreased colon cancer risk. However, this relationship may be due, at least in part, to other (nonfiber) components of fruits, vegetables, and grains (NRC 1989a). There is some evidence that dietary fiber may reduce the risk of adenomatous polyps of the colon, which are generally considered to be precursor lesions for colon cancer (Neugut et al. 1993). However, the data from animal studies are not consistent: some studies indicate protection whereas others indicate no effect or even enhanced cancer risk. In general, wheat bran exhibits the most consistent inhibiting effect (NRC 1989a). Recent studies suggest that some of the cancer-prevention effects of dietary fiber may be related to the lignan precursors and other phytoestrogens in whole grain foods rich in fiber (Thompson 1994).

Fat

Previous NRC committees (1982 and 1989) have concluded from epidemiologic studies that of all the dietary factors, fat exhibited the most consistent cancer-enhancing effect. However, a clear consensus on the strength of the relationship between dietary fat per se and cancer risk in humans remains elusive (Pariza and Boutwell 1987, Kritchevsky 1993, Willett 1994). For example, although many case-control studies have found positive associations between breast cancer and dietary fat intake, most cohort studies have failed to reproduce this finding (NRC 1989a, Willett 1994). Studies of colon cancer and the consumption of fat (including saturated fat) have been more consistent. However, the fat association is at least in part attributable to a strong association with red meat (Giovannucci et al. 1994). Such an association could reflect other carcinogenic constituents in these foods, such as the heterocyclic amines produced during cooking at high temperatures. A similar situation occurs in prostate cancer, which has been associated with high intake of saturated fats, but also with the high consumption of red meats (Kolonel et al. 1988, Giovannucci et al. 1993b, Le Marchand et al. 1994).

In contrast to the results of epidemiologic investigations, animal studies have produced a much more consistent pattern, because the diets of experimental animals can be readily controlled. Recent experimental studies have suggested that dietary fat and energy may interact in some manner to modify cancer. For example, high dietary fat enhanced mammary carcinogenesis in rats only when diets were freely fed (Welsch et al. 1990). Furthermore, when energy from fat and from carbohydrate were compared for their impact on carcinogenesis, calories from fat appeared to be somewhat more effective in enhancing carcinogenesis than calories from carbohydrates (Zhu et al. 1991, Birt et al. 1993). Thus, while at least some of the impact of fat on cancer appears due to its high caloric density, it also appears that certain properties of fat may enhance cancer, independent of energy.

Dietary fat has been extensively studied experimentally as a modulator in animal models of the multistage process of carcinogenesis. The data are strongest for an impact of dietary fat on events involved in cell proliferation and gene expression (NRC 1982).

Rancid fat contains peroxides and aldehyde mutagens that could initiate and/or promote carcinogenesis, but this possiblity has not been extensively studied (Ames 1983). It has also been proposed that fatty acid oxidation may be involved in tumor promotion within the colon (Ames 1983, Carroll 1985, Welsch 1987). Lane et al. (1985) reported that mammary tissue from mice fed diets high in corn oil had less malonaldehyde (a product of lipid peroxidation) than mice fed diets low in corn oil, even though the mice fed the high corn oil diet developed more mammary tumors after 7,12-dimethylbenzathracene was administered. Hence, while in situ lipid peroxidation may be important in enhancing the development of some forms of cancer (e.g., colon cancer), it does not appear to be involved in carcinogenesis at other sites (e.g., breast).

Linoleic Acid

Linoleic acid is the only fatty acid that has been shown unequivocally to enhance carcinogenesis in animal studies. The effect depends on levels of dietary linoleic acid and exhibits a linear dose response when the concentration is between 1% and 5%. Above 5%, the effect plateaus (Ip et al. 1985). At extremely high levels (>16%) of linoleic acid in the diet, there is a reduction in cell proliferation in the mammary gland. The implications for carcinogenesis in the mammary gland should be explored (Lok et al. 1988, 1990, 1992). Much of the reported effect on experimental carcinogenesis of "fat type" appears to be due to the linoleic acid effect.

Conjugated Linoleic Acid (CLA)

As linoleic acid is the only fatty acid shown unequivocally to enhance carcinogenesis, conjugated linoleic acid (CLA) is the only fatty acid shown unequivocally to inhibit carcinogenesis in experimental animals (Ha et al. 1987, 1990; Ip et al. 1991, 1994). In contrast, the data indicating that omega-3 fatty acids may inhibit carcinogenesis are ambiguous (Pariza 1988), although these fatty acids appear to play a role in reducing the risk of heart disease in human populations (NRC 1989a). The major dietary sources of CLA are foods derived from ruminant animals, for example dairy products and beef (Chin et al. 1992).

CLA is effective as an anticarcinogen when present in the diet of experimental animals at levels as low as 0.05% to 0.1% (Ip et al. 1994). It appears to act via signal transduction pathways and effects on prostaglandin metabolism. In this regard, it has recently been shown that CLA is a growth factor for rats, possibly because it also modulates the catabolic effects resulting from immune stimulation (Chin et al. 1994). There are similarities in the effects of CLA and the effects of omega-3 fatty acids on mammals and birds; in general, CLA appears to be more potent (Miller et al. 1994).

Bile Acids and Free Fatty Acids

Bile acids and free fatty acids are generated during normal digestion. They are toxic for cells of the colonic mucosa and may potentiate the development of colon cancer. It has been proposed that calcium may inhibit the effect by complexing with bile acids and free fatty acids (Scalmati et al. 1992). Epidemiologic data on the relationship of fecal bile acids and neutral steroids to the risk of colon cancer are inconsistent (Kolonel and Le Marchand 1986).

Protein

The major effect of dietary protein on carcinogenesis appears to be caloric (Clinton et al. 1992), although under conditions where protein is growth-limiting, fewer tumors develop (Topping and Visek 1976). Excessive dietary protein increases colonic ammonia levels; ammonia in turn may enhance the development of chemically induced colonic tumors (Clinton et al. 1988). However, few epidemiologic studies have implicated dietary protein in cancer risk

(NRC 1989a). Some studies show associations of colon and breast cancers with dietary protein, particularly animal protein (Lubin et al. 1986, Potter and McMichael 1986). This association could indirectly reflect high correlations between the intake of protein and fat or protein and red meat in the study populations.

Alcohol

Unlike other dietary macronutrients, alcohol refers to a single substance, ethyl alcohol. However, in epidemiologic investigations, it is generally not possible to isolate the effects of ethanol from those of the many congeners in alcoholic beverages. Excessive alcohol consumption has been linked to increased cancer risk at several sites in humans, particularly when combined with certain other factors including tobacco use, infection with Hepatitis B virus, and poor dietary habits (NRC 1989a). Animal experiments indicate that ethyl alcohol enhances cancer risk when administered in the diet or applied topically in conjunction with another carcinogenic agent. In humans, alcohol ingestion appears to increase the risk of cancer in susceptible individuals, but it does not appear to be a genotoxic carcinogen (Seitz and Simanowski 1988). A variety of mechanisms have been proposed to explain the enhancement of carcinogenesis by alcohol, including effects on cell membranes, DNA structure, and carcinogen metabolism.

EFFECT OF DIETARY MICRONUTRIENTS ON CARCINOGENESIS

As noted earlier, considerable epidemiologic and experimental evidence suggests that a number of micronutrients, including vitamins A, C, E, and selenium, contribute to cancer prevention. Conversely, diets deficient in these micronutrients have been associated with an increased risk of cancer. These micronutrients are antioxidants and evidence suggests that some of their anticancer effects may be through inhibition of oxidation; however, they may act through other mechanisms.

This section provides an overview of the micronutrients that have been most extensively studied in cancer cause and prevention. Much of the evidence that these micronutrients are important in cancer prevention comes from the association of fruits and vegetables with cancer prevention. It should be noted that supplemental nutrients have not been observed to be as effective as a diet rich in fruits and vegetables (NRC 1989a). It should be further noted that direct evidence for a specific effect of fruits and vegetables, based on intervention studies in humans, has not yet been reported. It is possible that diets rich in fruits and vegetables are associated with reduced cancer rates because of the lower fat and calorie intake associated with such diets. However, studies involving experimental animals, in which fat and energy intake are controlled, suggest that fruits and vegetables have inhibitory properties (Birt and Bresnick 1991). Furthermore, several epidemiologic studies have reported an inverse relationship between the intake of fruits and/or vegetables and specific cancers; the relationship was shown to be independent of fat or energy intake (Macquart-Moulin et al. 1986, Slattery et al. 1988, Hunter et al. 1993, Pohan et al. 1993, Omenn 1995).

Vitamin A

The naturally occurring forms of vitamin A (retinol, retinal, retinoic acid and its carotenoid precursors) have been extensively studied in animals and humans for their efficacy in cancer prevention. The strength of the inverse relationship between intakes of vitamin A (especially its precursors, the carotenoids) and reduced cancer at several sites led to the development of synthetic analogues of vitamin A which have been extensively studied in animals and recently used in breast cancer patients.

The most convincing evidence that vitamin A and its precursors, the carotenoids, prevent human cancer comes from prospective and retrospective epidemiologic studies associating low intakes of fruits and vegetables with elevated risk of cancer (Ziegler 1991). The data are particularly convincing with respect to lung cancer; however, studies also suggest that vegetable and fruit intake may reduce the risk of cancers at other sites (e.g., the oral cavity, pharynx, larynx, esophagus, colon, rectum, bladder, and cervix) (Ziegler 1991). Investigations suggest that β-carotene is the most effective carotenoid in cancer prevention. However, one study implicates other components of fruits and vegetables in cancer prevention (Le Marchand et al. 1989). In this study of the relationship between the intake of fruits and vegetables and lung cancer risk in humans, results indicated a negative dose-dependent relationship between dietary β-carotene and lung cancer risk, but no clear association for retinol, vitamin C, folic acid, iron, dietary fiber, or fruits. However, all vegetables showed a stronger inverse relationship with lung cancer risk than did β-carotene, suggesting that other constituents of vegetables, such as lutein, lycopene, and indoles, may have anticancer activity (Le Marchand et al. 1989).

The mechanism(s) of vitamin A inhibition of cancer have been extensively debated. Whatever the mechanism, it appears that the carotenoid precursors of vitamin A are responsible for at least some of its anticancer effects (Bendich and Olson 1989). Hypothesized mechanisms whereby carotenoids may inhibit cancer are diverse and include (1) inhibition of mutagenesis and protection against photo-damage, (2) enhancement of immune system responses, (3) reduction of nuclear damage by carcinogenic agents, (4) protection against neoplastic events in cells, and (5) the quenching of highly reactive singlet oxygen (Bendich and Olson 1989, Krinsky 1991). With respect to these mechanisms, β-carotene has been shown to protect against the mutagenic effects of 8-methoxypsoralen (xanthotoxin) and ultraviolet-A light in the presence of oxygen but not under anoxic conditions (Krinsky 1991). β-carotene and other carotenoids have also been shown to enhance immune system responses in cells and animals (Bendich and Olson 1989, Krinsky 1991). For example, addition of β-carotene or canthaxanthin to peripheral blood mononuclear cells results in an increase in cells with natural killer markers and with interleukin-2 receptors (Krinsky 1991). A study of the transformation of fibroblasts exposed to 3-methylcholanthrene or to x-rays found that β-carotene protected against nuclear damage at physiologic concentrations (Bendich and Olson 1989). Studies have also shown that vitamin A binds to nuclear receptors that are members of the steroid hormone receptor superfamily (Evans 1988).

In addition, experimental studies with vitamin A-deficient animals indicate an enhancement of lung cancer by 3-methylcholanthrene and of liver and colon cancer by aflatoxin B_1. While vitamin A may protect against the development of colon cancer, the presence of vitamin A deficiency inhibited N-methyl-N'-nitro-N-nitrosoguanidine induced colon cancer in animals (Birt 1986). The hypothesis that vitamin A protects against a number of human cancers is based on the similarities observed between morphological changes in vitamin A-deficient tissues and in premalignant lesions. Furthermore, vitamin A has been identified as a mammalian morphogen (Evans 1988).

The development of synthetic analogues of vitamin A was driven by the need for agents possessing its cancer-preventive properties, but without its inherent toxicity. A number of analogues have been developed that are effective in cell culture systems and laboratory animals (Moon 1989). Some of these compounds appear to involve interaction with the nuclear vitamin A receptors to modify gene transcription. Other mechanisms of action may involve induction of apoptosis or induction of growth factors that play a role in regulation of cell proliferation (Roberts and Sporn 1992). Preliminary evidence in human trials suggests that 13-cis-retinoic acid may prove useful against oral cancer (Borden et al. 1993). However, the toxicity of vitamin A and its analogues still remains a barrier to extensive use.

Ongoing clinical trials with β-carotene in the prevention of several forms of human cancer, including lung, oral cavity, and breast cancer, should help to determine whether the association between fruit and vegetable intake and reduced rates of cancer is due in part to the presence of β-carotene. In one recent report, neither β-carotene nor α-tocopherol supplements were effective in preventing lung cancer in Finnish men who were heavy smokers (Heinonen and Albanes 1994). These data may mean that β-carotene and α-tocopherol are not the active agents in fruits and vegetables that reduce cancer, or they may indicate that these smokers had a level of damage that could not be corrected by these supplements. Further research will be needed to determine the contribution, if any, of other carotenoids in cancer prevention. It is clear that dietary supplementation with vitamin A for cancer prevention is unlikely at this point because of its inherent toxicity. However, improving our understanding of its mechanism as a morphogen and the role it plays in the induction of differentiation may help us to develop a more effective analogues of vitamin A for future cancer prevention research.

Vitamin C (Ascorbic Acid)

Higginson (1966) reported an inverse association between consumption of foods rich in ascorbic acid and the appearance of certain cancers. Since then, a comprehensive review of epidemiologic studies has assessed the role of ascorbic acid in cancer and provided convincing evidence that ascorbic acid, an important component of fruits and vegetables, prevents cancer at a number of sites (Block 1991). An examination of the relationship between gastric cancer and ascorbic acid provides some of the strongest evidence for its anticancer effects (Mirvish 1983, Block 1991); ascorbic acid status is particularly important in the prevention of gastric cancer in populations with chronic gastric infection (Correa 1994). Cancers of the esophagus, larynx, oral cavity, pancreas, rectum, breast, and cervix are lower in people who consume diets rich in fruits and vegetables (Block 1991). There is also some evidence that inhibition of lung cancer may be related to the ascorbic acid content of these foods (Block 1991). Ascorbic acid was shown to be reduced in smokers, independent of dietary intake. The recommended daily dietary allowance for Vitamin C is 60 mg for adult men and women, while the daily requirement of ascorbic acid is estimated to be 200 mg for smokers (Schectman 1993).

It is believed that ascorbic acid exerts much of its anticarcinogenic effect by inhibiting the formation of N-nitroso compounds in the stomach (Mirvish 1983, Tannenbaum et al. 1991). By reducing nitrite to nitric oxide, ascorbic acid prevents the reaction between nitrite and amines. A reaction between nitrite and amines would result in the formation of nitroso-compounds (Tannenbaum et al. 1991). In addition, it has been demonstrated that sodium ascorbate (22.7 g/kg) and morpholine administered in the diet, along with sodium nitrite in the drinking water, inhibited the formation of N-nitrosomorpholene and liver cancer (Mirvish 1983). The inhibitory role of ascorbic acid in chemically induced carcinogenesis has also been studied in experimental animals at other sites (e.g., skin, trachea, lung, mammary gland, colon, kidney, and urinary bladder) (Birt 1986). Cancers of the skin and colon were reported to be enhanced and inhibited, cancer of the urinary bladder was enhanced, while cancers of the other organs were inhibited. Several mechanisms have been proposed to explain the ability of ascorbic acid to prevent chemically induced carcinogenesis. Mechanisms include its effects as an antioxidant, its role in enhancing cellular immunity, and its role in inhibiting the activation of chemical carcinogens. However, the role of ascorbic acid in chemically induced cancer prevention remains unclear (Block 1991).

Vitamin E (Tocopherols)

Vitamin E consists of a number of related tocopherols. In contrast to the studies of vitamins A and C, epidemiologic studies provide less consistent support for a role of vitamin E in cancer prevention. (Diplock 1991, Stähelin et al. 1991, Garland et al. 1993). The inconsistencies reported in the literature may relate to the poor stability of tocopherol in stored samples. Prospective studies require collection of a large number of samples, and often it is impossible to analyze all the samples at once (Diplock 1991). The 12-year follow-up in the Basel prospective study provided little evidence for an association between vitamin E and cancer at any site (Stähelin et al. 1991). Another prospective study reported that the serum concentration of vitamin E in cancer patients was lower than in controls when the patients were diagnosed within one year of the date of blood collection (Wald et al. 1987). However, these investigators suggested that the low levels of serum vitamin E were a consequence rather than a cause of cancer.

Experimental carcinogenesis studies have provided evidence that vitamin E plays a role in cancer prevention (Birt 1986). Topical administration of vitamin E resulted in inhibition of carcinogenesis when the skin was initially treated with 7-12-dimethyl-benz(a)anthracene (DMBA) followed by 12-0-tetradecanoylphorbol-13-acetate. Dietary administration of vitamin E resulted in inhibiting skin cancer induced by dibenzopyrene. In addition, DMBA-produced cancers of the hamster cheek pouch, mouse forestomach, and rat mammary gland were inhibited by oral treatment (gavage or dietary) with vitamin E (Birt 1986). However, consistent effects of vitamin E were not observed in colon carcinogenesis (Birt 1986).

Vitamin E, like ascorbic acid, inhibits nitrosation of amines. Vitamin E, however, is effective in the lipid compartments of cells, while vitamin C acts in aqueous environments (Newberne and Locaiskar 1990). Studies of its ability to quench the superoxide anion indicate that vitamin E, like vitamin A, may contribute to protection of biological systems from singlet oxygen (Di Mascio et al. 1991). Interestingly, α-tocopherol, generally the most abundant tocopherol in the plasma, is also the most effective form of vitamin E in quenching singlet oxygen (Di Mascio et al. 1991). In addition, considerable evidence suggests that vitamin E may inhibit free radicals formed by mitochondria (Ames et al. 1993).

Folic Acid

Folic acid is found abundantly in vegetables and fruits. Because the consumption of such foods has been associated with reduced cancer rates, and because adequate dietary folic acid is required for the regulation of normal gene expression (1994), folic acid has been implicated in cancer prevention. Considerable research has been conducted on the role of methyl deficiency (usually including deficiencies of folic acid, vitamin B-12, choline, and methionine), DNA methylation, and the induction of liver cancer in rodents (Dizik et al. 1991, Cravo et al. 1992). However, it was not clear if the methyl-deficient conditions induced in animals were applicable to human diets, although the prevalence of inadequate folate intakes has been documented (NRC 1989a). A case-control study of colon and rectum cancer was conducted in 1975-1986 (Freudenheim et al. 1991). Cancer patients (428 colon and 372 rectal cancer patients) were matched with controls, and all were interviewed about dietary practices. When data were adjusted for energy intake, odds ratios for rectal cancer patients with the highest folate intakes compared with those with the lowest intakes were 0.3 and 0.5 for men and women, respectively (Freudenheim et al. 1991). Risk of colon cancer was not associated with dietary folate intake. Furthermore, the difference in odds ratio was greatest for men with the highest alcohol intake, suggesting a possible interaction (Freudenheim et al. 1991). Although earlier studies suggested that folate might protect against cervical cancer, recent case-control studies uncovered no such relationship (Ziegler et al. 1990).

The relation between intake of folic acid, methionine and alcohol, and colon cancer was further investigated because hypomethylated DNA was observed in patients with colorectal carcinomas and because folic acid plays a role in DNA methylation (Giovannucci et al. 1993a). This investigation followed women in the Nurses' Health Study and men in the Health Professionals Follow-up Study after a 1-year dietary assessment. Adenomatous polyps were observed in 564 women and in 331 men. Dietary folate was inversely associated with risk of adenoma in women and men, while alcohol intake above 30 gm/day was positively associated with adenoma risk. Dietary methionine was inversely associated with risk of an adenoma one cm or larger (Giovannucci et al. 1993a). These results support the importance of methyl group availability in the prevention of colorectal cancer.

A recent study demonstrates that methyl-deficient diets (deficient in choline, methionine, and folic acid) in rats fed semipurified diets could result in imbalances in deoxynucleotide pools, which are known to produce mutagenic events (James et al. 1992). In addition, hypomethylation of cytosine, cytosine, guanine, guanine (CCGG, a sequence of nucleotides in DNA) sites have been demonstrated in animals with severe methyl deficiency (diets lacking choline, methionine, folic acid, and vitamin B-12). It is known that CCGG sites in genes, such as c-myc, c-fos and c-Ha-ras, are involved in cellular proliferation and cancer (Christman et al. 1993). Furthermore, folate deficiency has been associated with increases in chromosomal breaks (Ames et al. 1995). These observations support the role of folic acid in cancer prevention.

Vitamin D and Calcium

The role of dietary vitamin D and calcium in cancer prevention was first suggested because of the observation that people in increasingly northern latitudes had higher colon cancer mortality rates (Garland and Garland 1980). Such an association could be due to the impact of ultraviolet light on the synthesis of vitamin D in the skin, and subsequently, on the absorption of dietary calcium. This suggestion was pursued in a 19-year prospective study in Chicago, Illinois, which demonstrated a 50% reduction in colon cancer in men who had a daily intake of 3.75 µg vitamin D and a 75% reduction in men who had a daily intake of >1200 mg calcium (Garland et al. 1991). Evaluation of the levels of circulating 25-hydroxy vitamin D revealed higher values in controls (67-102 nmol/L) (Garland et al. 1991). A prospective study on women in Iowa further supports the hypothesis that vitamin D and/or calcium protect against colon cancer (Bostick et al. 1993).

An extensive series of experiments was conducted in rodents (Newmark and Lipkin 1992) to assess a diet that mimicked four of the suggested dietary risk factors for colon cancer: high fat and phosphate, and low calcium and vitamin D. Feeding this stress diet for 12 weeks resulted in hyperproliferation of cells in the sigmoid colon. Subsequent experiments demonstrated that increasing the level of dietary calcium could return colonic proliferation to normal values. Studies in human subjects at increased risk for colon cancer similarly found a reduction in hyperproliferation of the colonic epithelium when diets were supplemented with calcium (Newmark and Lipkin 1992). Studies of rats treated with 1,2-dimethylhydrazine (DMH) and fed graded levels of calcium and vitamin D showed that both nutrients reduced DMH-induced colon cancer and altered colonic cell kinetics (Beaty et al. 1993). Comparable studies on mammary carcinogenesis induced by 7,12-dimethylbenz(a)-anthracene (DMBA) suggested that high levels of dietary calcium and vitamin D protect against mammary carcinogenesis, while high levels of dietary phosphate increase susceptibility (Carroll et al. 1991).

Prostate cancer risk was recently reported to be inversely associated with exposure to ultraviolet light and it was hypothesized that this was another cancer related to vitamin D intake (Hanchette and Schwartz 1992). This hypothesis is supported by the presence of vitamin receptors in the prostate gland (Berger et al. 1988) and by the evidence supporting a role for vitamin D in the regulation of differentiation and gene expression (Minghetti and Norman 1988).

Selenium

The impact of dietary selenium on carcinogenesis has been the subject of considerable controversy. Early observations of selenium toxicity in animals indicated that excessive amounts were associated with the development of neoplastic alterations in the liver. However, under controlled experimental conditions selenium was a potent inhibitor of liver carcinogenesis, an observation that has been extended to a number of experimental models (El-Bayoumy 1991). Over the past 30 years, numerous investigations have probed the role of selenium in cancer epidemiology and in experimental carcinogenesis (El-Bayoumy 1991). There appears to be a particularly narrow range between the intake of dietary selenium that risks deficiency and those levels at which toxicity can occur.

The first investigation of the relationship between selenium and human cancer assessed the connection between forage selenium and cancer mortality (Clark et al. 1991). A strong inverse relationship between regional forage selenium and cancer mortality was observed. This association was re-examined recently, and cancers of the lung, breast, rectum, bladder, esophagus, and corpus uteri were shown to be elevated in areas with low forage selenium. The association between plasma selenium and esophageal cancer was examined in blacks living in rural areas of southern Africa (Jaskiewicz et al. 1988). Blacks living in areas of high esophageal cancer incidence had lower whole blood selenium levels (58-71 ng/ml) than blacks living in areas of low esophageal cancer incidence (114-177 ng/ml) (Jaskiewicz et al. 1988). In addition, the mean level of blood selenium was lower in patients with premalignant or malignant esophageal cytologic changes than in subjects without such lesions.

A prospective cohort study on lung cancer risk and selenium status (measured by toenail selenium) reported a 50% reduction in relative risk for the cancer among individuals with the highest toenail selenium levels (Van den Brandt et al. 1993). Interestingly, the protective effect of selenium against lung cancer was strongest in the individuals with lower intakes of vitamin C or β-carotene (Van den Brandt 1993). Interactions between selenium and other nutrients have also been observed in studies with animals (Birt 1986). Breast cancer risk was not found to be related to plasma selenium in a prospective study on Guernsey Island (Denmark) (Overvad et al. 1991), although numerous experimental studies in animals have shown that selenium treatment inhibits breast cancer (El-Bayoumy 1991). The association between urinary bladder cancer and serum selenium, a-tocopherol, lycopene, β-carotene, and retinol was reported in a 12-year follow-up of a prospective study in Washington County, Maryland (Helzlsouer et al. 1989). The results indicated the controls had lower plasma selenium concentrations (Helzlsouer et al. 1989).

Extensive investigations have been conducted on the impact of dietary selenium on carcinogenesis in laboratory animals (El-Bayoumy 1991). Induction of preneoplastic lesions in the liver and of liver carcinogenesis by a number of carcinogens was inhibited by selenium administration by dietary, gavage, intraperitoneal or subcutaneous route (El-Bayoumy 1991). Skin carcinogenesis was generally inhibited by topical and dietary selenium administration (El-Bayoumy 1991), but at high doses of selenium, or high doses of carcinogen, selenium was found to enhance skin carcinogenesis (Birt et al. 1989). Colon carcinogenesis was consistently inhibited in animals administered dietary selenium, but inconsistent effects were observed in the pancreas (El-Bayoumy 1991). Selenium was generally observed to be effective at inhibiting carcinogenesis at doses of 0.2 to 5 ppm in the diet. However, the association between cancer and selenium deficiency in animals has not been clearly demonstrated (El-Bayoumy 1991). Recent investigations are exploring novel seleno- compounds with increased efficacy in cancer prevention (El-Bayoumy 1991).

Numerous mechanisms have been explored to explain the modulation of carcinogenesis by selenium (Medina 1986, El-Bayoumy 1991). The best characterized function of selenium in mammalian cells is as a component of the seleno- enzyme, glutathione peroxidase. This enzyme is localized in the cytosol and mitochondrial matrix, and it eliminates organic peroxides from the cell (Medina 1986). However, available evidence suggests that the prevention of carcinogenesis by selenium is not related to its function in glutathione peroxidase (Medina 1986). Other seleno- proteins have been identified, but their impact on carcinogenesis is not defined (Medina 1986). There is some evidence that selenium may alter the metabolism of carcinogens or the interaction of chemical carcinogens with DNA, but there is considerable controversy in the literature (Medina 1986). Additional mechanistic studies suggest that selenium may alter cell proliferation and/or immunologic responses (Medina 1986, El-Bayoumy 1991). Further research is needed to understand the mechanisms whereby selenium prevents cancer.

Iron

Considerable controversy has surrounded the role of iron in carcinogenesis (Weinberg 1992), largely because of the policy of fortifying food with iron to prevent anemia. Recent reports have provided some evidence for the impact of iron status on the development of cancer. Results from a prospective study of 41,000 men and women in Finland indicated an elevated risk of colorectal and lung cancer for individuals with transferrin saturation in excess of 60% (Knekt et al. 1994). In contrast, the risk of stomach cancer was inversely related to serum iron and transferrin saturation in those cases occurring during the first 5 years of followup (Knekt et al. 1994). Studies conducted in South African populations with excessive iron intake and high levels of serum iron did not provide evidence of an elevated risk of cancer (Higginson and Oettle 1960). Further investigations are needed to understand the effect, if any, of iron on the development of cancer.

ENGINEERING AN OPTIMAL DIET

For thousands of years mankind has manipulated the quality of food to obtain improved flavor, color, odor, productivity, and safety. The work of Gregor Mendel in the last century provided the scientific basis for the discipline of plant breeding used so successfully in this century to improve our food plants. Animal breeders also have selected for superior characteristics in species used as food by man.

Conventional plant breeding is based on the cross breeding of different plants possessing desirable characteristics. Initially, the crossing involved individuals of the same species, but today sexually incompatible species of the same family often can successfully be crossed. In both cases, native DNA of one individual is mixed with the DNA of the second and stably preserved and expressed, producing offspring, some of which will have the characteristics of both parents.

These impressive achievements are now being supplemented and enhanced by numerous techniques described under the general term of biotechnology. Biotechnology can be applied to plants and animals, but plants are enjoying greater attention because of their extensive use as food, their less-complex genetics, and the lack of some of the ethical issues animal biotechnology sometimes raises. Plant genetic engineering is a form of biotechnology in which DNA of defined chemical composition bearing specific genetic information is introduced into the genome of a plant to express a new protein or alter the level of an endogenous gene. In this sense, genetically engineered (transgenic) plants are less randomly changed genetically than varieties produced by crossing because the genome of the engineered plant will have been modified by one or at most two or three genes. In traditional plant breeding, many unknown genes are introduced by crossing. The resulting great variability among the offspring requires extensive and time-consuming screening. The full consequences can be known only by detailed physical, chemical, and physiological analysis of the offspring, which is seldom performed. For a more complete discussion of traditional and newer methods of genetic modification, see IFBC (1990a).

The past decade has seen the production of transgenic plants of many crop species (Gasser and Fraley 1989, 1992). Much of the early effort was toward improved agronomic traits such as resistance to herbicides or increased yield. More recently, food plants are being studied to obtain improved quality in storage and transport (tomatoes), tolerance to cold and freezing (strawberries), nutritional improvement (lipids, sugars, amino acids, and proteins), and improved processing properties (Comai 1993). Today, knowledge of plant genetic engineering is sufficiently advanced that any character that is controlled by one or only a few genes probably can be transferred to a food plant. Therefore, the application of plant genetic engineering to the task of removing known carcinogens or increasing the amounts of known anticarcinogens in foods should be expected.

In theory, the removal of a deleterious substance or the increase of a desirable compound could occur in several ways. Thus, the deletion of a carcinogen from a plant food source could occur by using antisense DNA technology to inactivate the gene coding for the enzyme catalyzing the rate-limiting step in biosynthesis of the carcinogenic compound. Alternatively, the amount of a carcinogen might be decreased using gene enhancement to increase the activity of an endogenous enzyme known to convert the carcinogen to the next compound in the normal metabolism of the carcinogen. Introduction of a gene for an enzyme known to detoxify the carcinogen (e.g., a cytochrome P450) would accomplish the same purpose.

The reciprocal approach could be used for increasing the amounts of a desirable anticarcinogen. Thus, the enzyme catalyzing the rate-limiting step in biosynthesis of the anticarcinogen would need to be enhanced, while an enzyme catalyzing the further metabolism of the anticarcinogen should be diminished.

Certain mycotoxins (aflatoxins, fumonisins, and ochratoxins) are produced by fungal infection of plant and animal foods by species of *Aspergillus, Fusarium, Penicillium,* and *Alternaria* (CAST 1989, IFBC 1990a). In these cases, it is the infective organism rather than the plant that produces the carcinogen. Because genetic engineering of ubiquitous, phytopathogenic fungi is a daunting, if not impossible task, a secondary approach should be considered. A food plant serving as host provides a source of macro- and micro-nutrients (sugars, amino acids, vitamins, and growth factors) that are required by the fungus. If the concentrations of nutrients within the host plant can be lowered, the fungus would not be able to grow. Alternatively, plants possess genes that confer resistance to fungi; if those genes can be identified and enhanced, the fungi would be unable to infect the plant and produce the mycotoxin.

All of the genetic engineering described above is dependent on knowledge of the biochemical processes involved in the biosynthesis of the carcinogens, anticarcinogens, and growth factors. That is, the enzymes responsible for a key step in biosynthesis or the first step in catabolism of the compounds of interest need to be available for isolation of the appropriate genes. Regrettably, there is little detailed information on the typically multistep biosynthesis of many of the known carcinogens and anticarcinogens. To decrease the carcinogen directly, another approach might be used. In one recent example, the concentration of a toxic glucosinolate (mustard oil glucoside) was greatly diminished in a commercially significant canola plant, not by inactivating the last step in its biosynthesis, but by diverting the first compound (precursor) in the biosynthetic pathway leading to the glucosinolate. Tryptophan is known to be converted to indole glucosinolates by a sequence of six or seven reactions, only some of which are known precisely. In other plants, tryptophan can be decarboxylated by the enzyme tryptophan decarboxylase to form tryptamine. When the gene for tryptophan decarboxylase was isolated from the medicinal plant *Cantharus roseus* and introduced into *Brassica napus,* the transformed plants were greatly reduced in their content of indole glucosinolates (Chavadej et al. 1994).

It is only a matter of time until a wide variety of bioengineered foods will be available for public consumption. Concerns regarding the safety of genetically engineered food plants have been extensively discussed (Comai 1993, IFBC 1990a, WHO 1991, Kessler et al. 1992, OECD 1992), and most scientists agree that the transformation process introduces no inherently new categories of hazard and that existing procedures for testing and screening, properly employed, are adequate to ensure the safety of the products. The policies regulating genetically engineered foods have also been summarized by Harlander (1993). The basic regulatory principles are found in a statement by the FDA (1992), which indicates that no regulation other than those applied to foods obtained by classical plant breeding are necessary.

The first genetically engineered food to be marketed is the Flavr/Savr™ tomato developed by Calgene, Inc. Its safety has been extensively examined and documented for examination by the FDA (Redenbaugh et al. 1992). As with most other new technologies, public acceptance of this first bioengineered food will doubtless depend on whether the purchaser sees a benefit from the product of the new technology.

SUMMARY AND CONCLUSIONS

The human diet is enormously complex; it consists of variable mixtures of dietary components. Animal studies indicate that certain dietary components may be carcinogenic, while others may have anticarcinogenic effects. Indeed, in some instances a single constituent might be carcinogenic and anticarcinogenic under different circumstances.

Nutrients present in the diet contribute to the prevention of cancer. Considerable evidence in human and animal systems suggests that diets rich in a number of vitamins and minerals protect against cancer at a wide variety of sites. Such diets tend to contain an abundance of fruits and vegetables and are also associated with reduced rates of other chronic diseases. Ongoing cancer prevention trials will help to identify the importance of specific nutrients or other constituents and, in some cases, interactions between nutrients. However, until we have this information, it is of the utmost importance to continue recommending that the public consume diets rich in fruits and vegetables but low in fat and calories. The consumption of vitamins and minerals in a moderate, varied, and balanced diet—not as dietary supplements—continues to be one of our best strategies for cancer prevention in people.

REFERENCES

Adenis, L., A. Demaille, and J. Driessens. 1968. Pouvoir cancérigène de l'uréthane chez le rat Sprague. C.R. Soc. Biol. (Paris) 162:458-461.

Aguilar, F., C.C. Harris, T. Sun, M. Hollstein, and P. Cerutti. 1994. Geographic variation of p53 mutational profile in non-malignant human liver. Science 264:1317-1319.

Alink, G.M., M.G. Knize, N. H. Shen, S. P. Hesse, and J.S. Felton. 1988. Mutagenicity of food pellets from human diets in the Netherlands. Mutat. Res. 206:387-393.

Ames, B.N. 1983. Dietary carcinogens and anticarcinogens. Science 221:1256-1264.

Ames, B.N., L.S. Gold, and W.C., Willett. 1995. The causes and prevention of cancer. Proc. Natl. Acad. Sci. U.S.A. 92:5258-5265.

Ames, B.N., M. Profet, and L.S. Gold. 1990. Dietary pesticides

(99.99% all natural). Proc. Natl. Acad. Sci. U.S.A. 87:7777:7781.

Ames, B.N., M.K. Shigenaga, and T.M. Hagen. 1993. Oxidants, antioxidants, and the degenerative diseases of aging. Proc. Natl. Acad. Sci. U.S.A. 90(17):7915-7922.

Anonymous. 1970. Webster's New World Dictionary of the American Language, 2nd College ed., D.B. Guralnik, ed. New York: World Publishing Co.

Anonymous. 1966. Webster's Third New International Dictionary of the English Language, Unabridged. Chicago, IL: Merriam-Webster. Encyclopedia Britannica.

ApSimon, J. 1989. Phytoalexins as human and animal toxins: recent advances Pp. 229-241 in 1989 Annual Summer Toxicology Forum. Washington, DC: Toxicology Forum.

Argus, M.F., and C. Hoch-Ligeti. 1961. Comparative study of the carcinogenic activity of nitrosamines. J. Nat. Cancer Inst. 27:695.

Autrup, H., T. Seremet, J. Wakhisi, and A. Wasumma. 1987. Aflatoxin exposure measured by urinary excretion of aflatoxin B_1-guanine adduct and hepatitis B virus infection in areas with different liver cancer incidence in Kenya. Cancer Res. 47:3430-3433.

Bannasch, P., U. Benner, H. Enzmann, and H.J. Hacker. 1985. Tigroid cell foci and neoplastic nodules in the liver of rats treated with a sigle dose of aflatoxin B_1. Carcinogenesis 6:1641-1648.

Beaty, M.M., E.Y. Lee, and H.P. Glauert. 1993. Influence of dietary calcium and vitamin D on colon epithelial cell proliferation and 1,2-dimethylhydrazine-induced colon carcinogenesis in rats fed high fat diets. J. Nutr. 123:144-152.

Bendich, A. and J.A. Olson. 1989. Biological actions of carotenoids. FASEB J. 3:1927-1932.

Berenblum, I., and N. Haran-Ghera. 1957. A quantitative study of the systemic initiating action of urethane (ethyl carbamate) in mouse skin carcinogenesis. Brit. J. Cancer 11:77-84.

Berger, U., P. Wilson, R.A. McClelland, K. Colston, M.R. Haussler, and J.W. Pike. 1988. Immunocytochemical detection of 1,25-dihydroxyvitamin D receptors in normal human tissues. J. Clin. Endocrinol. Metab. 67:607-613.

Birt, D.F. 1986. Update on the effects of vitamins A, C and E and selenium on carcinogenesis. Pp. 311-320 in Proceedings of the

Society for Experimental Biology and Medicine.

Birt, D.F. and E. Bresnick. 1991. Chemoprevention by nonnutrient components of vegetables and fruits. Pp. 221-261 in Human Nutrition: A Comprehensive Treatise, R. Alfin-Slater and D. Kritchevsky, eds. New York: Plenum.

Birt, D.F., P.M. Pour, and J.C. Pelling. 1989. The influence of dietary selenium on colon, pancreas and skin tumorigenesis. Pp.297-304 in 4th International Symposium on Selenium in Biology and Medicine, A. Wendet, ed.

Birt, D.F., H.J. Pinch, T. Barnett, A. Phan, and K. Dimitroff. 1993. Inhibition of skin tumor promotion by restriction of fat and carbohydrate calories in SENCAR mice. Cancer Res. 53:27-31.

Block, G. 1991. Vitamin C and cancer prevention: The epidemiologic evidence. Am. J. Clin. Nutr. 53:270S-282S.

Block, G., B. Patterson, and A. Subar. 1992. Fruit, vegetables, and cancer prevention: A review of the epidemiological evidence. Nutr. Cancer 18:1-29.

Booth, A.N., O.H. Emerson, F.T. Jones, and F. DeEds. 1957. Urinary metabolites of caffeic and chlorogenic acids. J. Biol. Chem. 229:51-59.

Borden, E.C., R. Lotan, D. Levens, C.W. Young, and S. Waxman. 1993. Differentiation therapy of cancer: Laboratory and clinical investigations. Cancer Res. 53: 4109-4115.

Bostick, R.M., J.D. Potter, T.A. Sellers, D.R. McKenzie, L.H. Kushi, and A.R. Folsom. 1993. Relation of calcium, vitamin D, and dairy food intake to incidence of colon cancer among older women: The Iowa women's health study. Am. J. Epidemiol. 137:1302-1317.

Bulatao-Jayme, J., E.M. Almero, M.C.A. Castro, M.T.R. Jardeleza, and L.A. Salamat. 1982. A case-control dietary study of primary liver cancer risk from aflatoxin exposure. Int J. Epidemiol. 11:112-119.

Butler, W.H., M. Greenblatt, and W. Lijinsky. 1969. Carcionogenesis in rats by aflatoxins B_1, G_1, and B_2. Cancer Res. 29:2206-2211.

Carroll, K.K. 1985. Lipid oxidation and carcinogenesis. Pp. 237-244 in Genetic Toxicology of the Diet, I. Knudsen, ed. New York: Liss. 351 pp.

Carroll, K.K., E.A. Jacobson, L.A. Eckel, and H.L. Newmark. 1991. Calcium and carcinogenesis of the mammary gland. Am. J. Clin.

Nutr. 54(Suppl.):206S-208S.

Chavadej, S., N. Brisson, J.N. McNeil, and V. DeLuca. 1994. Redirection of tryptophan leads to production of low indole glucosinolate canola. Proc. Natl. Acad. Sci. 91:2166-2170.

Cheftel, J.C., J.-L. Cuq, and D. Lorient. 1985. Amino acids, peptides, and proteins. Pp. 245-369 in Food Chemistry, 2nd edition, O.R. Fennema, ed. New York: Marcel Dekker, Inc.

Chin, S.F., W. Liu, J.M. Storkson, Y.L. Ha, and M.W. Pariza. 1992. Dietary sources of conjugated dienoic isomers of linoleic acid, a newly recognized class of anticarcinogens. J. Food Comp. Analysis 5:185-197.

Chin, S.F., J.M. Storkson, K.J. Albright, M.E. Cook, and M.W. Pariza. 1994. Conjugated linoleic acid is a growth factor for rats as shown by enhanced weight gain and improved feed efficiency. J. Nutr. 124:2344-2349.

Christman, J.K., G. Sheikhnejad, M. Dizik, S. Abileah, and E. Wainfan. 1993. Reversibility of changes in nucleic acid methylation and gene expression induced in rat liver by severe dietary methyl deficiency. Carcinogenesis 14:551-557.

Clapp, N.K., A. W. Craig, and R.E. Toya, Sr. 1968. Pulmonary and hepatic oncogenesis during treatment of male RF mice with dimethylnitrosamine. J. Nat. Cancer Inst. 41:1213.

Clapp, N.K., and R.E. Toya, Sr. 1970. Effect of cumulative dose and dose rate on dimethylnitrosamine oncogenesis in RF mice. J. Nat. Cancer Inst. 45:495.

Clark, L.C., K.P. Cantor, and W.H. Allaway. 1991. Selenium in forage crops and cancer mortality in U.S. counties. Arch. Environ. Health 46:37-42.

Clarke, R.J., and R. Macrae, eds. 1985. Coffee, Volume 1, Chemistry. New York: Elsevier Applied Science. 306 pp.

Clinton, S.K., D.G. Bostwick, L.M. Olson, H.J. Manigan, and W.J. Visek. 1988. Effects of ammonium acetate and sodium cholate on N-methyl-N'nitro-N-nitrosoguanidine-induced colon carcinogenesis of rats. Cancer Res. 48:3035-3039.

Clinton, S.K., P.B. Imrey, H.J. Mangian, S. Nandkumar, and W.J. Visek. 1992. The combined effects of dietary fat, protein, and energy intake on azoxymethane-induced intestinal and renal carcinogenesis.

Cancer Res. 52:857-865.

Comai, L. 1993. Impact of plant genetic engineering on foods and nutrition. Annu. Rev. Nutr. 13:191-215.

Connolly, J.D. and R.A. Hill. 1991. Dictionary of terpenoids. Vols. 1-3. London: Chapman and Hall

Corpet, D.E., D. Stamp, A. Medline, S. Minkin, M.C. Archer, and W.R. Bruce. 1990. Promotion of colonic microadenoma growth in mice and rats fed cooked sugar or cooked casein and fat. Cancer Res. 50:6955-6958.

Correa, P. 1991. The epidemiology of gastric cancer. World J. Surg. 15:228-234.

Cravo, M.L., J.B. Mason, and Y. Dayal, M. Hutchinson, D. Smith, J. Selhub, and I.H. Rosenberg. 1992. Folate deficiency enhances the development of colonic neoplasia in dimethylhydrazine-treated rats. Cancer Res. 52:5002-5006.

Crosby, D.G. 1969. Natural toxic background in the food of man and his animals. J. Ag. and Food Chem. 17:(May-June)532-538.

Cusumano, V. 1991. Aflatoxins in sera from patients with lung cancer. Oncology 48:194-195.

Czok, V.G., W. Walter, K. Knoche, and H. Degener. 1974. Reabsorption of chlorogenic acid in the rat.(in German). Zeit. fur Ernahrungswissenschaft 13:108-112.

Davíâdek, J., J. Velâíśek, and J. Pokornây, J., eds. 1990. Chemical Changes During Food   Processing. New York: Elsevier. Pp. 100-119.

Della Porta, G., J. Capitano, W. Montipo, and L. Parmi. 1963a. Studio sull' azione cancerogena dell' uretano nel topo. Tumori 49:413-428.

Della Porta, G., J. Capitano, and P. Strambio de Castillia. 1963b. Studies on leukemogenesis in urethan-treated mice. Acta Un. Int. Cancer 29:783-785.

Den Engelse, L., P.A.J. Bentvelzen, and P. Emmelot. 1969/1970. Studies on lung tumours. I. Methylation of deoxyribonucleic acid and tumour formation following administration of dimethylnitrosamine to mice. Chem.-Biol. Interactions 1:394-406.

Di Mascio, P., M.E. Murphy, and H. Sies. 1991. Antioxidant defense systems: the role of carotenoids, tocopherols and thiols. Am. J. Clin.

Nutr. 53:194S-200S.

Dickey, R. 1989. Ciguatera: Toxin production in isolates of *Procentrum concavum* and *P. lima*. Pp. 247-252 in 1989 Annual Summer Toxicology Forum. Washington, DC: Toxicology Forum.

Diplock, A.T. 1991. Antioxidant nutrients and disease prevention: An overview. Am. J. Clin. Nutr. 53(Suppl.):189S-193S.

Dizik, M., J.K. Christman, and E. Wainfan. 1991. Alterations in expression and methylation of specific genes in livers of rats fed a cancer promoting methyl-deficient diet. Carcinogenesis 12:1307-1312.

Ehrlich, P.R., and P.H. Raven. 1964. Butterflies and plants: A study in coevolution. Evolution 18:586-608.

El-Bayoumy, K. 1991. The role of selenium in cancer prevention. Pp. 1-15 in Cancer Principles and Practice of Oncology, 4th edition, V. Davita, S. Helman, and S.A. Rosenberg, eds. Philadelphia, PA.

Epstein, S., B. Bartus, and E. Farber. 1969. Renal epithelial neoplasms induced in male Wistar rats by oral aflatoxin B_1. Cancer Res. 29:1045-1050.

Esumi, H., H. Ohgaki, E. Kohzen, S. Takayama, and T. Sugimura. 1989. Induction of lymphoma in CDF_1 mice by the food mutagen, 2-amino-1-methyl-6-phenylimidazo[4,5-*b*]pyridine. Jpn. J. Cancer Res. 80:1176-1178.

Evans, R.M. 1988. The steroid and thyroid hormone receptor superfamily. Science 240:889-895.

Farnsworth, N.R. 1994. Data were obtained from the NAPRALERT database on natural products, which covers the natural product literature from at least 1975 through October 1, 1994. NAPRALERT has the capability of restricting searches to plants used as foods and is available on line through the Scientific and Technical Network (STN) of Chemical Abstracts Services. Columbus, Ohio.

FDA (U.S. Food and Drug Administration). 1992. Statement of Policy: Foods derived from new plant varieties. Fed. Regist. 57:22984-23005 (29 May 1992).

Feeny, P. 1975. Coevolution of Animals and Plants: Symposium V, First International Congress of Systematic and Evolutionary Biology.

L.E. Gilbert and P.H. Raven, eds. Austin, TX: University of Texas Press.

Felton, J.S., M.G. Knize, N.H. Shen, B.D. Andersen, L.F. Bjeldanes, and F.T. Hatch. 1986. Identification of the mutagens in cooked beef. Environ. Health Perspec. 67:17-24.

Fraenkel, G.S. 1959. The *raison d'être* of secondary plant substances. Science 129:1466-1470.

Freudenheim, J.L., S. Graham, J.R. Marshall, B.P. Haughey, S. Cholewinski, and G. Wilkinson. 1991. Folate intake and carcinogenesis of the colon and rectum. Int. J. Epidemiol. 20:368-374.

Garland, C.F., and F.C. Garland. 1980. Do sunlight and vitamin D reduce the likelihood of colon cancer? Int. J. Epidemiol. 9:227-231.

Garland, C.F., F.C. Garland, and E.D. Gorham. 1991. Can colon cancer incidence and death rates be reduced with calcium and vitamin D. Am. J. Clin. Nutr. 54(Suppl.):193S-201S.

Garland, M., W.C. Willett, J.E. Manson, and D.J. Hunter. 1993. Antioxidant micronutrients and breast cancer. J. Am. Coll. Nutr. 12:400-411.

Geil, J.H., R.J. Stenger, R.M. Behki, and W.S. Morgan. 1968. Hepatotoxic and carcinogenic effects of dimethylnitrosamine in low dosage. Light and electron microscopic study. J. Nat. Cancer Inst. 40:713-730.

Gil, R., R. Callaghan, J. Boix, A. Pellin, and A. Llombart-Bosch. 1988. Morphometric and cytophotometric nuclear analysis of altered hepatocyte foci induced by N-nitrosomorpholine (NNM) and aflatoxin B_1 (AFB_1) in liver of Wistar rats. Virchows Arch. B Cell Pathol. 54:341-349.

Giovannucci, E., E.B. Rimm, G.A. Colditz, M.J. Stampfer, A. Ascherio, C.C. Chute, and W.C. Willett. 1993b. A prospective study of dietary fat and risk of prostate cancer. J. Natl. Cancer Inst. 85:1571-1579.

Giovannucci, E., M.J. Stampfer, G.A. Colditz, E.B. Rimm, D. Trichopoulos, B.A. Rosner, F.E. Speizer, and W.C. Willett. 1993a. Folate, methionine, and alcohol intake and risk of colorectal adenoma. J. Natl. Cancer Inst. 85:875-884.

Giovannucci, E, E.B. Rimm, M.J. Stampfer, G.A. Colditz, A. Ascherio, and W.C. Willett. 1994. Intake of fat, meat, and fiber in relation to risk of colon cancer in men. Cancer Res. 54:2390-2397.

Glasby, J.S. 1982. Encyclopedia of Terpenoids. Vols. 1 and 2. Chichester, New York: Wiley. 2646 pp.

Grasl-Kraupp, B., W. Bursch, B. Ruttkay-Nedecky, A. Wagner, B. Lauer, and R. Schulte-Hermann. 1994. Food restriction eliminates preneoplastic cells through apoptosis and antagonizes carcinogenesis in rat liver. Proc. Natl. Acad. Sci. USA 91:9995-9999.

Greenblatt, M.S., W.P. Bennett, M. Hollstein, and C.C. Harris. 1994. Mutations in the p53 tumor suppressor gene: Clues to cancer etiology and molecular pathogenesis. Cancer Res. 54:4855-4878.

Ha, Y.L., N.K. Grimm, and M.W. Pariza. 1987. Anticarcinogens from fried ground beef: Heat-altered derivatives of linoleic acid. Carcinogenesis 8:1881-1887.

Ha, Y.L., J. Storkson, and M.W. Pariza. 1990. Inhibition of benzo(a)pyrene-induced mouse forestomach neoplasia by conjugated dienoic derivatives of linoleic acid. Cancer Res. 50:1097-1101.

Hadjiolov, D., and D. Markow. 1973. Fine structure of hemangioendothelial sarcomas in the rat liver induced with N-nitrosodimethylamine. Arch. Geschwulstforsch. 42:120-126.

Hall, R.L. 1992. Food Additives. Pp. 280-283 in McGraw-Hill Encyclopedia of Science and Technology, 7th ed., Vol. 7. New York: McGraw-Hill, Inc.

Hall, S. 1989. Introduction to marine toxins and paralytic shellfish poisons. Pp. 242-246 in 1989 Annual Summer Toxicology Forum. Washington, DC: Toxicology Forum.

Hanchette, C.L., and G.G. Schwartz. 1992. Geographic patterns of prostate cancer mortality: Evidence for a protective effect of ultraviolet radiation. Cancer 70:2861-2869.

Harborne, J.B. 1988. The Flavonoids: Advances in Research Since 1980, vol. 2. London: Chapman and Hall. 900 pp.

Harborne, J.B. 1994. Introduction to Ecological Biochemistry, 4th edition. London: Academic Press. 400 pp.

Harborne, J.B., T.J. Mabry, and H. Mabry. 1975. The Flavonoids. Vols. 1 and 2. London: Chapman and Hall. 1204 pp.

Hart, R.W., and A. Turturro. 1995. Dietary restriction: An update. Pp. 1-12 in Dietary Restriction: Implications for the Design and

Interpretation of Toxicity and Carcinogenicity Studies. R.W. Hart, D.A. Neumann, and R.T. Robertson, eds. Washington, DC: ILSI Press.

Haseman, J.K., and G.N. Rao. 1992. Effects of corn oil, time-related changes, and inter-laboratory variability on tumor occurrence in control Fischer 344 (F344/N) rats. Toxicol. Pathol. 20:52-60.

Hawk, P.B. 1965. Hawk's Physiological Chemistry, 14th edition. B.L. Oser, ed. New York: McGraw-Hill. pp. 112.

Heinonen, O.P. and D. Albanes. 1994. The effect of vitamin E and beta carotene on the incidence of lung cancer and other cancers in male smokers. The Alpha-Tocopherol, Beta Carotene Cancer Prevention Study Group. N. Engl. J. Med. 330:1029-1035.

Helzlsouer, K.J., G.W. Comstock, and J.S. Morris. 1989. Selenium, lycopene, α-tocopherol, β-carotene, retinol, and subsequent bladder cancer. Cancer Res. 49:6144-6148.

Herrmann, K. 1989. Occurrence and content of hydroxycinnamic and hydroxybenzoic acid compounds in food. Crit. Rev. Food Sci. Nutr. 28:315-347.

Higginson, J. 1966. Etiological factors in gastrointestinal cancer in man. JNCI 37:527-545.

Higginson, J., and A.G. Oettle. 1960. Cancer incidence in the Bantu and "Cape Colored" races of South Africa: Report of a cancer survey in the Transvaal (1953-1955. JNCI 24:589-671.

Hirose, M., A. Masuda, S. Fukushims, and N. Ito. 1988. Effects of subsequent antioxidant treatment on 7,12-dimethylbenz[a]anthracene-initiated carcinogenesis of the mammary gland, ear duct and forestomach in Sprague-Dawley rat. Carcinogenesis 9:101-104.

Hirose, M.M. Mutai, S. Takahashi, M. Yamada, S. Fukushima, and N. Ito. 1991. Effects of phenolic antioxidants in low dose combination on forestomach carcinogenesis in rats pretreated with N-methyl-N'-nitrosoguanidine. Cancer Res. 51:824-827.

Hirose, M., M. Kawabe, M. Shibata, S. Takahashi, S. Okazaki, and N. Ito. 1992. Influence of caffeic acid and other o-dihydroxybenzene derivatives on N-methyl-N'-nitro-N-nitrosoguanidine-initiated rat forestomach carcinogenesis. Carcinogenesis 13:1825-1828.

Hölldobler, B. 1995. The chemistry of social regulation:

Multicomponent signals in ant societies. Proc. Nat. Acad. Sci. 92(1):19-22.

Hudson, B.J.E. 1990. Food Antioxidants. London: Elsevier Applied Science. 317 pp.

Hunter, D.J., J.E. Manson, G.A. Colditz, M.J. Stamper, B. Rosner, C.H. Hennekens, F.E. Speizer, and W.C. Willett. 1993. A prospective study of the intake of vitamins C, E, and A and the risk of breast cancer. N. Engl. J. Med. 329:234-240.

IARC (International Agency for Research on Cancer). 1974. IARC Monographs on the Evaluation of Carcinogenic Risk of Chemicals to Man. Some Anti-Thyroid and Related Substances, Nitrofurans, and Industrial Chemicals. Volume 7. Lyon, France: IARC.

IARC (International Agency for Research on Cancer). 1978. Chemicals with Sufficient Evidence of Carcinogenicity in Experimental Animals. IARC Monographs Volumes 1-17. (IARC Intern. Tech. Rep. No. 78/003). Lyon, France: IARC.

IARC (International Agency for Research on Cancer). 1987. IARC Monographs on the Evaluation of Carcinogenic Risks to Humans. Overall Evaluations of Carcinogenicity: An Updating of IARC Monographs Volumes 1 to 42, Supplement 7. Lyon, France: IARC.

IARC (International Agency for Research on Cancer). 1993. IARC Monographs on the Evaluation of Carcinogenic Risks to Humans. Some Naturally Occurring Substances: Food Items and Constituents, Heterocyclic Aromatic Amines and Mycotoxins. Vol. 56. Lyon France: IARC.

IFBC (International Food Biotechnology Council). 1990a. Biotechnologies and food: Assuring the safety of foods produced by genetic modification. Regul. Toxicol Pharmacol. 12:3(part 2) S1-S196.

IFBC (International Food Biotechnology Council). 1990b. Biotechnologies and food: Assuring the safety of foods produced by genetic modification. Regul. Toxicol Pharmacol. 12:3(part 2) S23.

IFBC (International Food Biotechnology Council). 1990c. Biotechnologies and food: Assuring the safety of foods produced by genetic modification. Regul. Toxicol Pharmacol. 12:3(part 2) S28-S29.

IFBC (International Food Biotechnology Council). 1990d.

Biotechnologies and food: Assuring the safety of foods produced by genetic modification. Regul. Toxicol Pharmacol. 12:3(part 2) S92-93.

ILSI (International Life Sciences Institute). 1995. Dietary Restriction: Implications for the Design and Interpretation of Toxicity and Carcinogenicity Studies. R.W. Hart, D.A. Neumann, and R.T. Robertson, eds. Washington, D.C.: ILSI Press.

Inoue, S., K. Ito, K. Yamamoto, and S. Kawanishi. 1992. Caffeic acid causes metal-dependent damage to cellular and isolated DNA through H_2O_2 formation. Carcinogenesis 13:1497-502.

Ip, C., C.A. Carter, and M.M. Ip. 1985. Requirement of essential fatty acid for mammary tumorigenesis in the rat. Cancer Res. 45:1997-2001.

Ip, C., S.F. Chin, J.A. Scimeca, and M.W. Pariza. 1991. Mammary cancer prevention by conjugated dienoic derivative of linoleic acid. Cancer Res. 51:6118-6124.

Ip, C., M. Singh, H.J. Thompson, and J.A. Scimeca. 1994. Conjugated linoleic acid suppresses mammary carcinogenesis and proliferative activity of the mammary gland in the rat. Cancer Res. 54:1212-1215.

Ito, N., and M. Hirose. 1987. The role of antioxidants in chemical carcinogenesis. Jpn. J. Cancer Res (Gann) 78:1011-1026.

Ito, N., and M. Hirose. 1989. Antioxidants—Carcinogenic and chemopreventive properties. Adv. Cancer Res. 53:247-302.

Ito, N., R. Hasegawa, M. Sano, S. Tamano, H. Esumi, S. Takayama, and T. Sugimura. 1991. A new colon and mammary carcinogen in cooked food, 2-amino-1-methyl-6-phenylimidazo[4,5-*b*]-pyridine (PhIP). Carcinogenesis 12:1503-1506.

Iverson, F. 1989. A toxicological perspective on the 1987 domoic acid mussel poisoning incident in Eastern Canada. Pp. 253-268 in 1989 Annual Summer Toxicology Forum. Washington, DC: Toxicology Forum.

James, S.J., D.R. Cross, and B.J. Miller. 1992. Alterations in nucleotide pools in rats fed diets deficient in choline, methionine and/or folic acid. Carcinogenesis 13:2471-2474.

Jaskiewicz, K., W.F.O. Marasas, J.E. Rossouw, F.E. Van Niekerk, and E.W. Heine Tech. 1988. Selenium and other mineral elements in populations at risk for esophageal cancer. Cancer 62:2635-2639.

Jenner, A. 1973. Food: Fact and Folklore. Pp. 1-37. Toronto:

McClelland and Stewart, Ltd.

Kalengayi, M.M.R., G. Ronchi, and V.J. Desmet. 1975. Histochemistry of gamma-glutamyl transpeptidase in rat liver during aflatoxin B_1-induced carcinogenesis. J. Natl Cancer Inst. 55:579-588.

Klein, M. 1962. Induction of lymphocytic neoplasms, hepatomas, and other tumors after oral administration of urethan in infant mice. J. Nat. Cancer Inst. 29:1035-1046.

Klein, M. 1966. Influence of age on induction with urethan of hepatomas and other tumors in infant mice. J. Nat. Cancer Inst. 36:1111-1120.

Knekt, P., A. Reunanen, H. Takkunen, A. Aromaa, M. Helivaara, and T. Hakulinen. 1994. Body iron stores and risk of cancer. Int. J. Cancer 56:379-382.

Kolonel, L.N. and L. Le Marchand. 1986. The epidemiology of colon cancer and dietary fat. Pp. 69-91 in Progress in Clinical and Biological Research, Vol. 222: Dietary Fat and Cancer, C. Ip, D. Birt, A.E. Rogers, and C. Mettlin, eds. New York: Alan R. Liss, Inc.

Kolonel, L.N., C.N. Yoshizawa, and J.H. Hankin. 1988. Diet and prostatic cancer: A case-control study in Hawaii. Am. J. Epidemiol. 127:999-1012.

Kowalewski, K., and E.F. Todd. 1971. Carcinoma of the gallbladder induced in hamsters by insertion of cholesterol pellets and feeding dimethylnitrosamine. Proc. Soc. Exp. Biol. Med. (NY) 136:482-486.

Krinsky, N.I. 1991. Effects of carotenoids in cellular and animal systems. Am. J. Clin. Nutr. 53:238S-246S.

Kritchevsky, D. 1993. Undernutrition and chronic disease: Cancer. Proc. Nutr. Soc. 52:39-47.

Kroto, H.W., J.R. Heath, S.C. O'Brien, R.F. Curl, and R.E. Smalley. 1985. C60: Buckminsterfullerene. Nature 318:162-163.

Lane, H.W., J.S. Butel, C. Howard, F. Shepherd, R. Halligan, and D. Medina. 1985. The role of high levels of dietary fat in 7,12-dimethyl-benzanthracene-induced mouse mammary tumorigenesis: Lack of an effect on lipid peroxidation. Carcinogenesis 6:403-407.

Laranjinha, J.A., L.M. Almeida, and V.M. Madeira. 1992. Lipid peroxidation and its inibition in low density lipoproteins: quenching of cis-parinaric acid fluorescence. Archives Biochem Biophys

297:147-154.

Laranjinha, J.A., L.M. Almeida, and V.M. Madeira. 1994. Reactivity of dietary phenolic acids with peroxyl radicals: antioxidant acitvity upon low density lipoprotein peroxidation. Biochem Pharmacol. 48:487-94.

Le Marchand, L., C.N. Yoshizawa, L.N. Kolonel, J.H. Hankin, and M.T. Goodman. 1989. Vegetable consumption and lung cancer risk: A population-based case-control study in Hawaii. JNCI 81:1158-1164.

Le Marchand, L., L.N. Kolonel, L.R. Wilkens, B.C. Myers, and T. Hirohata. 1994. Animal fat consumption and prostate cancer: A prospective study in Hawaii. Epidemiol. 5:276-82.

Le Page, R.N., and G.S. Christie. 1969a. Induction of liver tumours in the rabbit by feeding dimethylnitrosamine. Brit. J. Cancer. 23:125.

Le Page, R.N., and G.S. Christie. 1969b. Induction of liver tumours in the guinea pig by feeding dimethylnitrosamine. Pathology 1:49.

Li, Y., and M.A. Trush. 1994. Reactive oxygen-dependent DNA damage resulting from the oxidation of phenolic compounds by a copper-redox cycle mechanism. Cancer Research 54(Suppl 7):1895s-1898s.

Li, P., H.Z. Wang, X.Q. Wang, and Y.N. Wu. 1994. The blocking effect of phenolic acid on N-nitrosomorpholine formation in vitro. Biomed. Environ. Sci. 7:68-78.

Lijinsky, W. and A.E. Ross. 1967. Production of carcinogenic polynuclear hydrocarbons in the cooking of food. Food Cosmet. Toxicol. 5:343-347

Lok, E., E.A. Nera, F. Iverson, F. Scott, Y. So, and D.B. Clayson. 1988. Dietary restriction, cell proliferation, and carcinogenesis: A preliminary study. Cancer Letters 38:249-255.

Lok, E., W.M. Ratnayake, F.W. Scott, R. Mongeau, S. Fernie, E.A. Nera, S. Malcolm, E. McMullen, P. Jee, and D.B. Clayson. 1992. Effect of varying the type of fat in a semi-purified AIN-76A diet on cellular proliferation in the mammary gland and intestinal crypts in female Swiss Webster mice. Carcinogenesis 13(10):1735-1741.

Lok, E., F.W. Scott, R. Mongeau, E.A. Nera, S. Malcolm, and D.B. Clayson. 1990. Calorie restriction and cellular proliferation in various tissues of the female Swiss Webster mouse. Cancer Letters

51:67-73.

Lubin, F., Y. Wax, and B. Modan. 1986. Role of fat, animal protein, and dietary fiber in breast cancer etiology: A case-control study. J. Natl. Cancer Inst. 77:605-612.

Macquart-Moulin, G., E. Riboli, J. Cornee, B. Charnay, P. Berthezene, and N. Day. 1986. Case-control study on colorectal cancer and diet in Marseilles. Int. J. Cancer 38:183-191.

Magee, P.N., and J.M. Barnes. 1956. The production of malignant primary hepatic tumours in the rat by feeding dimethylnitrosamine. Brit. J. Cancer 10:114.

Magee, P.N., and J.M. Barnes. 1959. The experimental production of tumours in the rat by dimethylnitrosamine (N-nitroso-dimethylamine). Acta. Un. Int. Cancer 15:187.

Magee, P.N., and J.M. Barnes. 1962. Induction of kidney tumours in the rat with dimethylnitrosamine (N-nitroso-dimethylamine). J. Path. Bact. 84:19.

Maarse, H., and C.A. Visscher, eds. 1989. Volatile Compounds in Foods. Qualitative and Quantitative Data. The Netherlands: TNO-CIVO Food Analysis Institute.

Mattocks, A.R. 1986. Chemistry and toxicology of pyrrolizidine alkaloids. Orlando, FL: Academic Press. 393 pp.

Medina, D. 1986. Selenium and murine mammary tumorigenesis. Pp. 23-41 in Diet, Nutrition, and Cancer: A Critical Evaluation, B.S. Reddy and L.A. Cohen, ed. Boca Raton, FL: CRC Press, Inc.

Meinwald, J., and T. Eisner. 1995. The chemistry of phyletic dominance. Proc. Nat. Acad. of Sci. 92(1):14-18.

Miller, C.C., Y. Park, M.W. Pariza, and M.E. Cook. 1994. Feeding conjugated linoleic acid to animals partially overcomes catabolic responses due to endotoxin injection. Biochem. Biophys. Res. Commun. 198:1107-1112.

Minghetti, P.P. and A.W. Norman. 1988. 1,25(OH)2-vitamin D3 receptors: Gene regulation and genetic circuitry. FASEB J. 2:3043-3053.

Mirvish, S.S. 1983. The etiology of gastric cancer: Intragastric nitrosamide formation and other theories. J. Natl. Cancer Inst. 71:629-647.

Moon, R.C. 1989. Comparative aspects of carotenoids and retinoids as chemopreventive agents for cancer. J. Nutr. 119:127-134.

Moore, M.R., H.C. Pitot, E.C. Miller, and J.A. Miller. 1982. Cholangiocellular carcinomas induced in Syrian golden hamsters administered aflatoxin B_1 in large doses. J. Natl Cancer Inst. 68:271-278.

Morgan, E.D. 1984. Insect Communication (pp. 169-194), Lewis, T., ed. New York: Academic Press.

Nagao, M., and T. Sugimura. 1993. Carcinogenic factors in food with relevance to colon cancer development. Mutat. Res. 290:43-51.

Nakayama, T. 1994. Suppression of hydroperoxide-induced cytotoxicity by polyphenols. Cancer Research 54(Suppl 7):1991s-1993s.

Nawar, W.W. 1985. Lipids. Pp. 139-244 in Food Chemistry, 2nd edition, O.R. Fennema, ed. New York: Marcel Dekker.

Neugut, A.I., G.C. Garbowski, W.C. Lee, T. Murray, J.W. Nieves, K.A. Forde, M.R. Treat, J.D. Waye, and C. Fenoglio-Preiser. 1993. Dietary risk factors for incidence and recurrence of colorectal adenomatous polyps. Ann. Intern. Med. 118:91-95.

Newberne, P.M., and M. Locniskar. 1990. Roles of micronutrients in cancer prevention: Recent evidence from the laboratory. Prog. Clin. Biol. Res. 346:119-134.

Newmark, H.L. and M. Lipkin. 1992. Calcium, vitamin D, and colon cancer. Cancer Res. 52(Suppl.):2067s-2070s.

Nishizumi, M., R.E. Albert, F.J. Burns, and L. Bilger. 1977. Hepatic cell loss and proliferation induced by N-2-fluorenylacetamide, diethylnitrosamine, and aflatoxin B_1 in relation to hepatoma induction. Br. J. Cancer 36:192-197.

NRC (National Research Council). 1975. Underexploited Tropical Plants with Promising Economic Value (pp. 1-8). Washington, DC: National Academy Press.

NRC (National Research Council). 1977. Arsenic. Washington, DC: National Academy Press.

NRC (National Research Council). 1981. The Health Effects of Nitrite, Nitrate, and N-Nitroso Compounds. Washington, DC: National Academy Press.

NRC (National Research Council). 1982. Diet, Nutrition and Cancer. Washington, DC: National Academy Press.

NRC (National Research Council). 1988. Designing foods. Animal Product Options in the Marketplace. Washington, DC: National Academy Press. 367 pp.

NRC (National Research Council). 1989a. Diet and Health: Implications for Reducing Chronic Disease Risk. Food and Nutrition Board, Committee on Diet and Health. Washington, DC: National Academy Press. 749 pp.

NRC (National Research Council). 1989b. Dietary intake and nutritional status: trends and assessment. Pp. 41-84 in Diet and Health: Implications for Reducing Chronic Disease Risk, Food and Nutrition Board, ed. Committee on Diet and Health. Washington, DC: National Academy Press.

NRC (National Research Council). 1989c. Recommended Dietary Allowances, 10th edition. Washington, DC: National Academy Press, p. 44.

NTP (National Toxicology Program). 1994. Seventh Annual Report on Carcinogens 1994 - Summary. National Toxicology Program, Research Triangle Park, NC, and Bethesda, MD.

Ochiai, M., K. Ogawa, K. Wakabayashi, T. Sugimura, S. Nagase, H. Esumi, and M. Nagao. 1991. Induction of intestinal adenocarcinomas by 2-amino-1-methyl6-phenylimidazo[4,5-b]pyridine in Nagase analbuminemic rats. Jpn. J. Cancer Res. 82:363-366.

Otsuka, H., and A. Kuwahara. 1971. Hemangiomatous lesions of mice treated with nitrosodimethylamine. Gann 62:147.

Overvad, K., D.Y. Wang, J. Olsen, D.S. Allen, E.B. Thorling, R.D. Bulbrook, and J.L. Hayward. 1991. Selenium in human mammary carcinogenesis: A case-cohort study. Eur. J. Cancer 27:900-902.

Paracelsus (Philippus Theophrastus Aureolus Bobastus von Hohenheim. 1564. Third defense in Septem Defensiones. Arnold Bryckmann. Cologne.

Pariza, M.W. 1988. Dietary fat and cancer risk: Evidence and research needs. Annu. Rev. Nutr. 8:167-183.

Pariza, M.W., and R.K. Boutwell. 1987. Historical perspective: Calories and energy expenditure in carcinogenesis. Am. J. Clin. Nutr. 45(Suppl):151-156.

Parkin, D.M., P. Srivatanakul, M. Khlat, D. Chenvidhya, P. Chotiwan,

S. Insiripong, S., K.A. L'Abbé, and C.P. Wild. 1991. Liver cancer in Thailand. I. A case-control study of cholangiocarcinoma. Int. J. Cancer 48:323-328.

Peers, F.G., X. Bosch, J. Kaldor, C.A. Linsell, and M. Pluijmen. 1987. Aflatoxin exposure, hepatitis B virus infection and liver cancer in Swaziland. Int. J. Cancer 39:545-553.

Pelletier, S.W. 1983-1992. Alkaloids: Chemical and Biological Properties. Vols. 1-6. New York: Wiley.

Pitt, J.I., A.D. Hocking, K. Bhudasamai, B.F. Miscamble, K.A. Wheeler, and P. Tanbook-Ek. 1993. The normal mycoflora of commodities from Thailand. I. Nuts and oilseeds. Int. J. Food Microbiol. 20:211-226.

Pohan, T.E., G.R. Howe, C.M. Friedenrich, M. Jain, and A.B. Miller. 1993. Dietary fiber, vitamins A, C, and E, and risk of breast cancer: A cohort study. Cancer Causes and Control 4:29-37.

Potter, J.D. and A. J. McMichael. 1986. Diet and cancer of the colon and rectum: A case-control study. NJCI 76:557-569.

Prival, M.J. 1985. Carcinogens and mutagens present as natural components of food or induced by cooking. Nutrition and Cancer 6:236-253.

Pyke, M. 1968. Food and Society. London: John Murray. 178 p.

Qian, G.S., R.K. Ross, M.C. Yu, J.M. Yuan, Y.T. Gao, B.E. Henderson, G.N. Wogan, and J.D. Groopman. 1994. A follow-up study of urinary markers of aflatoxin exposure and liver cancer risk in Shanghai, People's Republic of China. Cancer Epidemiol. Biomarkers Prev. 3:3-10.

Ray, J.S., M.L. Harbison, R.M. McClain, and J.I. Goodman. 1994. Alterations in the methylation status and expression of the *raf* oncogene in phenobarbital-induced and spontaneous B7C3F1 mouse liver tumors. Molecular Carcinogenesis 9:155-166.

Riopelle, J.L., and G. Jasmin. 1969. Nature, classification and nomenclature of kidney tumors induced in the rat by dimethylnitrosamine. J. Nat. Cancer Inst. 42:643.

Roberts, A.B., and M.B. Sporn. 1992. Mechanistic interrelationships between two superfamilies: The steroid/retinoid receptors and transforming growth factor-beta. Cancer Surv. 14:205-220.

Rodricks, J.V., and A.E. Pohland. 1981. Food Hazards of Natural

Origin Pp. 181-237 in Food Safety, H.R. Roberts, ed. New York: Wiley.

Ross, R.K., J.M. Yuan, M.C. Yu, G.N. Wogan, G.S. Qian, J.T. Tu, J.D. Groopman, Y.T. Gao, and B.E. Henderson. 1992. Urinary aflatoxin biomarkers and risk of hepatocellular carcinoma. Lancet 339:943-946.

Rozin, E. 1973. The Flavor Principle Cookbook. New York: Hawthorn Books, Inc.

Safe, S.H. 1995. Environmental and dietary estrogens in human health: Is there a problem. Environmental Health Perspectives 103:346-351.

Scalmati, A., M. Lipkin, and H. Newmark. 1992. Relationships of calcium and vitamin D to colon cancer. Pp. 249-262 in Cancer Chemoprevention, L. Wattenberg, M. Lipkin, C.W. Boone, and G.J. Kelloff, eds. Boca Raton, FL: CRC Press.

Schectman, G. 1993. Estimating ascorbic acid requirements for cigarette smokers. Ann. NY Acad. Sci. 686:335-345.

Schmähl, D., and R. Preussmann. 1959. Cancerogene Wirkung von Nitrosodimethylamin bei Ratten. Naturwissenschaften 46:175.

Schwartz, A.G. and L.L. Pashko. 1994. Role of adrenocortical steroids in mediating cancer-preventive and age-retarding effects of food restriction in laboratory rodents. J. Gerontol. 49:B37-B41.

Seitz, H.K., and U.A. Simanowski. 1988. Alcohol and carcinogenesis. Annu. Rev. Nutr. 8:99-119.

Shabad, L.M., and L.A. Savluchinskaya. 1971. Some results of studying the blastomogenic action of nitrosamines on mice. Biull. éksp. Biol. Med. 71:76.

Shinohara, Y., M. Arai, K. Hirao, S. Sugihara, K. Nakanishi, H. Tsunoda, and N. Ito. 1976. Combination effect of citrinin and other chemicals on rat kidney tumorigenesis. Gann 67:147-155.

Sieber, S.M., P. Correa, D.W. Dalgard, and R.H. Adamson. 1979. Induction of osteogenic sarcomas and tumors of the hepatobiliary system in nonhuman primates with aflatoxin B. Cancer Res. 39:4545-4554.

Simic, M.G., and M. Karel. 1980. Autoxidation in food and biological systems. New York: Plenum Press. 659 pp.

Slattery, M.L., A.W. Sorenson, A.W. Mahoney, T.K. French, D.

Kritchevsky, and J.C. Street. 1988. Diet and colon cancer: Assessment of risk by fiber type and food source. J. Natl. Cancer Inst. 80:1474-1480.

Soffritti, M., and E.E. McConnell. 1988. Liver foci formation during aflatoxin B_1 carcinogenesis in the rat. Ann. N.Y. Acad. Sci. 534:531-540.

Srivatanakul, P., D. M. Parkin, Y.-Z. Jiang, M. Khlat, U.-T. Kao-Ian, S. Sontipong, and C.P. Wild. 1991a. The role of infection by *Opisthorchis viverrini*, hepatitis B virus, and aflatoxin exposure in the etiology of liver cancer in Thailand. A correlation study. Cancer 68:2411-2417.

Stähelin, H.B., K.F. Gey, M. Eichholzer, E. Lüdin, F. Bernasconi, J. Thurneysen, and G. Brubacher. 1991. Plasma antioxidant vitamins and subsequent cancer mortality in the 12-year follow-up of the prospective basel study. Am. J. Epidemiol. 133:766-775.

Stich, H.F. 1991. The beneficial and hazardous effects of simple phenolic compounds. Mutat. Res. 259:307-324.

Stich, H.F. 1992. Teas and tea components as inhibitors of carcinogen formation in model systems and man. Preventive Medicine 21:377-84.

Stryer, L. 1975. Biochemistry. San Francisco: W.H. Freeman and Company. 877 p.

Sugimura, T. 1985. Carcinogenicity of mutagenic heterocyclic amines formed during the cooking process. Mutat. Res. 150:33-41.

Sugimura, T., M. Nagao, and K. Wakabayashi. 1994. Heterocyclic amines in cooked foods: Candidates for causation of common cancers. Journal of the National Cancer Institute 86:2-4.

Takahashi, M., K. Toyoda, Y. Aze, K. Furuta, K. Mitsumori, and Y. Hayashi. 1993. The rat urinary bladder as a new target of heterocyclic amine carcinogenicity: Tumor induction by 3-amino-1-methyl-5H-pyrido[4,3-b]indole acetate. Jpn. J. Cancer Res. 84:852-858

Takayama, S., and K. Oota. 1965. Induction of malignant tumours in various strains of mice by oral administration of N-nitrosodimethylamine and N-nitrosodiethylamine. Gann 56:189.

Tanaka ,T., T. Kojima, T. Kawamori, A. Wang, M. Suzui, K. Okamoto, and H. Mori. 1993. Inhibition of 4-nitroquinoline-1-oxide-induced rat tongue carcinogenesis by the naturally occurring plant phenolics caffeic, ellagic, chlorogenic and ferulic acids. Carcinogenesis 14:1321-5.

Tannahill, R. 1973. Food in History. New York: Stein and Day. 448p.

Tannenbaum, S.R., J.S. Wishnok, and C.D. Leaf. 1991. Inhibition of nitrosamine formation by ascorbic acid. Am. J. Clin. Nutr. 53(Suppl.):247S-250S.

Taylor, H.W., W. Lijinsky, P. Nettesheim, and C.M. Snyder. 1974. Alteration of tumor response in rat liver by carbon tetrachloride. Cancer Res. 34:3391-3395.

Terracini, B., P.N. Magee, and J.M. Barnes. 1967. Hepatic pathology in rats on low dietary levels of dimethylnitrosamine. Brit. J. Cancer 21:559.

Terracini, B., G. Palestro, M. Ramella Gigliardi, and R. Montesano. 1966. Carcinogenicity of dimethylnitrosamine in Swiss mice. Brit. J. Cancer 20:871.

Thompson, L.U. 1993. Potential health benefits and problems associated with antinutrients in foods. Food Res. Internatl. 26:131-149.

Thompson, L.U. 1994. Antioxidants and hormone mediated health benefits of whole grains. Crit. Rev. Food Sci. Nutr. 34:473-497.

Toda, S., M. Kumura, and M. Ohnishi. 1991. Effects of phenolcarboxylic acids on superoxide anion and lipid peroxidation induced by superoxide anion. Planta Med. 57:8-10.

Tomatis, L., P.N. Magee, and P. Shubik. 1964. Induction of liver tumors in Syrian golden hamsters by feeding dimethylnitrosamine. J. Nat. Cancer Inst. 33:341.

Topping, D.C. and W.J. Visek. 1976. Nitrogen intake and tumorigenesis in rats injected with 1,2-dimethylhydrazine. J. Nutrit. 106:1583-1590.

Toth, B., and I. Boreisha. 1969. Tumorigenesis with isonicotinic acid hydrazide adn urethan in the Syrian golden hamster. Europ. J. Cancer 5:165-171.

Toth, B., G. Della Porta, and P. Shubik. 1961a. The occurrence of malignant lymphomas in urethan-treated Swiss mice. Brit. J. Cancer 15:322-326.

Toth, B., L. Tomatis, and P. Shubik. 1961b. Multipotential carcinogenesis with urethan in the Syrian golden hamster. Cancer Res. 21:1537-1541.

Toth, B., P.N. Magee, and P. Shubik. 1964. Carcinogenesis study with dimethylnitrosamine administered orally to adult and subcutaneously to newborn BALB/c mice. Cancer Res. 24:1712-1721.

Ueno, Y. 1987. Tricothecenes in Food. Pp. 123-147 in Mycotoxins in Food. P. Krogh, ed. Chapter 6. New York: Academic Press.

Underwood, E.J. 1973. Trace elements. Pp. 48-49 in Toxicants Occurring Naturally in Foods. National Resarch Council. Washington, DC: National Academy Press.

van den Brandt, P.A., R. A. Goldbohm, P. van't Veer, P. Bode, E.Dorant, R.J.J. Hermus, and F. Sturmans. 1993. A prospective cohort study on selenium status and the risk of lung cancer. Cancer Res. 53:4860-4865.

van't Veer, P., F.J. Kok, H.A.M. Brants, T. Ockhuizen, F. Sturmans, and R.J.J. Hermus. 1990. Dietary fat and the risk of breast cancer. Int. J. Epidemiol. 19:12-18.

Visser, J.H., and A.K. Minks, ed. 1982. Proceedings of the Fifth International Symposium on Insect-Plant Relationships. Wageningen, The Netherlands: Pudoc. 464 pp.

Wald, J., S.G. Thompson, J.W. Densem, J. Boreham, and A. Bailey. 1987. Serum vitamin E and subsequent risk of cancer. Br. J. Cancer 56:69-72.

Watson, D.H. 1985. Toxic fungal metabolites in food. CRC Crit. Rev. Food Sci. Nutr. 22:177-198.

Wattenberg, L.W., J.B. Coccia, and L.K.T. Lam. 1980. Inhibitory effects of phenolic compounds on benzo[a]pyrene-induced neoplasia. Cancer Res. 40:2820-2823.

Weinberg, E.D. 1992. Roles of iron in neoplasia. Promotion, prevention, and therapy. Biol. Trace Elem. Res. 34:123-140.

Welsch, C.W. 1987. Enhancement of mammary tumorigenesis by dietary fat: Review of potential mechanisms. Am. J. Clin. Nutr. 45:192-202.

Welsch, C.W., J.L. House, B.L. Herr, S.J. Eliasberg, and M.A. Welsch. 1990. Enhancement of mammary carcinogenesis by high levels of dietary fat: A phenomenon dependent on ad libitum feeding. JNCI 82:1615-1620.

Whistler, R.L., and J.R. Daniel. 1985. Carbohydrates. Pp. 69-137 in Food Chemistry, 2nd edition, O.R. Fennema, ed. New York: Marcel Dekker, Inc.

Willett, W.C. 1994. Diet and health: What should we eat? Science 264:532-537.

Willett, W.C., M.J. Stampfer, G.A. Colditz, B.A. Rosner, and F.E. Speizer. 1990. Relation of meat, fat, and fiber intake to the risk of colon cancer in a prospective study among women. N. Engl. J. Med. 323:1664-1672.

Wogan, G.N. 1969. Metabolisma and biochemical effects of aflatoxins. Pp. 151-186 in Aflatoxin. Scientific Background, Control, and Implications, L.A. Goldblatt, ed. New York: Academic Press.

Wogan, G.N. 1992. Aflatoxins as risk factors for hepatocellular carcinomas in humans. Cancer Res. 52:2114S-2118S.

Wogan, G.N., and P.M. Newberne. 1967. Dose-response characteristics of aflatoxin B_1 carcinogenesis in the rat. Cancer Res. 27:2370-2376.

Wogan, G.N., G.S. Edwards, and P.M. Newberne. 1971. Structure-activity relationships in toxicity and carcinogenicity of aflatoxins and analogs. Cancer Res. 31:1936-1942.

Yeh, F.-S., J.-C. Yu, C.-C. Mo, S. Luo, M.J. Tong, and B.E. Henderson. 1989. Hepatitis B virus, aflatoxins, and hepatocellular carcinoma in southern Guangxi, China. Cancer Res. 49:2506-2509.

Zak, F.G., J.H. Holzner, E.J. Singer, and H. Popper. 1960. Renal and pulmonary tumors in rats fed dimethylnitrosamine. Cancer Res. 20:96.

Zawirska, B., and W. Bednarz. 1981. The particular traits of carcinogenesis induced in Wistar rats by aflatoxin B_1. III. Porphyrins and the activity of gamma-glutamyltranspeptidase in primary hepatomas and in their tissue of origin. Neoplasma 28:35-49.

Zhou, Y.-C., and R.-L. Zheng. 1991. Phenolic compounds and an analog as superoxide anion scavengers and antioxidants. Biochem. Pharmacol. 42:1177-1179.

Zhu, P., E. Frei, B. Bunk, M.R. Berger, and D. Schmahl. 1991. Effect of dietary calorie and fat restriction on mammary tumor growth and hepatic as well as tumor glutathione in rats. Cancer Lett. 57:145-152.

Ziegler, R.G. 1991. Vegetables, fruits, and carotenoids and the risk of cancer. Am. J. Clin. Nutr. 53(Suppl.):251S-259S.

Ziegler, R.G., L.A. Brinton, R.F. Hamman, H.F. Lehman, R.S. Levine, K. Mallin, S.A. Norman, J.F. Rosenthal, A.C. Trumble, and R.N. Hoover. 1990. Diet and the risk of invasive cervical cancer among white women in the United States. American J. of Epidemiology 132(3):432-445.

Zwicker, G.M., W.W. Carlton, and J. Tuite. 1972. Carcinogenic activity of toxigenic penicillia (Abstract). Lab. Invest. 26:497.

3

Synthetic Carcinogens
in the Diet

This chapter addresses two principal questions. First, do naturally occurring and synthetic chemicals, considered as general classes, differ in their chemical and physical properties, e.g., extent of halogenation, lipophilicity, environmental or biological half-life? Second, can the principles and techniques used to evaluate synthetic chemicals as potential carcinogens be used to evaluate naturally occurring chemicals? It should be emphasized that the purpose of this chapter is comparative. It discusses general principles and does not review in detail the wealth of material available on the universe of synthetic chemicals. Instead, it examines how synthetic chemicals have been addressed by the toxicological and regulatory communities, and considers whether naturally occurring chemicals, as a group, may differ in their potential hazardous properties, as a group, from synthetic chemicals.

The public, the scientific community, and, consequently, the regulatory agencies have been concerned with synthetic chemicals for some time. Although food additives are regulated, many synthetic additives, both intentional and incidental, can be found in the diet. Some of the incidental ones, such as cyclamate, are at the center of current controversies regarding their possible carcinogenicity. In the past, the public has been exposed to other synthetic additives before they were regulated and/or removed from the diet.

It is axiomatic that a specific chemical, whether it is of natural or synthetic origin, is the same in its physical, chemical, and toxicological properties. However, it is uncertain whether naturally occurring chemicals, as a class, differ in some important way from chemicals of synthetic origin. Do they, for example, persist in the environment in the same way? Thus, knowledge of synthetic chemicals may be invaluable in assessing the potential carcinogenicity of naturally occurring chemicals.

A characteristic of synthetic chemicals often deemed desirable for commercial purposes is chemical stability. This is often achieved by halogenation, particularly chlorination, although other techniques are also available, such as the replacement of ester bonds by ether linkages. Chemical stability usually gives rise to persistence in the environment, to bioaccumulation, and to recalcitrance to metabolism. For example, highly chlorinated chemicals such as PCBs, PBBs, and the pesticides DDT and mirex have been shown to be persistent and hazardous. In addition, TCDD, a byproduct of combustion and other processes, is a stable, environmentally persistent chemical that bioaccumulates and causes severe acute and chronic effects in animals.

Naturally occurring chemicals, unlike synthetics, have not been intentionally altered to achieve chemical stability. A number of halogenated compounds are natural products; however, their degree of chlorination and, therefore, their resistance to metabolism, is generally not as great as that of synthetic chemicals. In addition, naturally occurring chemicals usually exist as a single stereoisomer; synthetics, on the other hand, are frequently a mixture of two or more stereoisomers. Further, naturally occurring chemicals are more likely to appear in the diet as conjugates than are synthetic chemicals. Such conjugates include glucuronides, glucosides, methylated compounds, glutathione conjugates, and others. Many of these conjugates will be hydrolyzed, either in the gastrointestinal tract or in mammalian tissues, and the resulting hydrolysis products may be toxic if indeed the chemical in question is toxic. Furthermore, it should be noted that the toxicokinetics following the ingestion of a conjugate may influence the rate of delivery of the toxic moiety to the active site.

SYNTHETIC FOOD ADDITIVES

Tables 3-1 and 3-2 list examples of direct and indirect synthetic food additives, respectively. *Direct* (intentional) additives include antioxidants, colorants, flavor ingredients, artificial sweeteners, solvents, and humectants. *Indirect* additives include pesticides, solvents, and packaging-derived chemicals. Table 3-3 lists sources of nonintentional food additives, some natural, some synthetic, that may have toxicologic significance. Depending upon circumstances of processing or packaging, the same chemical can be a direct, indirect, or nonintentional food additive.

Direct, or intentional, food additives are chemicals or compounds, natural or synthetic, added deliberately to make some change in the food product, e.g., to add color, to preserve, or to provide a nutritional supplement (see Table 3-1).

Indirect additives are chemicals or compounds present but not added deliberately to change a product. Pesticides can be classified based on their use. Table 3-2 lists examples of indirect synthetic food additives, including pesticides, according to their use category. Representative chemical classes are presented. Over the past several decades, pesticides from many of these categories have been banned or otherwise regulated because of a concern for their carcinogenic potential or other risk to human health or the environment.

Table 3-2 also provides examples of chemicals derived from packaging materials, including vinyl chloride (a known human carcinogen), acrylonitrile (a known animal and suspected human carcinogen), as well as dyes used for printing. Recent attention has focused on several phthalate esters used as plasticizers since these compounds are known peroxisome proliferators in rodents.

Table 3-3 lists sources of nonintentional food additives with possible toxicological significance. These chemicals may enter foods indirectly in trace amounts during production, processing, packaging, and storage from a wide variety of sources, both natural and synthetic.

Table 3-1 Selected Direct Food Additives

Appearance modifiers	Glazes, waxes, polishes. Clouding and crystallization agents and inhibitors (e.g., methyl glucoside-coconut oil ester, oxystearin), colors and coloring adjuncts (e.g., FD & C Yellow No. 5 (tartrazine, a pyrazolone dye)), FD & C Yellow No. 6 (Sunset Yellow, a monoazophenyl naphthalene dye)), and surface finishing agents (e.g., oxidized polyethylene and polyvinyl-pyrrolidone)
Curing and pickling agents	Sodium nitrite, salt, sodium tripolyphosphate, and ascorbic acid
Nutrient replacements	Microemulsified protein (natural) and sucrose polyesters
Nutrient supplements	All essential nutrients (e.g., vitamin A and other vitamins, iron and other minerals, amino acids, and essential fatty acids)
pH control agents	Acids (e.g., acetic, tartaric, and hydrochloric), bases (e.g., sodium bicarbonate and sodium hydroxide), and buffering agents (e.g., sodium citrate)
Processing aids	Fermentation and malting aids (e.g., gibberellic acid and potassium bromate), formulation aids (e.g., starch as a binder), freezing agents (e.g., liquid nitrogen and carbon dioxide), lubricants and release agents (e.g., mineral oil), and washing, peeling, and vegetable-cleaning agents (e.g., sodium hydroxide and sodium n-alkyl benzene sulfonate)

Table 3-1 Continued

Product stability and safety aids	Antioxidants (e.g., BHA), preservatives and antimicrobials (e.g., sodium benzoate and potassium sorbate), sequestrants (e.g., EDTA and sodium metaphosphate), synergists (e.g., citric acid), oxidizing and reducing agents (e.g., hydrogen peroxide), and inert gases (e.g., nitrogen and combustion gas)
Solvents, vehicles, bulking agents, dispensing aids	Solvents (e.g., alcohol and propylene glycol), bulking agents (e.g., microcrystalline cellulose), and dispensing aids (e.g., nitrogen)
Sweeteners	Nutritive (e.g., sucrose and glucose (natural)) and reduced calorie (e.g., saccharin, cyclamate, acetsulfam, and aspartame)
Taste and flavor modifiers (except sweeteners, salt, and pH control agents)	Flavoring ingredients (e.g., vanillin), flavoring adjuncts (e.g., triethyl citrate (solvent and fixative)), flavor enhancers (e.g., msg (natural) and ethyl maltol)
Texture and consistency control agents	Anticaking agents (e.g., calcium stearate and silica aerogel), dough conditioners and strengtheners (e.g., potassium bromate and acetone peroxide), drying agents (e.g., anhydrous dextrose), emulsifiers (e.g., mono- and diglycerides and polysorbates), firming agents (e.g., calcium salts), flour-treating agents (e.g., benzoyl peroxide), humectants (e.g., sorbitol), leavening agents (e.g., sodium carbonate and sodium acid phosphate), masticatory substances (e.g., paraffin and

Table 3-1 Continued

Texture and consistency control agents (continued)	glycerol esters of wood rosin), stabilizers and thickeners (e.g., modified food starches), surface-active agents (e.g., sodium lauryl sulfate and dimethyl polysiloxane), and texturizers (e.g., glycerine and modified food starch)

Sources: Adapted from Hall 1979, Hodgson and Levi 1987, U.S. GPO 1991.

OCCURRENCE AND EXPOSURE

This section discusses chemical additives found in drinking water and the diet, foodstuffs containing the most important additives, and concentrations of additives in representative foodstuffs and drinking water. The large amount of exposure data on synthetic chemicals in the diet precludes detailed enumeration. For the great majority of constitutive chemicals so far identified (see Chapter 2), virtually no data exist on the extent of human exposure. However, among these are approximately 2,000 constitutive chemicals with recognized commercial value, including nutrients, some colors, and many flavoring ingredients, which are either isolated from natural sources or duplicated by synthesis for intentional addition to foods. For these substances there are extensive data on exposure, both from natural and intentional addition (NRC 1973, 1975, 1976, 1978, 1979, 1984, 1989; Stofberg and Kirschman 1985; Stofberg 1987).

Drinking Water

Whether consumed directly or used in food processing and preparation, drinking water is a source of potential exposure to a large

Table 3-2 Selected Indirect Synthetic Food Additives and Additives Used in Packaging[a]

Use Category	Chemical Class or Broad Category
Pesticides	
Acaricides	Organosulfur compounds, formamidines, dinitrophenols, and organochlorines (DDT analogs)
Algicides	Organotins
Fungicides	Dicarboximides, chlorinated aromatics, dithiocarbamates, and mercurials
Herbicides	Amides, acetamides, bipyridyls, carbamates, thiocarbamates, phenoxy compounds, dinitrophenols, dinitroanilines, substituted ureas, and triazines
Insecticides	Chlorinated hydrocarbons, chlorinated alicyclics, cyclodienes, chlorinated terpenes, organophosphates, carbamates, thiocyanates, dinitrophenols, fluoroacetates, botanicals (nicotinoids, rotenoids, and pyrethroids), juvenile hormone analogs, growth regulators, inorganics (arsenicals and fluorides), and microbials
Insecticide synergists	Methylenedioxyphenyls, and dicarboximides
Molluscicides	Chlorinated hydrocarbons
Nematocides	Halogenated alkanes
Rodenticides	Anticoagulants, botanicals (alkaloids and glycosides), fluorides, inorganics, and thioureas

Table 3-2 Continued

Packaging

Adhesives and pressure-sensitive adhesives	A wide variety of solvents, resins, polymers, glues, preservatives, and miscellaneous additives
Adjuvants (emulsifiers, antistatic agents, lubricants, plasticizers, colorants, filtering aids, etc.)	A wide variety of chemical classes
Antioxidants and stabilizers	Substituted phenols, triazenes, organotin stabilizers, other free-radical acceptors, inorganic compounds, and adjuvants
Coatings (for metals, plastics, paperboard, etc.	A wide variety of polymers, copolymers, resins, rosins, drying oils, glycerides, fatty acids, catalysts, colorants, solvents, and adjuncts
Components of paper and paperboard	A wide variety of polymers, copolymers, catalysts, olefins, esters, inorganic compounds, chelating agents, defoaming agents, preservatives, solvents, and adjuncts
Substances used as basic components of articles in contact with food (containers, utensils, films, membranes)	Polymers, copolymers, resins, fibers, lubricants, colors, and adjuvants

Substances used to control the growth of micro-organisms	Hydrogen peroxide and other peroxides, iodine and chlorine compounds, quaternary ammonium compounds, sulfonated detergents, other surface-active agents, and solvents
Prior-sanctioned substances[b]	
GRAS substances (substances generally recognized as safe for use in or on foods)[c]	

Sources: Adapted from Hodgson and Levi 1987, U.S. GPO 1991.

[a]The indirect additive regulations, in general, make no distinction between natural and synthetic ingredients, except that at several points a regulation expressly authorizes the synthetic equivalents of certain naturally occurring substances, such as fatty acids. Furthermore, the distinction between natural and synthetic is often not clear for these substances. The majority are doubtless synthetic.

[b]Nearly all of the regulations covering indirect additives (components and constituents) used in packaging, also permit, as a class, and unless otherwise restricted, all "prior sanctioned" substances, i.e., those authorized by FDA or USDA for use in food prior to 1958. Those known by the agency to be prior sanctioned are listed in CFR 21, Part 181.

[c]Packaging regulations also consistently permit, unless otherwise restricted, any GRAS substances used in or on food. There is no one listing of GRAS substances. The two major lists are those published by the FDA (CFR 21, Parts 182, 184, and 186, and lists published by the Flavor and Extract Manufacturers' Association (Smith, R.L., and R.A. Ford, 1993). Beyond the published lists, however, the law permits private, unpublished determination of GRAS status, subject to challenge by the FDA. The number of such private GRAS substances is presumably not large but is unknown. Most GRAS substances would not be suitable for use in packaging.

Table 3-3   Sources of Nonintentional Food Additives of Possible Toxicological Significance

During Production

1. Antibiotics and other agents used for prevention and control of disease
2. Growth-promoting substances
3. Microorganisms of toxicologic significance
4. Parasitic organisms
5. Pesticide residues (insecticides, fungicides, herbicides, etc.)
6. Toxic metals and metallic compounds
7. Radioactive compounds

During Processing

1. Microorganisms and their toxic metabolites
2. Processing residues and miscellaneous foreign objects
3. Radionuclides

During Packaging and Storage

1. Labeling and stamping materials
2. Microorganisms and their toxic metabolites
3. Migrants from packaging materials
4. Toxic chemicals from external sources

number of synthetic chemicals. However, it is difficult to quantify the number of chemicals or the amounts to which a particular individual might be exposed via drinking water. The U.S. Environmental Protection Agency has published two surveys with information for assessing potential exposure, though one must observe the caveats provided by the agency (EPA 1992).

One of these sources of information is a database established by the EPA in response to the Safe Drinking Water Amendments of 1986, which mandated that community water systems and nontransient, noncommunity water systems be monitored for 34 to 51 volatile organic compounds, identified as "unregulated contaminants." The database was designed to assist the agency in estimating the occurrence of these compounds and their seasonal variations. A summary report presenting results as of July 31, 1992, had data from 43 states on systems using ground and surface water sources for drinking water (EPA 1992a). The trihalomethanes (chloroform, bromodichloromethane, dibromochloromethane, and bromoform), which are formed as the result of the chlorination process, were reported as being present most frequently. All other unregulated contaminants occurred in less than 5% of the water samples. Of the 32 states that reported positive data on specific chemicals, over half found that the trihalomethanes, ethylbenzene, toluene, tetrachloroethylene (perchloroethylene), xylene (all isomers combined), cis/trans-1,2-dichloropropene, 1,1-dichloroethane, dichloromethane, and fluorotrichloromethane occurred at least once. However, the agency cautions that no national inferences can be made from these data nor can the actual concentrations to which any individual is exposed be calculated using these data.

The second source of information for assessing potential exposure to synthetic chemicals is the National Survey of Pesticides in Drinking Water Wells, the results and interpretation of which were reported in two phases (EPA 1990, 1992b). The data represent measurements on a statistically representative sample of wells. In the study 1,349 samples from community water system wells and rural domestic water wells were analyzed for the presence of 101 pesticides, 25 pesticide degradation products, and nitrate. The samples were collected between 1988 and 1990. Phase I involved the national estimates of frequency and concentrations of the pesticides, while Phase II, entitled *Another Look: National Survey of Pesticides in Drinking Water Wells, Phase II Report* (EPA 1992b), was concerned with the presence of the pesticides and correlations with local factors such as patterns of use and ground water vulnerability. It should be noted that the survey was restricted to drinking water from wells and did not study drinking water from ground and surface water sources.

In the survey the number of wells found to contain any particular pesticide was low. Of the 127 analytes, only 17 were detected and only 13 of these exceeded the minimum reporting limits (MRL) established by the primary laboratories involved in the study. In extrapolating to the approximately 38,300 community water systems employing about 94,600 wells and 10.5 million rural domestic wells, EPA estimated that about 10.4% of the community wells and 4.2% of the rural domestic wells contained at least one pesticide at a level above the MRL. None of the community water system wells were predicted to have levels above the Health Advisory Limit (HAL) or the Maximum Contaminant Level (MCL). For the rural wells, 0.2% were expected to exceed the HAL and 0.6% the MCL. The most common findings were acid metabolites of dimethyl tetrachloroterephthlate (DCPA) and atrazine. All DCPA metabolite detections were at a small fraction (0.2% or less) of the HAL. The median atrazine levels were also low. Five pesticides (alachlor, atrazine, dibromochloropropane, ethylene dibromide, and γ-hexachlorohexane [lindane]) were detected in a small number of samples at levels above their MCLs. In contrast, over half the community water system wells and rural domestic wells exceeded the MRL for nitrate, with 1.2% of the community wells and 2.4% of the rural domestic wells exceeding the MCL. It is estimated that community wells serve about 3 million people and rural wells serve about 1.5 million people. EPA cautions that the data represent a one-time snapshot of the wells, and the results would be expected to vary with season and location.

In considering each of these surveys, it should be emphasized that they examine only a select group of chemicals , i.e., select volatile organic compounds or pesticides.

Foods

In comparing the possible carcinogenic risks associated with dietary exposure to natural and to synthetic chemicals, it is important that the consumption of both types be put into perspective. Scheuplein (1990) divided food chemicals into seven categories, and reported estimates of the amounts ingested per day in a typical U.S. diet (see Table 5-7). Traditional foods (e.g., grains, fruits, vegetables, and meat) comprise the bulk of the diet. Items such as sugar and salt are the most frequently used direct food additives; these are GRAS (generally recognized as safe) items. Used in much smaller amounts are other direct additives (e.g., artificial sweeteners, colors, and preservatives), spices and flavors (e.g., mustard, pepper, cinnamon, poppy seed, and vanilla). Indirect food additives, such as those chemicals that migrate into food from pesticides and packaging materials, represent over 2,000 other chemicals, many of which may be present in food below the level of detection.

Pesticides have been of more concern to the public and to regulatory agencies than any other indirect food additives. Pesticides in food are generally derived from agricultural residues that remain on foodstuffs but may also be derived from chemicals used in storage facilities or from water used in food preparation. Several previous NRC studies have considered the effect of pesticides in the diet, including: *Diet, Nutrition and Cancer* (1982); *Diet, Nutrition and Cancer, Directions for Research* (1983); and *Pesticides in the Diets of Infants and Children* (1993). These studies should be consulted for an in-depth analysis.

It is clear from these and other reports that pesticide residues are common, but below allowable tolerances, on many foodstuffs in the U.S. diet. Federal agencies concerned with residues in food include the EPA, USDA (Food Safety and Inspection Service and Agricultural Marketing Service), and the FDA. Most of the data about residues is generated by FDA in connection with enforcement of tolerance levels. However, there is no single, comprehensive, reliable source of information on pesticide residues in foods. This is due in part to analytical and sampling problems. For example, sampling for compliance emphasizes suspected high samples. Also, the effect of postharvest processing is seldom adequately investigated. In addition to data from federal agencies, data generated by states are subject to the same uncertainties.

An FDA survey covering the period from 1988 to 1989 (FDA 1994) studied the frequency of occurrence of 46 pesticides (primarily insecticides, with a very small number of herbicides and fungicides). This survey found that occurrence varied from 0.1% (dichlorvos, ethoprop, carbophenothion) to 24.3% (for daminozide) and 28.5% (for benomyl). It should be noted that chemicals were eliminated from the survey if the sample size was too small to be representative (less than 100 samples, compared with more than 45,000 for the most sampled chemical, chlorpyrifos).

Hazard assessment and epidemiologic studies of pesticides show that many, if not all, have the potential to produce toxicity in humans, particularly in studies of occupational or accidental high dose exposures. In addition to cancer (Blair et al. 1985, 1993; Blair and Zahm 1990, 1991; Brown et al. 1990), toxic effects may include neurological ones (Deapen and Henderson 1986, Ecobichon et al. 1990, Tanner and Langston 1990, Rosenstock et al. 1991) and reproductive ones (Gordon and Shy 1981, Schwartz and Logerfo 1988). Despite this potential, accurate estimations of risk from pesticides in the diet are subject to many uncertainties. Epidemiologic studies, almost without exception, involve occupational exposure and are complicated by multiple, sequential exposures as well as routes of exposure other than dietary. The use of tolerance levels in risk estimates is a further complication, since these levels are seldom approached, and even less often exceeded. Extrapolation from rodent assays is also problematic in part because the levels of pesticides in foods are frequently at or below the level of detection. Nevertheless, results from epidemiologic studies of farm families and farm workers occupationally exposed to pesticides suggest that the risk of cancer and other illnesses such as Parkinson's disease (Tanner and Langston 1990) should be further studied.

MECHANISMS OF CARCINOGENESIS

Although detailed molecular mechanisms of carcinogenesis are not known, several factors involved in the process have been determined (Cohen and Ellwein 1990, 1991; Stanbridge 1990; Bishop 1991; Weinstein et al. 1995). It has become increasingly clear that cancer arises as a result of genetic alterations, either inherited or resulting from the mutation of somatic cells. It is also apparent that more than one genetic error is required for the expression of the malignant phenotype. For genetic errors to become permanent, cell replication is required. The defect must occur in a stem cell (variably defined, but basically a pluripotential cell) population. On the basis of these premises, it is apparent that the likelihood of cancer development in a given cell population can be increased by directly damaging DNA during cell replication or by increasing the number of replication cycles taking place in the cells. Cell births can be increased by direct mutagenesis or by regeneration following cytotoxicity; cell deaths can be increased by inhibiting apoptosis or by altering gene expression and differentiation. Agents that enhance cell DNA damage or cell replication in appropriate cell populations will increase the cancer risk, whereas agents that decrease cell DNA damage or cell proliferation should decrease the risk.

Chemicals can generally be divided into those that directly affect DNA (genotoxic) and those that do not (nongenotoxic), although the genotoxicity of some chemicals remains poorly defined (Williams and Weisburger 1986, Tennant et al. 1987, Rosenkrantz and Klopman 1990). Some chemicals can exert both types of activities, and some chemicals may lead to indirect damage to DNA via, for example, the formation of oxygen radicals.

Genotoxic chemicals, either directly or after metabolic activation, form DNA adducts, some of which lead to mutations (Williams and Weisburger 1986, Tennant et al. 1987, Reitz et al. 1988, Harris 1990, Rosenkrantz and Klopman 1990). A spectrum of mutation patterns in specific genes has been ascertained for some carcinogens, such as aflatoxin (Harris 1993). Several methods have been developed for assessing exposure of individuals to chemicals based on their formation of specific DNA adducts (Choy 1993, Weinstein et al. 1995). These methods, which include ^{32}P post-labeling, immunochemical assays, and mass spectroscopy, have led to the quantitation of potency in animals and in humans. In addition, surrogate markers have also been used to estimate exposures of individuals to various chemicals. Examples of these markers include adduct formation with various proteins, particularly hemoglobin and to a lesser extent albumin. When enzymes involved in the metabolic activation and inactivation of these chemicals are modified, the compounds show considerable variability in their potential for mutagenicity and carcinogenicity. This variability has been specifically defined in only limited cases and is a major area for continued investigation (Sipes and Gandolfi 1986).

Nongenotoxic chemicals may affect the carcinogenic process by modifying the number of cell divisions per unit time, but other mechanisms may also play a role. This modification can be accomplished by any of several mechanisms, including direct mitogenesis, cytotoxicity followed by regenerative hyperplasia, inhibiting apoptosis, inhibiting differentiation, or a combination of these processes (Cohen and Ellwein 1990, 1991, 1992). The DNA errors arising during cell replication can occur secondarily to a variety of possible endogenous mechanisms, including oxidative damage, depurination and depyrimidination, deamination, formation of exocyclic adducts (possibly secondary to oxidative damage or lipid peroxidation), defects in DNA repair, indirect chromosomal aberrations, and other mechanisms yet to be defined. Nongenotoxic chemicals can be more broadly divided into those that interact with specific receptors on cells, such as hormones, dioxin, and phorbol esters, and those that interact with cells through nonreceptor-mediated processes, such as phenobarbital, sodium saccharin, or d-limonene (Cohen and Ellwein 1990). Many of the nongenotoxic chemicals, especially those acting through specific receptors, alter signal transduction and gene expression. Chemicals that alter gene expression tend to be tissue-specific and frequently species-specific. Chemicals can clearly have more than one of the effects described above.

Because multiple genetic errors are required before malignancy will develop, several multistage models of carcinogenesis have been developed. The first of these models was the initiation-promotion model of Berenblum and Shubik (1947), which was later modified to include the stage of progression (Boutwell 1964). On the basis of this model, the effects of a chemical have been classified in terms of initiation, promotion, or progression. However, when they are completely evaluated, chemicals usually exhibit more than one of these effects, and even single doses of potent carcinogens, such as aflatoxin B_1 or diethylnitrosamine, can induce cancer in rodent models. Although the terms initiation, promotion, and progression continue to be used in the field of carcinogenesis, it is difficult to define these stages in many model systems, in studies involving chemical mixtures, or in human carcinogenesis. Nevertheless, numerous authors use the term initiation to mean genotoxicity and promotion to mean nongenotoxic events.

Other multistage models of carcinogenesis have been presented. Armitage and Doll (1954) postulated a sequence of multiple genetic events occurring over time, with the incidence increasing proportionally to an exponent of time, the exponent being defined by one less than the number of stages in the carcinogenic process. Although this model was derived from epidemiologic studies and fits well with most human cancer types, it does not fit the age-specific mortality data for some cancers, such as childhood cancers, Hodgkin's disease, and breast cancer.

To account for these latter anomalies, models involving not only genetic errors but cell populations and replication have been developed (Knudson 1971, Moolgavkar and Knudson 1981, Greenfield et al. 1984, Cohen and Ellwein 1990, 1991). Numerous examples of multiple genetic errors in carcinogenesis have been established in animal models and in humans with the use of powerful molecular biological techniques. Also, it is still unclear which genes are directly involved in carcinogenesis and which are related to increased susceptibility to the development of the critical DNA mistakes that occur in carcinogenesis (Cohen and Ellwein 1990, 1991, 1992).

The evidence to date suggests that the processes of carcinogenesis are similar for natural and synthetic chemicals. A combination of approaches used in cell and molecular biology, pharmacokinetics, biochemistry, and in chemistry should continue to provide insight into the overall carcinogenic process in animals and in humans. The committee accepts the concept of multistage carcinogenesis, but because of the difficulties associated with the initiation-promotion-progression model, especially in applying it to human carcinogenesis, we have chosen to use the terms genotoxic and non-genotoxic in referring to specific agents.

METABOLISM

The biotransformation of xenobiotics involves phase I (oxidation, reduction, and hydrolysis) or phase II (conjugative) reactions (Bridges and Chasseaud 1976, Testa and Jenner 1976, Jenner and Testa 1981). In many cases, the parent compound may not undergo phase I biotransformation if it has a functional group available for conjugation. For example, glucuronidation is the major metabolic pathway for acetaminophen and naturally occurring morphine. Similarly, reactions such as mercapturic acid formation and sulfation are common in humans. It should be noted that interspecies variations are extensive, as are interindividual variations, particularly in humans. Furthermore, it has been apparent for many years that metabolism of xenobiotics may be a detoxication event or, through the production of reactive intermediates, an activation event that increases toxicity.

Cytochrome P450 is the principal enzyme involved in the phase I metabolism of xenobiotics. It is located in the endoplasmic reticulum and is found in many living organisms. Over two hundred isozymes have been identified (Degtyarenko and Archakov 1993, Nelson et al. 1993). These isozymes have broad but different specificities that frequently overlap. Isozyme distribution differs between species, organs, and developmental stages. A unique feature of the cytochrome system is its induction by specific chemicals. Other phase I enzymes include the flavin-containing monooxygenase, also located in the endoplasmic reticulum, the molybdenum hydroxylases (e.g., aldehyde oxidase and xanthine oxidase), alcohol and aldehyde dehydrogenases, esterases and amidases, and peroxidases and epoxide hydrolase. Xenobiotics may also be co-oxidized by prostaglandin synthetase (Hodgson and Levi 1994). It should be noted that Phase I reactions may result in the formation of free radical and other reactive intermediates.

Phase II reactions involve the conjugation of endogenous intermediates with phase I metabolites or the conjugation of the parent compound itself. Phase II enzymes include UDP-glucuronyl-transferase, UDP-glucosyltransferase, sulfotransferase, acetyl-transferase, methyltransferase, acyltransferases (which affect amino acid conjugation) and glutathione S-transferase (Dauterman 1994).

It is not surprising that the metabolic pathways involved in the biotransformation of both synthetic and naturally occurring chemicals are similar. It is possible that these pathways developed in response to naturally occurring chemicals and offered some selective advantage to organisms capable of detoxifying xenobiotics. However, it must be stressed that biotransformation reactions may lead to bioactivation, especially to the formation of reactive metabolites that may alkylate DNA, thereby initiating the carcinogenic process.

An example of a reaction leading to both detoxication and activation is the metabolism of ethanol, a natural product of fermentation, to acetaldehyde by alcohol dehydrogenase. This metabolism terminates the action of ethanol on the central nervous system. However, the metabolite acetaldehyde may cause some of the other toxic effects associated with ethanol before it, in turn, is metabolically detoxified to acetate. This same enzyme, alcohol dehydrogenase, is involved in the metabolism of other simple alcohols and glycols such as the antifreeze ethylene glycol. A variety of esterases are also important in the metabolism of both natural and synthetic compounds, including drugs (e.g., aspirin, meperidine, acetanilide, and procaine), and pesticides (e.g., permethrin, malathion, and paraoxon) (Hayes and Laws 1991), chemicals of environmental concern such as plasticizers (e.g., diethylhexylphthalate), and natural compounds (e.g., the alkaloid arecoline) (Testa and Jenner 1976).

Most phase I metabolic reactions involve microsomal monooxygenases. Ring hydroxylations, such as those associated with benzene and its derivatives (e.g., the moth repellent p-dichlorobenzene), and with drugs like the barbiturate phenobarbital and the antipyretic acetanilide, are extremely common. Side chain oxidations are also common phase I reactions. Examples include the hydroxylation of the N-methyl group of the pesticide carbaryl and the metabolic schemes for pentobarbital, riboflavin (vitamin B_2), and pyrethrin, a natural pesticide.

Other common, metabolic pathways shared by natural and synthetic chemicals include epoxidations and dealkylations (Oritz de Montellano 1985). With respect to the first, epoxides may subsequently be metabolized to diols by epoxide hydrolases. A number of epoxides or diol epoxides have been shown to bind to DNA to form adducts. For example, aflatoxin B_1 undergoes metabolic activation to an epoxide that can bind to DNA or protein, or can react with glutathione, a detoxification process (IARC 1993). Naphthalene is an example of another aromatic compound that undergoes metabolic activation to a reactive intermediate. Epoxidations can also occur with double bonds in non-aromatic rings such as with the marihuana constituent Δ^9-tetrahydrocannabinol (Testa and Jenner 1976). Other chemicals that undergo side chain or alkene epoxidations include the synthetic chemicals 4-vinylcyclohexene (Smith et al. 1990), butadiene (Malvoisin and Roberfroid 1982), and naturally occurring d-limonene (IARC 1993). In addition, resulting epoxides may then undergo further phase II conjugation reactions. It should be noted, however, that not all epoxides are reactive. Dieldrin, the epoxide metabolite of aldrin, is quite stable.

Examples of dealkylations, the other common reaction shared by natural and synthetic compounds, include atrazine, one of the most widely used herbicides in the United States, which is N-dealkylated, nicotine, which is dealkylated to nornicotine, and the drug tamoxifen, which is also N-dealkylated (Jansen and de Fluiter 1992). O-Dealkylations encompass a wide range of compounds, including synthetics such as p-nitroanisole, phenacetin, and the pesticide methoxychlor, and the naturally occurring compounds scoparone (6,7-dimethylcoumarin), rotenone, and thebaine (Testa and Jenner 1976).

Less common reactions include deamination and dehydroxylation. Chemicals that undergo deamination include amphetamine and mescaline (Testa and Jenner 1976). Dehydroxylation is postulated to occur in vivo by gut bacteria. Such reactions are important in the metabolism of catechols such as the naturally occurring caffeic acid (IARC 1993), which can also be detoxified via glucuronide conjugation. Many other reactions can occur but are of lesser importance and are not covered here.

One of the factors that tends to make chemicals resistant to metabolism by mammalian organisms is the presence of chlorine groups. However, dechlorination can occur (such as with the pesticide DDT or with the herbicide atrazine), even in mammalian systems. Of particular concern are highly halogenated synthetic chemicals such as hexachlorobenzene and the PCBs (polychlorinated biphenyls). Dechlorination of these chemicals can be very slow. Structure-activity relationships indicate that PCBs with vicinal-substituted carbons are highly resistant to epoxidation by metabolizing enzymes. Similar arguments can be made for other chlorinated chemicals, such as the dibenzo-p-dioxins and dibenzofurans.

A number of halogenated compounds are natural products (Neidleman and Geigert 1986, Gribble 1992, Willes et al. 1993). Over 1500 halogenated compounds have been identified in marine organisms, more than 250 in red algae alone. Chlorinated compounds are formed in bacteria, algae, fungi, ferns, higher plants, and even lower animals. These compounds, chlorinated via chloroperoxidases, may be quite complex (e.g., chlortetracycline), but the degree of chlorination and, therefore, resistance to metabolism is generally not as great as for synthetic chemicals.

TOXICOLOGICAL COMPARISONS

In this section, toxicological comparisons are made between chemically related synthetic and naturally occurring chemicals, some of which are known to be carcinogenic. Classes of related compounds discussed include peroxisome proliferators, nitrosamines, hydrazines, phenolic antioxidants, methylene dioxyphenyl (benzodioxole) compounds, sodium salts, aromatic amines and related chemicals, and α_{2u}-globulin binding compounds.

Nitrosamines

Several nitrosamines occur naturally in our environment. Others can be formed endogenously (IARC 1978, 1982). For example, ingested nitrites interact with amines in the acid conditions of the mammalian stomach to form nitrosamines (Sander et al. 1968). Nitrates are reduced to nitrites by bacteria, especially in saliva.

Nitrites from swallowed saliva or from the diet can produce nitrosa-mines in the stomach (NRC 1981, Kyrtopoulos 1989, Leaf et al. 1989). Because of this, the use of nitrites and nitrates as additives to foods such as meat and fish is strictly regulated. Secondary and tertiary amines, N-alkylamides (including peptides), ureas, carba-mates, and guanidines can all be nitrosated (Mirvish 1975, Shep-herd and Lutz 1989). Some of these compounds occur ubiquitously in nature, while others are synthetic agricultural chemicals and drugs. For example, the drug aminopyrine reacts readily with traces of nitrosating agents, including gaseous nitrogen oxides, resulting in the formation of dimethylnitrosamine, traces of which have been found in the drug itself (Eisenbrand et al. 1978). The amount of N-nitroso compounds (nitrosamines and nitrosamides) formed by nitrosation depends upon nitrite concentration, the concentration and basicity of the amine or amide, and pH. The presence of nucleophilic ions such as thiocyanates increases the rate of N-nitrosamine formation (Fan and Tannenbaum 1973, NRC 1981). In contrast, ascorbic acid, α-tocopherol, and various pheno-lic compounds inhibit the formation of N-nitrosamines (Mirvish 1975, 1981, 1994; Morgens et al. 1978). Nitroso compounds are also contaminants in foodstuffs, alcoholic beverages, and cosmetics (Tricker et al. 1989). Tobacco contains several nitrosamines and nitrosatable amines, which are formed during the curing and burn-ing of the product. These compounds appear to be significant carcinogens in the induction of various cancers in humans exposed to tobacco smoke and other tobacco products (Hecht and Hoffman 1989). Nitrosation also occurs in soils, organic waste, and water, where industrial and other discharges contain large amounts of amines.

Nitrosamines require metabolic activation for expression of mu-tagenic and carcinogenic activity. The cytochrome P-450s are re-sponsible for this activation by hydroxylation at the α-carbon of the alkyl substituents (Okada 1984, Yang et al. 1984, Archer 1989). The alkyldiazohydroxide intermediates that are formed readily alkylate proteins and nucleic acids. The possibility that traces of ni-trosamines pose a cancer risk for humans has yet to be proved, but certain correlations suggest that target N-nitroso compounds are involved in the etiology of gastric, esophageal, and nasopharyngeal cancers and possibly others (Magee 1989). Childhood leukemia and brain cancer were recently associated with nitrite-preserved hot dogs consumed by children or their parents, but it was unclear whether hot dogs were the primary factor or merely a factor indica-tive of a low socio-economic status (Bunin et al. 1994, Peters et al. 1994, Sarasua and Savitz 1994). Many target organs in a variety of animal species are susceptible to the carcinogenic action of N-ni-troso compounds. Human tissues and cytochrome P-450s can bioactivate nitrosamines to mutagenic intermediates that form adducts with tissue constituents (Hoffman and Hecht 1985). Of the variety of alkyl products formed, the O-alkylations of guanine and thymine are mutagenic, and their formation is associated with the carcinogenic potential of the compound or with the mutagenic susceptibility of the specific organ (Singer 1985).

Although certain nitrosamines have been synthesized for com-mercial use, they may also occur naturally. For example, dimethyl-nitrosamine was used in the synthesis of dimethylhydrazine, but it has also been found in a variety of food products (as discussed above). There is no evidence to suggest differences in the properties of naturally occurring versus synthetic nitrosamines.

Hydrazines

Humans are exposed to naturally occurring and synthetic hydra-zines with known mutagenic and carcinogenic potential (Toth 1975). Exposure to these chemicals occurs because of their wide-spread use by the agricultural, pharmaceutical, aerospace and petro-leum industries, and because a number of hydrazine derivatives occur naturally. For example, Toth (1991) reported on 11 hydra-zine analogs that were identified in 22 species of mushrooms, one of which is cultivated. Another natural source of hydrazine is tobacco and tobacco smoke, which have been shown to contain hydrazine and 1,1-dimethylhydrazine.

The carcinogenic properties of natural and synthetic hydrazines are similar with respect to organotropism (Toth 1980). For example, when administered orally to mice, phenylhydrazine (synthetic) and 4-methylphenylhydrazine (natural) produce tumors of the lungs and blood vessels. Methylhydrazine, which is produced synthetically but also occurs naturally, produces pulmonary adenocarcinomas in Swiss mice and histiocytomas of the liver and tumors of the cecum in Syrian golden hamsters (Toth 1984). Tissue localization depends upon the animal species tested, the route of administration, the dose, and the hydrazine derivative.

The carcinogenic properties of hydrazines may be a result of their enzymatic activation. A number of enzyme systems have been shown to metabolize hydrazine derivatives. These include cytochrome P450, the flavin-containing monooxygenase, and monoamine oxidase. The substituents on the hydrazine moiety determine its metabolic fate. For example, monosubstituted hydrazines and 1,2-disubstituted hydrazines are predominantly metabolized by cytochrome P450 (Prough and Maloney 1985). The metabolism of 1,1-disubstituted hydrazines is catalyzed largely by the flavin-containing monooxygenase (Prough and Maloney 1985).

The metabolism of hydrazine derivatives can lead to a variety of chemically reactive species, including diazines, diazonium ions, and carbon-centered radicals (Gannett et al. 1991, Albano et al. 1993). It has been postulated that radicals formed during the enzymatic activation of hydrazine and hydrazine derivatives may subsequently bind to DNA to form adducts (Gannett et al. 1991). Such alterations can result in miscoding upon DNA replication. The enzymatic activation of N-methyl-N-formylhydrazine, a naturally occurring hydrazine, results in the formation of such radicals (Gannett et al. 1991). Thus the formation of DNA adducts may be the initial event in the carcinogenicity of N-methyl-N-formylhydrazine.

Like synthetic hydrazines, naturally occurring hydrazines have been shown to be mutagenic. The role of metabolic activation in the mutagenicity of hydrazines (natural or synthetic) is questionable, since many hydrazines are mutagenic in the absence of S-9 mix. In fact, the mutagenicity of many hydrazines is inhibited by the presence of S-9 mix or bovine serum albumin (Matsushita et al. 1993).

Methylenedioxyphenyl Compounds

Methylenedioxyphenyl (benzodioxole) compounds (MDPs) occur widely in plants. Among the dietary sources of MDPs are parsnips, carrots, nutmeg, sesame seeds (and sesame seed oil), pepper, and sassafras. Synthetic derivatives of these compounds are used commercially for insecticide synergists. The principal synthetic MDP used as a synergist is piperonyl butoxide (Hodgson and Philpot 1974). Although it is not widely used on crops, it is frequently included in aerosol preparations for household use.

In mammals, MDPs affect multiple enzyme pathways; the effect on the cytochrome P450 system has been the most studied (Goldstein et al. 1973, Hodgson and Philpot 1974). MDPs have been shown to inhibit P450-mediated metabolism and to induce several P450 isozymes (Fujii et al. 1970, Wagstaff and Short 1971, Hodgson and Philpot 1974, Thomas et al. 1983, Yeowell et al. 1985, Lewandowski et al. 1990). As inhibitors of P450 activity, MDPs have been used extensively with the pyrethroid and carbamate insecticides; the metabolism of these insecticides is, in large part, P450-mediated (Haley 1978). It has been postulated that inhibition of P450 activity leads to the formation of a stable inhibitory complex between the heme iron of P450 and the carbene species formed when water is cleaved from the hydroxylated methylene carbon of the MDP (Dahl and Hodgson 1979). While the 3,4-methylenedioxyphenyl group is essential for activity, the relative effectiveness varies with the nature of the side chains in the 1 and

6 positions, a long, lipophilic side chain favoring the formation of a more stable inhibitory complex. Thus the development of commercial synergists involves the addition of a lipophilic side chain to naturally occurring MDPs.

Naturally occurring MDPs and their synthetic derivatives induce various isozymes of the P450 system. In studies conducted with mice, MDPs have been shown to induce P450 1A2 by an Ah receptor-independent mechanism as well as P450 2B10. They also induce P450 1A1, but only at doses higher than those necessary for the first two inductions named. Although extensive structure-activity studies have not been carried out, it appears that the MDP group is essential for this particular pattern of induction; however, the extent of induction varies with other molecular characteristics (Cook and Hodgson 1985, 1986; Murray et al. 1985; Adams et al. 1994).

Some naturally occurring and synthetic MDPs are known to be carcinogenic at high-dose levels. Safrole (5-(2-propenyl)-1,3-benzodioxole), a naturally occurring MDP found in black pepper and oil of sassafras, has been used in flavoring and perfume. It has been shown to be a hepatocarcinogen in animal studies, causing liver tumors at a dietary concentration of 0.5 percent. The active metabolite appears to be the sulfate ester of the 1'-hydroxy derivative (Homberger et al. 1961, Long et al. 1963, Ioannides et al. 1981).

Piperonyl butoxide (alpha(2-(2-butoxyethoxy)ethoxy)-4,5-methylenedioxy-2-propyltoluene) tested negative in early tests for carcinogenicity and mutagenicity, but recent long-term feeding studies have demonstrated hepatocellular carcinoma in both male and female F344 rats. However, the lowest effective dose was 1.2% of the diet, some 400,000 times the ADI for humans (Takahashi et al. 1994).

In summary, naturally occurring and synthetic MDPs appear to be attractive models for comparing natural and synthetic carcinogens. There are, however, significant data gaps and unanswered questions. These include the following: 1) Is the MDP group irrelevant to the carcinogenicity of safrole and piperonyl butoxide, with side chain substituents being of greater, or sole, importance? 2) Is suitability for metabolism to a sulfate ester the critical parameter? 3) Does rendering the molecule more lipophilic and, therefore, more persistent, make the potential for carcinogenicity greater? 4) Do the high-dose levels required make this an inappropriate model? 5) Given the wide distribution of MDP compounds and the potential for additive effects, are high doses likely to be reached in any case? In spite of these data gaps and unanswered questions, two factors suggest that these compounds require further study: one, the potential for human exposure to naturally occurring and synthetic MDPs and two, MDPs induce and inhibit P450 isozymes, which are often involved in the early stages of carcinogeneses.

Aromatic Amines and Related Chemicals

Aromatic amines are among the earliest class of chemicals suggested to be potential human carcinogens. This idea was based on observations by Rehn in 1895 that workers in the aniline dye industry in Germany had an increased risk of developing bladder cancer (Miller and Miller 1983). Subsequently, several aromatic amines were identified as human bladder carcinogens, including 2-naphthylamine, benzidine, and 4-aminobiphenyl, as well as related chemicals such as benzidine dyes and phenacetin. Much of what is known today about the metabolic activation and inactivation of chemical carcinogens is the result of investigations conducted on 2-acetylaminofluorene.

More recently, numerous polycyclic, heterocyclic aromatic amines have been identified as pyrolysis products resulting from the cooking of foods at very high temperatures (Wakabayashi et al. 1992). Aromatic amines, such as 4-aminobiphenyl and o-toluidine, have also been detected in cigarette smoke (Vineis et al. 1994).

The metabolism of the synthetic and naturally occurring aromatic amines are similar (Miller and Miller 1983, Wakabayashi et al. 1992, Snyderwine et al. 1993, Vineis et al. 1994). Enzymatic activation occurs through N-hydroxylation. The metabolic intermediates thus formed may then undergo phase II conjugation to form various esters, such as sulfates, glucuronides, and acetyl derivatives, and they may covalently bind to DNA (usually to C8 of guanine) to form adducts.

The mutagenic potential of many aromatic amines has been demonstrated in vitro using prokaryotic assays, and several amines have subsequently been shown to be carcinogenic in rodent bioassays and in nonhuman primates. Among the pyrolysis products are included 2-amino-3-methylimidazo[4,5-f]quinoline (IQ) and 2-amino-1-methyl-6-phenylimidazo[4,5-b]pyridine (PhIP).

Depending on the chemical, route of administration, species, and strain, these chemicals produce tumors predominantly of liver, mammary gland, bladder, and colon in rodents, the urinary bladder in dogs, and the liver in nonhuman primates. Epidemiologic studies have associated them only with the formation of urinary bladder cancer in humans, but recent animal experimental evidence suggests that aromatic amines may also be associated with other tumor types, such as colon cancer (Ito et al. 1991). Evidence indicates that naturally occurring and synthetic aromatic amines have similar potencies in both in vitro assays and rodent carcinogenicity bioassays.

Peroxisome Proliferators

Several compounds of diverse chemical structure (Reddy and Rao 1992, Gibson 1993) are known to induce peroxisome proliferation. These include fibric acid derivatives such as clofibrate, gemfibrizol, and ciprofibrate which are used as hypolipidemic agents; other unrelated drugs such as valproic acid and chlorcyclizine; phthalate ester plasticizers, notably di-2-ethylhexylphthalate; herbicides such as 2,4-dichlorophenoxyacetic acid; and simple compounds such as trichloroacetic acid (Moody et al. 1991). While these agents cause morphological effects in a number of tissues, the primary target organ is the liver, where they cause hypertrophy, hyperplasia, and peroxisome proliferation. The latter is preceded by an increase in the enzymes involved in fatty acid ß-oxidation and, to a lesser extent, in catalase (Lock et al. 1989). In addition, peroxisomal proliferators also induce drug metabolizing enzymes (most notably glucuronyl transferase, epoxide hydrolase, and cytochrome P450 4A1), stimulate growth factors, and activate oncogenes (Bieri 1993).

Hepatocarcinogenicity is the primary toxicity of concern associated with peroxisomal proliferators, especially in rodents such as rats and mice. The mechanism responsible for hepatocarcinogenicity is not clear because these chemicals are routinely negative in genotoxicity tests. The pleiotropic response following the administration of peroxisome proliferators appears to be related to their activation of a novel steroid hormone receptor, the peroxisome proliferator-activated receptor (PPAR). Tumorigenicity may ultimately be related to the oxidative stress that results from the enhanced peroxisomal fatty acid oxidation and the concomitant hydrogen peroxide synthesis. Alternatively, these chemicals may enhance cellular replication of hepatocytes, especially cells in foci, since in some studies the degree of sustained DNA replication has been found to be highly correlated with tumorigenicity rather than with peroxisome proliferation (Green et al. 1992).

A limited number of natural products, such as phytol—a decomposition product of chlorophyll—have been investigated for their potential to induce peroxisome proliferation (Watanabe and Suga 1983, Van den Branden et al. 1986). High fat diets, vitamin E deficiency, and diabetes can also produce peroxisome proliferation in rodents (Moody et al. 1991). The role of peroxisomal proliferators in human carcinogenesis is not clear, since peroxisome proliferation does not occur in humans (Blumcke et al. 1983, Hanefeld et al. 1983). Nevertheless, humans do respond to these agents (e.g., with hypolipidemia following treatment with the fibric acid derivatives) and they, like rodents, possess PPARs that are sensitive to activation.

Phenolic Antioxidants

Butylated hydroxyanisole (BHA) and butylated hydroxytoluene (BHT) are synthetic chemicals used as food antioxidants. They have been widely used to preserve foods, particularly oils, fats, and shortenings, which are subject to oxidative deterioration and rancidity (Verhagen et al. 1991). Although BHA and BHT are compounds with low acute toxicity, they are known to alter the activities of enzymes involved in the activation/detoxification of xenobiotics. For example, the activities of glutathione-S-transferase, epoxide hydrolase, glucuronyl transferase, and cytochrome P-450 are all increased in rats and/or mice after BHA or BHT is administered. Because these enzymes are often involved in the activation and detoxification of chemicals, it is not surprising that they have been shown to modify the toxicological response of a variety of chemicals. BHA reduces liver damage caused by bromobenzene, acetaminophen, and CCl_4 in mice, and protects the rat adrenal gland from dimethylbenz[a]anthracene-induced necrosis (Kahl 1984, Stich 1991). Many similar types of protective effects have been observed in other tissues. Most relevant to this discussion are the tumorigenic and antitumorigenic actions of these antioxidants.

BHA suppresses the development of DMBA-initiated tumors of the lung, forestomach, and mammary gland (Kahl 1984, Stich 1991). It has also been shown to suppress skin tumors initiated by DMBA and promoted by TPA. In several studies, BHA and BHT have been shown to be effective against other carcinogens. For example, both chemicals inhibited the hepatocarcinogenesis of concurrently-administered aflatoxin B_1 (Williams et al. 1986). BHT also reduced the incidence of N-hydroxy-N-2-fluorenylacetamide-induced hepatomas (in male rats) and mammary cancer (in female rats) (Ulland et al. 1973). However, these potentially beneficial effects of BHA and other synthetic antioxidants became questionable when it was reported that they induced carcinomas of the forestomach in rats and hamsters (Ito et al. 1983, 1985). A subsequent study showed that feeding of high dose levels of BHA to rats enhanced the development of N-methyl-N'-nitro-N-nitrosoguanidine-initiated squamous cell neoplasms of the forestomach (Ito et al. 1985).

Naturally occurring antioxidants produce similar types of effects. Caffeic acid, a phenolic antioxidant found in several fruits and vegetables, is both tumorigenic and antitumorigenic, as discussed in Chapter 2 (IARC 1993, Stich 1991). Dietary administration of caffeic acid at doses comparable to those used with BHA resulted in squamous cell papillomas and carcinomas of the forestomachs of mice and rats. Caffeic acid also increased the incidence of papillomas of the forestomach in rats treated with DMBA as an initiating agent (Hirose et al. 1988). In another study, when caffeic acid was administered before and with benzo(a)pyrene, it decreased the incidence of forestomach tumors induced by benzo[a]pyrene (Wattenberg et al. 1980). Similar effects have been reported for other naturally occurring antioxidants. For example, catechol induces cell proliferation and is active as a glandular stomach carcinogen (Stich 1991).

The above discussion documents that synthetic and naturally occurring antioxidants behave similarly when tested at high doses for tumorigenic and antitumorigenic effects. The ultimate outcome depends on the amount of exposure the animals received. *However, it is clear that synthetic and naturally occurring phenolic antioxidants are tumorigenic in rodents, when given at high doses.* The implications for human risk, however, remain poorly defined, although a recent expert panel questioned the relevance of the BHA rodent carcinogenesis results to humans (FASEB 1994).

Sodium Salts and Rodent
Urinary Tract Carcinogenesis

Sodium saccharin (Ellwein and Cohen 1990) is an artificial sweetener which was found to produce urothelial carcinomas in rats when high doses were given beginning at birth or earlier. It did not produce cancer when administration started at 6-8 weeks of age (as in a standard 2-year bioassay). The male rat appeared to be more susceptible than the female and no proliferative or tumorigenic effects were found in mice, hamsters, guinea pigs, or monkeys. IARC has found the evidence for carcinogenicity to animals for saccharin sufficient; however, the evidence for effects in humans is inconclusive (IARC 1987) and is consistent with two possibilities, first that it does not cause human bladder cancer, and second that it is a very weak cause cause of human bladder cancer (Armstrong 1985)

Research on saccharin (Ellwein and Cohen 1990) indicates that it is not metabolized, is nucleophilic rather than electrophilic (pKa of approximately 2.0), and is absorbed and largely excreted in the urine within hours of consumption. At the level of approximately 1.0% of the diet, it has been shown to have no effect on proliferation, tumor enhancement, or carcinogenicity. Acidification of the urine below pH 6.5 results in inhibiting the proliferative and tumorigenic effects of saccharin. Similarly, administration of certain forms of saccharin, such as calcium or acid saccharin, which produce acidic urine, has no effect on the rat urothelium. However co-administration of calcium saccharin with alkalinizing substances results in the appearance of proliferative effects. The proliferative and tumorigenic effects associated with high doses of sodium saccharin appear due to the formation of a urinary amorphous precipitate. This precipitate is largely calcium phosphate, but it also contains saccharin, protein, silicates, potassium, chloride, and acidic mucopolysaccharides (Cohen et al. 1991, 1993). It is not clear how the precipitate is formed or how it causes its toxic effect. In addition, studies of how sodium saccharin acts in the rat have raised questions about the underlying assumptions of cancer risk assessment, including the basic assumptions of high to low-dose extrapolation and interspecies extrapolation from rodents to humans (Fukushima et al. 1986, Cohen and Ellwein 1990, 1991).

Most sodium salts, administered at high doses, produce urothelial proliferative and tumorigenic effects in the male rat similar to those of sodium saccharin, providing that the urinary pH is approximately 6.5 or greater (Ellwein and Cohen 1990, Cohen and Ellwein 1992). For example, sodium ascorbate, which has been extensively studied, produces effects similar to those produced by sodium saccharin at comparable doses (approximately 5% of the diet), including effects of urinary acidification and alkalinization (Ellwein and Cohen 1990). Other sodium salts which have produced similar effects in male rats at comparably high doses include glutamate (DeGroot et al. 1988), aspartate, citrate, erythorbate, succinate, phosphate, bicarbonate (Lina et al. 1994), and to a limited extent, chloride. All produce a urinary amorphous precipitate similar to that seen with sodium saccharin (Cohen et al. 1995). Lack of effects can also be similar.

Like sodium saccharin, sodium ascorbate does not affect the urothelium of the mouse (Tamano et al. 1993). It should be noted that all these substances other than saccharin are naturally occurring, and several are essential to human survival. Several are also generated endogenously as part of intermediary metabolism. Urinary concentrations of the anion when the salt is administered as 5% of the diet are approximately 200 mM. Under normal circumstances, these ions are present in the urine at lower, though still substantial, amounts. For example, serum bicarbonate is normally approximately 26 mM and tightly regulated, whereas urinary concentration can range from less than 1 mM to greater than 100 mM depending on pH (Thier 1981). Urinary chloride can range from 10 to 100 mM in rats and 40 to 250 mM in humans. Urinary sodium ranges from 10 to 250 mM in rats compared with 1 to 300 mM in humans, depending on degree of hydration and numerous other factors (Cohen 1995). It is not surprising that diet greatly influences responsiveness to these chemicals. For example, administration of an AIN-76A semisynthetic diet, which produces acidic urine, completely inhibits the proliferative and tumorigenic effects of sodium saccharin (Okamura et al. 1991).

An apparent exception to the urothelial effects of the sodium salts is sodium hippurate. When administered at high levels in the diet, it produces no urothelial proliferative or tumorigenic effects in any of the species tested, including the rat (Fukushima et al. 1983, Schoenig et al. 1985). However, this lack of effect may be due to the fact that the urinary pH is consistently below 6.5 in rats fed diets high in sodium hippurate.

It also appears that potassium salts produce similar effects as the sodium salts when administered at high doses, although they are somewhat less potent (Ellwein and Cohen 1990). Most notably, potassium bicarbonate was recently shown to be carcinogenic to the rat bladder in a 30-month bioassay (Lina et al. 1994).

All of the substances discussed above are nongenotoxic and appear to produce their tumorigenic effects on the rat urothelium secondary to increased proliferation. Several other substances are known to produce bladder tumors in rats, and occasionally in mice, when administered at high doses in the diet, by causing calculi in the urine (Cohen and Ellwein 1990, 1991, 1992). The calculi cause an erosive toxicity of the urothelium with prominent regenerative hyperplasia. Calculus-forming substances that produce cancer in rodents include numerous synthetic compounds, such as melamine, but they also include numerous, common, naturally occurring substances. Many of the latter are nutritionally essential or are products of intermediary metabolism, such as calcium phosphate, calcium oxalate, glycine, and uracil (Clayson 1974; Cohen and Ellwein 1990, 1991, 1992; Clayson et al. 1995, in press). All these compounds must be administered at doses sufficiently high to generate calculus formation in the urine and ultimately increase cell proliferation and tumorigenicity. A weak association between calculi and bladder tumors has also been suggested in humans (Burin et al. 1995, in press). The implication is that there is a threshold dose below which calculi, on precipitate, will not form in the urine. Because of physical-chemical and physiologic determinants, there is a threshold for tumorigenicity for all nongenotoxic sodium salts, whether they are naturally occurring or synthetic.

α_{2u}-Globulin Binding Compounds

α_{2u}-Globulin interacts with certain chemicals, resulting in protein droplet formation, and ultimately in renal carcinogenesis and nephropathy. This low molecular weight protein is synthesized under androgenic control in high amounts in the liver of male rats (Borghoff et al. 1990). It also forms a reversible binding complex with certain chemicals, thus inhibiting the hydrolysis of the protein by lysosomal degradation in the proximal convoluted tubule cells of the kidney. The protein is thus accumulated and causes cellular necrosis. It is postulated that this cell death leads to a compensatory cell division and subsequently to renal tumor formation (Borghoff et al. 1990, Swenberg et al. 1989, Flamm and Lehman-McKeeman 1991). However, this process has not been observed in female rats (Alden 1986), male NCI-Black-Reiter rats (Dietrich and Swenberg 1991), mice, guinea pigs, dogs, or monkeys (Alden 1986), all of which are known to be deficient in the production of the α_{2u}-globulin.

Chemicals, both synthetic and naturally occurring, which some have hypothesized act through this mechanism include unleaded gasoline (Olson et al. 1987) and 2,2,4-trimethylpentane as a surrogate (Charbonneau et al. 1987), p-dichlorobenzene (Charbonneau et al. 1989), decalin (Kanerva et al. 1987), pentachloroethane (Goldsworthy et al. 1988), perchloroethylene (Green et al. 1990), isophorone (Strasser et al. 1988), and tetralin (Serve et al. 1988). Of particular interest is the monoterpene d-limonene, which is found in high amounts in citrus fruits, is the major component of oil of orange, and has been used extensively as a flavoring agent. In a two-year bioassay, it was found to cause renal tumors in male F344 rats but not in female rats or mice of either sex (NTP 1990). It has been shown to be metabolized to d-limonene-1,2-oxide which binds reversibly with α_{2u}-globulin (Lehman-McKeeman et al. 1989). However, since it has been recognized that the formation of the α_{2u}-globulin is specific to the male rat, these results cannot extrapolated to humans (Borghoff et al. 1990, Olson et al. 1990, Flamm and Lehman-McKeeman 1991, Borghoff et al. 1993, Hard et al. 1993). Although a number of proteins have been identified in the serum and urine of humans which share some amino acid homology with α_{2u}-globulin, they are produced in comparatively small amounts. Furthermore, they are similar to those found in female rats and mice which, when exposed to α_{2u}-globulin binding compounds, do not form renal tumors. Lehman-McKeeman and Caudill note that α_{2u}-globulin may be the only member of this lipocalin protein superfamily that binds protein droplet-inducing agents (1992). An alternate hypothesis on the role of chemically induced protein droplet α_{2u}-globulin nephropathy in renal carcinogenesis has been proposed by Melnick (1992).

SUMMARY AND CONCLUSIONS

The principles and techniques developed to evaluate the carcinogenic potential of synthetic chemicals can serve as a guide for evaluating naturally occurring chemicals found in the human diet.

Overall, the mechanisms involved in the entire process of carcinogenesis, from exposure of the organism to the expression of tumors, are similar, if not identical, between synthetic and naturally occurring carcinogens. Similar too are problems associated with extrapolation between species and extrapolation between high and low doses.

Although there are differences between specific groups of synthetic and naturally occurring chemicals with respect to properties such as lipophilicity, degree of conjugation, recalcitrance to metabolism, and persistence in the body and environment, it is unlikely that information on these properties, if available, will enable predictions to be made of the degree of carcinogenicity of a naturally occurring or synthetic chemical in the diet. Both categories of chemicals—naturally occurring and synthetic—are large and diverse. Predictions based on chemical or physical properties are problematic, due to the likely overlap of values between the categories.

Given the vast number of naturally occurring chemicals, it is clear that if evaluation for carcinogenicity is to be carried out, priorities must be established. The most significant priority will be based on association with, or presence of a chemical in, foods associated with diets or life styles believed to be deleterious; however, refinements are possible based on our knowledge of synthetic carcinogens. For example, naturally occurring chemicals meeting the criteria of association with deleterious foods could be accorded a higher priority for testing if 1) they fall in the same chemical class as known carcinogens; 2) they contain chemical groups also found in known carcinogens; 3) based on structural comparisons with known carcinogens, they are likely to form reactive intermediates, in vivo; or 4) based on structural comparisons with known carcinogens, they are likely to be stable in vivo. It should be noted that all of the above aspects are susceptible to evaluation by modern QSAR (Quantitative Structure-Activity Relationship) techniques.

REFERENCES

Adams, N.H., P.E. Levi, and E. Hodgson. 1994. Regulation of cytochrome P450 isozymes by methylenedioxyphenyl compounds.

Chem. Biol. Interact. 86:255-274.

Albano, E., L. Goria-Gatti, P. Clot, A. Jannone, and A. Tomasi. 1993. Possible role of free radical intermediates in hepatotoxicity of hydrazine. Toxicology and Industrial Health 9(3):529-538.

Alden, C.L. 1986. A review of unique male rat hydrocarbon nephropathy. Toxicol. Pathol. 14:109-111.

Archer, M.C. 1989. Mechanisms of action of N-nitroso compounds. Cancer Surveys 8:241-250.

Armitage, P., and R. Doll. 1954. The age distribution of cancer and a multi-stage theory of carcinogenesis. Br. J. Cancer 8:1-12.

Armstrong, B.K. 1985. Saccharin/cyclamates: Epidemiologic evidence. Pp. 129-143 in Interpretation of Negative Epidemiological Evidence for Carcinogenicity, N.J. Wald and R. Doll, eds. IARC Scientific Publications No. 65. Lyon: International Agency for Research in Cancer.

Berenblum, I., and P. Shubik. 1947. A new, quantitative, approach to the study of the stages of chemical carcinogenesis in the mouse's skin. Br. J. Cancer 1:383-391.

Bieri, F. 1993. Peroxisome proliferators and cellular signaling pathways. A review. Biol. Cell 77:43-46.

Bishop, J.M. 1991. Molecular themes in oncogenesis. Cell 64:235-248.

Blair, A., M. Dosemeci, and E.F. Heineman. 1993. Cancer and other causes of death among male and female farmers from twenty-three states. Am. J. Ind. Med. 23:729-742.

Blair, A., H. Malker, K. Cantor, L. Burmeister, and K. Wiklund. 1985. Cancer among farmers: A review. Scand. J. Work Environ. Health 11:397-407.

Blair, A., and S.H. Zahm. 1990. Methodologic issues in exposure assessment for case-control studies of cancer and herbicides. Am. J. Ind. Med. 18:285-293.

Blair, A., and S.H. Zahm. 1991. Cancer among farmers. Pp. 335-54 in Occupational Medicine: State of the Art Reviews, D.H. Cordes, and D.F. Rea, eds. Hanley and Belfus.

Blumcke, S., W. Schwartzkopff, H. Lobeck, N.A. Edmondson, D.E. Prentice, and G.F. Blane. 1983. Influence of fenofibrate on cellular and subcellular liver structure in hyperlipidemic patients.

Atherosclerosis 46:105-116.

Borghoff, S.J., L.D. Lehman-McKeeman, B.G. Short, G.C. Hard, and J.A. Swenberg. 1993. Critique of R. Melnick's "An alternative hypothesis on the role of chemically induced protein droplet (α2u-globulin) nephropathy in renal carcinogenesis." Reg. Toxicol. Pharmacol. 18:357-364.

Borghoff, S.J., B.G. Short, and J.A. Swenberg. 1990. Biochemical mechanisms and pathobiology of α2u-globulin nephropathy. Annu. Rev. Pharmacol. Toxicol. 30:349-367.

Boutwell, R.K. 1964. Some biological aspects of skin carcinogenesis. Progr. Exp. Tumor Res. 4:207-250.

Bridges, J.W., and L.F. Chasseaud. 1976. Progress in Drug Metabolism. Vol. 1. London: John Wiley & Sons.

Brown, L.M., A. Blair, R. Gibson, G.D. Everett, K.P. Cantor, L.M. Schuman, L.F. Burmeister, S.F. Van Lier, and F. Dick. 1990. Pesticide exposures and other agricultural risk factors for leukemia among men in Iowa and Minnesota. Cancer Res. 50(20):6585-6591.

Bunin, G.R., R.R. Kuijten, C.P. Boesel, J.D. Buckley, and A.T. Meadows. 1994. Maternal diet and risk of astrocytic glioma in children: A report from the Childrens Cancer Group (United States and Canada). Cancer Causes Control 5:177-187.

Burin, G.I., H.I. Gibb, and R.N. Hill. 1995. Human bladder cancer: Evidence for a potential irritation-induced mechanism. Food Chem. Toxicol. 33:785-796.

Charbonneau, M., E.A. Lock, J. Strasser, M.G. Cox, M.J. Turner, and J.S. Bus. 1987. 2,2,4-Trimethylpentane-induced nephrotoxicity. 1. Metabolic disposition of TMP in male and female Fischer 344 rats. Toxicol. Appl. Pharmacol. 91:171-181.

Charbonneau, M., J. Strasser Jr., E.A. Lock, M.J. Turner, and J.A. Swenberg. 1989. Involvement of reversible binding to α2u-globulin in 1,4-dichlorobenzene-induced nephrotoxicity. Toxicol. Appl. Pharmacol. 99:122-132.

Choy, W.N. 1993. A review of the dose-response induction of DNA adducts by aflatoxin B1 and its implications to quantitative cancer-risk assessment. Mutat. Res. 296:181-198.

Clayson, D.B. 1974. Bladder carcinogenesis in rats and mice: Possibility of artifacts. J. Natl. Cancer Inst. 52:1685-1689.

Clayson, D.B., L. Fishbein, and S.M. Cohen. 1995. The effects of physical factors on the induction of rodent bladder cancer. Food Chem. Toxicol. 33:771-784.

Cohen, S.M. 1995. The role of urinary physiology and chemistry in bladder carcinogenesis. Food Chem. Toxicol. 33:715-730.

Cohen, S.M., M. Cano, R.A. Earl, S.D. Carson, and E.M. Garland. 1991. A proposed role for silicates and protein in the proliferative effects of saccharin on the male rat urothelium. Carcinogenesis 12:1551-1555.

Cohen, S.M., and L.B. Ellwein. 1990. Cell proliferation in carcinogenesis. Science 249:1007-1011.

Cohen, S.M., and L.B. Ellwein. 1991. Genetic errors, cell proliferation, and carcinogenesis. Cancer Res. 51:6493-6505.

Cohen, S.M., and L.B. Ellwein. 1992. Risk assessment based on high-dose animal exposure experiments. Chem. Res. Toxicol. 5:742-748.

Cohen, S.M., E.M. Garland, J.M. Wehner, L.S. Johnson, and M. Cano. 1993. Relationship between bladder changes produced in male rats by sodium saccharin treatment and formation of an insoluble, amorphous material in the urine. Proc. Am. Assoc. Cancer Res. 34:174.

Cohen, S.M., M. Cano, E.M. Garland, M. St John and L.L. Arnold. 1995. Urinary and urothelial effects of sodium salts in male rats. Carcinogenesis 16(2):343-348.

Cook, J.C., and E. Hodgson. 1985. The induction of cytochrome P-450 by isosafrole and related methylenedioxyphenyl compounds. Chem. Biol. Interact. 54:299-315.

Cook, J.C., and E. Hodgson. 1986. Induction of cytochrome P-450 in congenic C57BL/6J mice by isosafrole: Lack of correlation with the Ah locus. Chem. Biol. Interact. 58:233-240.

Dahl, A.R., and E. Hodgson. 1979. The interaction of aliphatic analogs of methylenedioxyphenyl compounds with cytochromes P-450 and P-420. Chem. Biol. Interact. 27:163-175.

Dauterman, W.C. 1993. Metabolism of toxicants: Phase II reactions. Pp. 113-132 in Introduction to Biochemical Toxicology, 2nd edition, E. Hodgson and P.E. Levi, eds. Norwalk, CT: Appleton and Lange.

Deapen, D.M., and B.E. Henderson. 1986. A case-control study of amyotrophic lateral sclerosis. Am. J. Epidemiol. 123(5):790-799.

DeGroot, A.P., V.J. Feron, and H.R. Immel. 1988. Induction of hyperplasia in the bladder epithelium of rats by a dietary excess of acid or base: Implications for toxicity/carcinogenicity testing. Food Chem. Toxicol. 26:425-434.

Degtyarenko, K.N., and A.I. Archakov. 1993. Molecular evolution of P450 superfamily and P450-containing monoxygenase systems. FEBS Lett. 332:1-8.

Dietrich, D.R., and J.A. Swenberg. 1991. NCI-Black-Reiter (NBR) male rats fail to develop renal disease following exposure to agents that induce α-2u-globulin (α2u) nephropathy. Fundam. Appl. Toxicol. 16:749-762.

Ecobichon, D.J., J.E. Davis, J. Doull, M. Ehrich, R. Joy, D. McMillan, R. MacPhail, L.W. Reiter, W. Slikker, and H. Tilson. 1990. Pp. 131-199 in The Effect of Pesticides on Human Health. Baker, S. R. and C. F. Wilkinson, eds. Princeton, NJ: Princeton Scientific Publishing Co.

Eisenbrand, G., B. Spiegelhalder, C. Janzowski, J. Kann, and R. Preussman. 1978. Volatile and non-volatile N-nitroso compounds in foods and other environmental media. Pp. 311-324 in Environmental Aspects of N-Nitroso Compounds, E.A. Walker, M. Castegnaro, L. Griciute, and R.E. Lyle, eds. Lyon: IARC Scientific Publications No. 19.

Ellwein, L.B., and S.M. Cohen. 1990. The health risks of saccharin revisited. Crit. Rev. Toxicol. 20:311-326.

EPA (U.S. Environmental Protection Agency). 1990. National Survey of Pesticides in Drinking Water Wells, Phase I Report. EPA570990015. Washington, D.C.: U.S. Environmental Protection Agency

EPA (U.S. Environmental Protection Agency). 1992b. Another Look: National Survey of Pesticides in Drinking Water Wells. Phase II Report. EPA570991020. Washington, D.C.: U.S. Environmental Protection Agency.

Fan, T.-Y., and S.R. Tannenbaum. 1973. Factors influencing the rate of formation of nitrosomorpholine from morpholine and nitrite: acceleration by thiocyanate and other anions. J. Agric. Food Chem. 21:237-240.

FASEB (Federation of American Societies for Experimental Biology).

1994. Evaluation of Evidence for the Carcinogenicity of Butylated Hydroxyanisole (BHA). FDA Contract No. 223-92-2185. Task Order No. 2.

FDA (U.S. Food and Drug Administration). 1994. Food and Drug Administration pesticide program: Residue monitoring 1993. J. Assoc. Official Analyt. Chem. Internat. 77:A161-A185.

Flamm, W.G., and L.D. Lehman-McKeeman. 1991. The human relevance of the renal tumor-inducing potential of d-limonene in male rats: Implications for risk assessment. Regul. Toxicol. Pharmacol. 13:70-86.

Fujii, K., H. Jaffe, Y. Bishop, E. Arnold, D. Mackintosh, and S.S. Epstein. 1970. Structure-activity relations for methylenedioxyphenyl and related compounds on hepatic microsomal enzyme function, as measured by prolongation of hexobarbital narcosis and zoxazolamine paralysis in mice. Toxicol. Appl. Pharmacol. 16:482-494.

Fukushima, S., A. Hagiwara, T. Ogiso, M. Shibata, and N. Ito. 1983. Promoting effects of various chemicals in rat urinary bladder carcinogenesis initiated by N-nitroso-n-butyl-(4-hydroxybutyl)amine. Food Chem. Toxicol. 21:59-68.

Fukushima, S., M.-A. Shibata, T. Shirai, S. Tamano, and N. Ito. 1986. Roles of urinary sodium ion concentration and pH in promotion by ascorbic acid of urinary bladder carcinogenesis in rats. Cancer Res. 46:1623-1626.

Gannett, P.M., C. Garrett, T. Lawson, and B. Toth. 1991. Chemical oxidation and metabolism of N-methyl-N-formylhydrazine. Evidence for diazenium and radical intermediates. Food Chem. Toxicol. 29(1):49-56.

Gibson, G.G. 1993. Peroxisome proliferators: Paradigms and prospects. Toxicol. Lett. 68:193-201.

Goldstein, J.A., P. Hickman, and R.D. Kimbrough. 1973. Effects of purified and technical piperonyl butoxide on drug-metabolizing enzymes and ultrastructure of rat liver. Toxicol. Appl. Pharmacol. 26:444-458.

Goldsworthy, T.L., O. Lyght, V.L. Burnett, and J.A. Popp. 1988. Potential role of α-2u-globulin, protein droplet accumulation, and cell replication in the renal carcinogenicity of rats exposed to trichloroethylene, perchloroethylene, and pentachloroethane.

Toxicol. Appl. Pharmacol. 96:367-379.

Gordon, J.E., and C.M. Shy. 1981. Agricultural chemical use and congenital cleft lip and/or palate. Arch. Environ. Health 36:213-221.

GPO (U.S. Government Printing Office). 1991. Code of Federal Regulations: 21 Food and Drugs, Parts 10 to 199. Revised April 1, 1991. Washington, DC: GPO.

Green, T., J. Odum, J.A. Nash, and J.R. Foster. 1990. Perchloroethylene-induced rat kidney tumors: An investigation of the mechanisms involved and their relevance to humans. Toxicol. Appl. Pharmacol. 103:77-89.

Green, S., J.D. Tugwood, and I. Issemann. 1992. The molecular mechanism of peroxisome proliferator action: A model for species differences and mechanistic risk assessment. Toxicol. Lett. 64/65:131-139.

Greenfield, R.E., L.B. Ellwein, and S.M. Cohen. 1984. A general probabilistic model of carcinogenesis: Analysis of experimental urinary bladder cancer. Carcinogenesis 5:437-445.

Gribble, G.W. 1992. Naturally occurring organohalogen compounds - a survey. J. Nat. Prod. 55:1353-1395.

Hall, R.L. 1979. Food ingredients and additives, and sources cited therein. Pp. 116-150 in Food Science and Nutrition: Current Issues and Answers, F.S. Clydesdale, ed. Englewood Cliffs, NJ: Prentice-Hall.

Haley, T.J. 1978. Piperonyl butoxide, alpha[2-(2-butoxyethoxy)ethoxy]-4,5-methylenedioxy-2-propyl toluene. A review of the literature. Ecotoxicol. Environ. Safety 2:9-31.

Hanefeld, M., C. Kemmer, and E. Kadner. 1983. Relationship between morphological changes and lipid-lowering action of p-chlorphenoxyisobutyric acid (CPIB) on hepatic mitochondria and peroxisomes in man. Atherosclerosis 46:239-246.

Hard, G.C., I. Rodgers, K.P. Baetcke, W.L. Richards, R.E. McGaughy, and L.R. Valcovic. 1993. Hazard evaluation of chemicals that cause accumulation of α2u-globulin, hyaline droplet nephropathy, and tubule neoplasia in the kidneys of male rats. Environ. Health Perspect. 99:313-349.

Harris, C.C. 1990. Interindividual variation in human chemical carcinogenesis: Implications for risk assessment. Pp. 235-251 in

Scientific Issues in Quantitative Cancer Risk Assessment. Moolgavkar, S.H., ed. Birkhaeuser Boston, Inc., Boston MA.

Harris, C.C. 1993. p53: At the crossroads of molecular carcinogenesis and risk assessment. Science 262:1980-1981.

Hayes, W.J., Jr., and E.R. Laws, Jr. 1990. Handbook of Pesticide Toxicology. San Diego, CA: Academic Press. 1576 p.

Hecht, S.S., and D. Hoffman. 1989. The relevance of tobacco-specific nitrosamines to human cancer. Cancer Surv. 8:273-294.

Hirose, M., A. Masuda, S. Fukushima, and N. Ito. 1988. Effects of subsequent antioxidant treatment on 7,12-dimethylbenz[a]anthracene-initiated carcinogenesis of the mammary gland, ear duct and forestomach in Sprague-Dawley rat. Carcinogenesis 9:101-104.

Hodgson, E., and P.E. Levi. 1987. A Textbook of Modern Toxicology. Elsevier Science Publishing Company, New York. 500 p.

Hodgson, E., and P.E. Levi. 1994. Metabolism of toxicants: Phase I reactions. Pp. 75-112 in Introduction to Biochemical Toxicology, 2nd edition, E. Hodgson and P.E. Levi, eds. Norwalk, CT: Appleton and Lange.

Hodgson, E., and R.M. Philpot. 1974. Interactions of methylenedioxyphenyl (1,3-benzodioxole) compounds with enzymes and their effects on mammals. Drug. Metab. Rev. 3:231-301.

Hoffman, D., and S.S. Hecht. 1985. Nicotine-derived N-nitrosamines and tobacco-related cancer: Current status and future directions. Cancer Res. 45:935-944.

Homberger, F., T. Kelley, Jr., G. Friedler, and A.B. Russfield. 1961. Toxic and possible carcinogenic effects of 4-allyl-1,2-methylenedioxybenzene (safrole) in rats on deficient diets. Med. Exptl. 4:1-11.

IARC (International Agency for Research on Cancer). 1978. IARC Monographs on the evaluation of carcinogenic risk of chemicals to humans, some N-nitroso compounds, Vol. 17. Lyon, France: IARC.

IARC (International Agency for Research on Cancer). 1982. IARC Monographs on the evaluation of carcinogenic risk of chemicals to humans, some aromatic amines, anthraquinones and nitroso compounds, and inorganic fluorides used in drinking water and dental preparations, Vol. 27. Lyon, France: IARC.

IARC (International Agency for Research on Cancer). 1987. IARC Monographs on the Evaluation of Carcinogenic Risks to Humans. Overall Evaluations of Carcinogenicity: An Updating of IARC Monographs Volumes 1 to 42, Supplement 7. Lyon, France: IARC.

IARC (International Agency for Research on Cancer). 1993. IARC Monographs on the Evaluation of Carcinogenic Risks to Humans. Some Naturally Occurring Substances: Food Items and Constituents, Heterocyclic Aromatic Amines and Mycotoxins, Vol 56. Lyon, France: IARC.

Ioannides, C., M. Delaforge, and D.V. Parke. 1981. Safrole: Its metabolism, carcinogenicity and interactions with cytochrome P-450. Food Cosmet. Toxicol. 19:657-666.

Ito, N., S. Fukushima, A. Hagiwara, M. Shibata, and T. Ogiso. 1983. Carcinogenicity of butylated hydroxyanisole in F344 rats. J. Natl. Cancer Inst. 70(2):343-352.

Ito, N., S. Fukushima, and H. Tsuda. 1985. Carcinogenecicity and modification of the carcinogenic response by BHA, BHT, and other antioxidants. CRC Critical Reviews in Toxicology, Vol. 15(2), pp. 109-150.

Ito, N., R. Hasegawa, M. Sano, S. Tamano, H. Esumi, S. Takayama, and T. Sugimura. 1991. A new colon and mammary carcinogen in cooked food, 2-amino-1-methyl-6-phenylimidazo[4,5-b]pyridine (PhIP). Carcinogenesis 12:1503-1506.

Jansen, E.H., and P. de Fluiter. 1992. Detection of the enzymatic activity of cytochrome P-450 enzymes by high-performance liquid chromatography. J. Chromatogr. 580:325-346.

Jenner, P.A., and B. Testa. 1981. Concepts in Drug Metabolism. New York: Marcel Dekker, Inc. 424 p.

Kahl, R. 1984. Synthetic antioxidants: Biochemical actions and interference with radiation, toxic compounds, chemical mutagens and chemical carcinogens. Toxicology 33:185-228.

Kanerva, R.L., G.M. Ridder, L.C. Stone, and C.L. Alden. 1987. Characterization of spontaneous and decalin-induced hyaline droplets in kidneys of adult male rats. Food Chem. Toxicol. 25:63-82.

Knudson, A.G., Jr. 1971. Mutation and cancer: Statistical study of retinoblastoma. Proc. Natl. Acad. Sci. 68:820-823.

Leaf, C.D., J.S. Wishnok, and S.R. Tannenbaum. 1989. Mechanisms of endogenous nitrosation. Cancer Surv. 9:323-334.

Lehman-McKeeman, L.D., and D. Caudill. 1992. $\alpha 2u$-Globulin is the only member of the lipocalin protein superfamily that binds to hyaline droplet inducing agents. Toxicol. Appl. Pharmacol. 116:170-176.

Lehman-McKeeman, L.D., P.A. Rodriguez, R. Takigiku, D. Caudill, and M.L. Fey. 1989. d-Limonene-induced male rat-specific nephrotoxicity: Evaluation of the association between d-limonene and $\alpha 2u$-globulin. Toxicol. Appl. Pharmacol. 99: 250-259.

Lewandowski, M., Y.C. Chui, P.E. Levi, and E. Hodgson. 1990. Differences in induction of hepatic cytochrome P450 isozymes by mice in eight methylenedioxyphenyl compounds. J. Biochem. Toxicol. 5:47-55.

Lina, B.A.R., V.M.H. Hollanders, and M.H.M. Kuijpers. 1994. The role of alkalizing and neutral potassium salts in urinary bladder carcinogenesis in rats. Carcinogenesis 15:523-527.

Lock, E.A., A.M. Mitchell, and C.R. Elcombe. 1989. Biochemical mechanisms of induction of hepatic peroxisome proliferation. Annu. Rev. Pharmacol. Toxicol. 29:145-163.

Long, E.L., A.A. Nelson, O.G. Fitzhugh, and W.H. Hansen. 1963. Liver tumors produced in rats by feeding safrole. Arch. Pathol. 75:595-604.

Malvoisin, E., and M. Roberfroid. 1982. Hepatic microsomal metabolism of 1,3-butadiene. Xenobiotica 12:137-144.

Magee, P.N. 1989. The experimental basis for the role of nitroso compounds in human cancer. Cancer Surv. 8:207-239.

Matsushita, H. Jr., O. Endo, H. Matsushita, M. Yamamoto, and M. Mochizuki. 1993. Mutagenicity of alkylhydrazine oxalates in Salmonella typhimurium TA100 and TA102 demonstrated by modifying the growth conditions of the bacteria. Mutat. Res. 301(4):213-222.

Melnick, R.L. 1992. An alternative hypothesis on the role of chemically induced protein droplet ($\alpha 2u$-globulin) nephropathy in renal carcinogenesis. Reg. Toxicol. Pharmacol. 16:111-125.

Miller, J.A., and E.C. Miller. 1983. Some historical aspects of N-aryl carcinogens and their metabolic activation. Environ. Health

Perspect. 49:3-12.

Mirvish, S.S. 1975. Formation of N-nitroso compounds: Chemistry, kinetics, and *in vivo* occurrence. Toxicol. Appl. Pharmacol. 31:325-351.

Mirvish, S.S. 1994. Experimental evidence for inhibition of N-nitroso compound formation as a factor in the negative correlation between vitamin C consumption and the incidence of certain cancers. Proc. Fourth Internat. Conf.: Mechanisms of Antimutagenesis and Radiation Protection. Cancer Res. 54:1948s-1951s.

Moody, D.E., J.K. Reddy, B.G. Lake, J.A. Popp, and D.H. Reese. 1991. Peroxisome proliferation and nongenotoxic carcinogenesis: Commentary on a symposium. Fundam. Appl. Toxicol. 16:233-248.

Moolgavkar, S.H., and A.G. Knudson, Jr. 1981. Mutation and cancer: A model for human carcinogenesis. J. Natl. Cancer Inst. 66:1037-1052.

Morgens, P.N., J.J. Kamin, H.L. Newmark, W. Fiddler, and J. Pensabine. 1978. Alpha-tocopherol: Uses in preventing nitrosamine formation. Pp. 199-212 in Environmental Aspects of N-Nitroso Compounds, E.A. Walker, M. Castegnaro, L. Griciute, and R.E. Lyle, eds. IARC Scientific Publication No. 19. Lyon, France: IARC.

Murray, M., C.F. Wilkinson, and C.E. Dube. 1985. Induction of rat hepatic microsomal cytochrome P-450 and aryl hydrocarbon hydroxylase by 1,3-benzodioxole derivatives. Xenobiotica 15:361-368.

Neidleman, S.L., and J. Geigert. 1986. Biohalogenation: Principles, Basic Roles and Applications. Chichester: Ellis Horwood Limited.

Nelson, D.R., T. Kamataki, D.J. Waxman, F.P. Guengerich, R.W. Estabrook, R. Feyereisen, F.J. Gonzalez, M.J. Coon, I.C. Gunsalus, O. Gotoh, K. Okuda, and D.W. Nebert. 1993. The P450 superfamily: Update on new sequences, gene mapping, accession numbers, early trivial names of enzymes, and nomenclature. DNA and Cell Biology 12:1-51.

NRC (National Research Council). 1973. A Comprehensive Survey of Industry on the Use of Food Chemicals Generally Recognized as Safe. National Technical Information Service (NTIS) PB-221949.

NRC (National Research Council). 1976. Estimating Distribution of

Daily Intakes of Certain GRAS Substances. National Technical Information Service (NTIS) PB-299-381.

NRC (National Research Council). 1978. Resurvey of the Annual Poundage of Food Chemicals Generally Recognized as Safe. National Technical Information Service (NTIS) PB288-081.

NRC (National Research Council). 1979. The 1977 Survey of Industry on the Use of Food Additives. National Technical Information Service (NTIS) PB80-113418.

NRC (National Research Council). 1981. The health effects of nitrate, nitrite and N-nitroso compounds. National Academy Press: Washington, DC.

NRC (National Research Council). 1982. Diet, Nutrition and Cancer. National Academy Press, Washington DC.

NRC (National Research Council). 1983. Diet, Nutrition and Cancer: Directions for Research. National Academy Press, Washington DC.

NRC (National Research Council). 1984. Poundage Update of Food Chemicals. National Technical Information Service (NTIS) PB91-127266.

NRC (National Research Council). 1989. 1987 Poundage and Technical Effects Update of Substances Added to Food. National Technical Information Service (NTIS) PB91-127266.

NRC (National Research Council). 1993. Pesticides in the Diets of Infants and Children. National Academy Press, Washington DC.

NTP (National Toxicology Program). 1990. NTP Technical Report on Toxicology and Carcinogenesis Studies of d-Limonene in F-344/N Rats and B6C3F1 Mice. NTP Technical Report TR 347. Research Triangle Park, N.C.: National Toxicology Program.

Okada, M. 1984. Comparative metabolism of N-nitrosamines in relation to their organ and species specificty. Pp. 401-409 in, N-nitroso Compounds: Occurrence, Biological Effects and Relevance to Human Cancer, I.K. O'Neill, R.C. Von Borstet, C.T. Miller, J. Long, and H. Bartsch, eds. IARC Scientific Publication No. 57. Lyon, France: IARC.

Okamura, T., E.M. Garland, T. Masui, T. Sakata, M. St. John, and S.M. Cohen. 1991. Lack of bladder tumor promoting activity in rats fed sodium saccharin in AIN-76A diet. Cancer Res. 51:1778-1782.

Olson, M.J., B.D. Garg, C.V. Ramana Murty, and A.K. Roy. 1987.

Accumulation of α2u-globulin in the renal proximal tubules of male rats exposed to unleaded gasoline. Toxicol. Appl. Pharmacol. 90:43-51.

Olson, M.J., J.T. Johnson, and C.A. Reidy. 1990. A comparison of male rat and human urinary proteins: Implications for human resistance to hyaline droplet nephropathy. Toxicol. Appl. Pharmacol. 102:524-536.

Ortiz de Montellano, P.R. 1985. Alkenes and alkynes. Pp. 121-155 in Bioactivation of Foreign Compounds, M.W. Anders, ed. Orlando, FL: Academic Press, Inc.

Peters, J.M., S. Preston-Martin, S.J. London, J.D. Bowman, J.D. Buckley, and D.C. Thomas. 1994. Processed meats and risk of childhood leukemia (California, USA). Cancer Causes Control 5:195-202.

Prough, R.A., and S.J. Moloney. 1985. Hydrazines. Pp. 433-449 in Bioactivation of Foreign Compounds. M.W. Anders, ed. Academic Press, Inc.

Reddy, J.K., and M.S. Rao. 1992. Peroxisome proliferation and hepatocarcinogenesis. Pp. 225-235 in Mechanisms of Carcinogenesis in Risk Assessment. H. Vainio, P.N. Magee, D.B. McGregor, and A.J. McMichael, eds. Lyon, France: IARC.

Reitz, R.H., A.L. Mendrala, C.N. Park, M.E. Andersen, and F.P. Guengerich. 1988. Incorporation of in vitro enzyme data into the physiologically-based pharmacokinetic (PB-PK) model for methylene chloride: Implications for risk assessment. Toxicol. Lett. 43:97-116.

Rosenkranz, H.S., and G. Klopman. 1990. Prediction of the carcinogenicity in rodents of chemicals currently being tested by the US National Toxicology Program: Structure-activity correlations. Mutagenesis 5:425-432.

Rosenstock, L., M. Keifer, W.E. Daniell, R. McConnell, K. Claypoole, and the Pesticides Health Effects Study Group. 1991. Chronic central nervous system effects of acute organophosphate pesticide intoxication. Lancet 338:223-227.

Sander, J., F. Schweinsberg, and H.-P. Menz. 1968. Utersuchungen uber die entstahung cancerogener nitrosamine in magen. Hoppe-Seyler's Z. Physiol. Chem. 349:1691-1697.

Sarasua, S., and D.A. Savitz. 1994. Cured and broiled meat

consumption in relation to childhood cancer: Denver, Colorado (United States). Cancer Causes Control 5:141-148.

Scheuplein, R.J. 1990. Perspectives on toxicological risk - an example: Food-borne carcinogenic risk. Pp. 351-371 in Progress in Predictive Toxicology. D.B. Clayson, I.C. Munro, P. Shubik, and J.A. Swenberg, eds. Amsterdam: Elsevier Publishers B.V.

Schoenig, G.P., E.I. Goldenthal, R.G. Geil, C.H. Frith, W.R. Richter, and F.W. Carlborg. 1985. Evaluation of the dose response and in utero exposure to saccharin in the rat. Food Chem. Toxicol 23:475-490.

Schwartz, D.A., and J.P. LoGerfo. 1988. Congenital limb reduction defects in the agricultural setting. Am. J. Public Health 78:654-659.

Serve, M.P., C.T. Olson, B.M. Llewelyn, R.H. Bruner, K.O. Yu, and D.W. Hobson. 1988. The metabolism and nephrotoxicity of tetralin in Fischer 344 rats. Toxicologist 8,180.

Shephard, S.E., and W.K. Lutz. 1989. Nitrosation of dietary precursors. Cancer Surv. 8:401-421.

Singer, B. 1985. *In vivo* formation and persistence of modified nucleosides resulting from alkylating agents. Environmental Health Perspectives 62:41-48.

Sipes, I.G., and A.J. Gandolfi. 1986. Biotransformation of toxicants. Pp. 64-98 in Casarett and Doull's Toxicology: The Basic Science of Poisons. C.D. Klaassen, M.O. Amdur, and J. Doull, eds. New York: Macmillan.

Smith, B.J., I.G. Sipes, J.C. Stevens, and J.R. Halpert. 1990. The biochemical basis for the species difference in hepatic microsomal 4-vinylcyclohexene epoxidation between female mice and rats. Carcinogenesis 11:1951-1957.

Snyderwine, E.G., M.H. Buonarati, J.S. Felton, and K.W. Turteltaub. 1993. Metabolism of the food-derived mutagen/carcinogen 2-amino-1-methyl-6-phenylimidazo[4,5-b]pyridine (PhIP) in nonhuman primates. Carcinogenesis 14:2517-2522.

Stanbridge, E.J. 1990. Human tumor suppressor genes. Annu. Rev. Genet. 24:615-657.

Stich, H.F. 1991. The beneficial and hazardous effects of simple phenolic compounds. Mutat. Res. 259:307-324.

Stofberg, J. 1987. Consumption ratio and food predominance of flavoring materials. Perfumer & Flavorist 12(4):27-68.

Stofberg, J., and J.C. Kirschman, 1985. The consumption ratio of flavouring materials: A mechanism for setting priorities for safety evaluation. Food Chem. Toxicol. 23(9):857-860.

Strasser, J., Jr., M. Charbonneau, S.J. Borghoff, M.J. Turner, and J.A. Swenberg. 1988. Renal protein droplet formation in male Fischer 344 rats after isophorone (IPH) treatment. Toxicologist 8:136.

Swenberg, J.A., B. Short, S. Borghoff, J. Strasser, and M. Charbonneau. 1989. The comparative pathobiology of α2u-globulin nephropathy. Toxicol. Appl. Pharmacol. 97:35-46.

Takahashi, O., S. Oishi, T. Fujitani, T. Tanaka, and M. Yoneyama. 1994. Chronic toxicity studies of piperonyl butoxide in F344 Rats: Induction of hepatocellular carcinoma. Fund. Appl. Toxicol. 22:293-303.

Tamano, S., E. Asakawa, P. Boomyaphiphat, T. Masui, and S. Fukushima. 1993. Lack of promotion of N-butyl-N-(4-hydroxybutyl)nitrosamine initiated urinary bladder carcinogenesis in mice by rat cancer promoters. Teratog. Carcinog. Mutagen. 13:89-96.

Tanner, C.M., and J.W. Langston. 1990. Do environmental toxins cause Parkinson's disease? A critical review. Neurology 40:17-30.

Tennant, R.W., B.H. Margolin, M.D. Shelby, E. Zeiger, J.K. Haseman, J. Spalding, W. Caspary, M. Resnick, S. Stasiewicz, B. Anderson, and R. Minor. 1987. Prediction of chemical carcinogenicity in rodents from in vitro genetic toxicity assays. Science 236:933-941.

Testa, B., and P. Jenner. 1976. Drug Metabolism: Chemical and Biochemical Aspects. New York: Marcel Dekker, Inc.

Thier, S.O. 1981. The kidney. Pp. 799-920 in Pathophysiology, The Biological Principles of Disease. L.H. Smith and S.O. Thier, eds. Philadelphia, PA: W. B. Saunders.

Thomas, P.E., L.M. Reik, D.E. Ryan, and W. Levin. 1983. Induction of two immunochemically related rat liver cytochrome P-450 isozymes, cytochromes P-450c and P-450d, by structurally diverse xenobiotics. J. Biol. Chem. 258:4590-4598.

Toth, B. 1975. Synthetic and naturally occurring hydrazines as possible cancer causative agents. Cancer Res. 35:3693-3697.

Toth, B. 1980. Actual new cancer-causing hydrazines, hydrazides, and hydrazones. J. Cancer Res. Clin. Oncol. 97:97-108.

Toth, B. 1991. Carcinogenic fungal hydrazines. In Vivo 5(2):95-100.

Tricker, A.R., B. Spiegelhalder, R. Preussmann. 1989. Environmental exposure to preformed nitroso compounds. Cancer Surv. 8:251-272.

Ulland, B.M., J.H. Weisburger, R.S. Yamamoto, and E.K. Weisburger. 1973. Antioxidants and carcinogenesis: Butylated hydroxytoluene, but not diphenyl-p-phenylenediamine, inhibits cancer induction by N-2-fluorenyl-acetamide and by N-hydroxy-N-2-fluorenylacetamide in rats. Food Cosmet. Toxicol. 11: 199-207.

Van den Branden, C., J. Vamecq, I. Wybo, and F. Roels. 1986. Phytol and peroxisome proliferation. Pediatr. Res. 20:411-415.

Verhagen, H., P.A. Schilderman, and J.C. Kleinjans. 1991. Butylated hydroxyanisole in perspective. Chem. Biol. Interact. 80:109-134.

Vineis, P., H. Bartsch, N. Caporaso, A.M. Harrington, F.F. Kadlubar, M.T. Landi, C. Malaveille, P.G. Shields, P. Skipper, G. Talaska, and S.R. Tannenbaum. 1994. Genetically based N-acetyltransferase metabolic polymorphism and low-level environmental exposure to carcinogens. Nature 369:154-156.

Wagstaff, D.J., and C.R. Short. 1971. Induction of hepatic microsomal hydroxylating enzymes by technical piperonyl butoxide and some of its analogs. Toxicol. Appl. Pharmacol. 19:54-61.

Wakabayashi, K., M. Nagao, H. Esumi, and T. Sugimura. 1992. Food-derived mutagens and carcinogens. Cancer Res. 52:2092s-2098s.

Watanabe, T., and T. Suga. 1983. Effects of phytol, a branched, long chain aliphatic alcohol on biochemical values and on hepatic peroxisomal enzymes of rats. Chem. Pharm. Bull. 31:2756-2761.

Wattenberg, L.W., J.B. Coccia, and L.K.T. Lam. 1980. Inhibitory effects of phenolic compounds on benzo[a]pyrene-induced neoplasia. Cancer Res. 40:2820-2823.

Weinstein, I.B., R.M. Santella, and F. Perera. 1995. Molecular Biology and Epidemiology of Cancer. Pp. 83-110 in Cancer Prevention and Control, P. Greenwald, B.S. Kramer, and D.L. Weed, ed. New York: Marcel Dekker, Inc.

Willes, R.F., E.R. Nestmann, P.A. Miller, J.C. Orr, and I.C. Munro. 1993. Scientific principles for evaluating the potential for adverse effects from chlorinated organic chemicals in the environment. Regul. Toxicol. Pharmacol. 18:313-356.

Williams, G.M., T. Tanaka, and Y. Maeura. 1986. Dose-related inhibition of aflatoxin B₁ induced hepatocarcinogenesis by the phenolic antioxidants, butylated hydroxyanisole and butylated hydroxytoluene. Carcinogenesis 7(7):1043-1050.

Williams, G.M., and J.H. Weisburger. 1991. Chemical carcinogens. Pp. 127-200 in Casarett and Doull's Toxicology: The Basic Science of Poisons, C.D. Klaassen, M.O. Amdur, and J. Doull, eds. New York: Macmillan.

Yang, C.S., Y.Y. Tu, J. Hong, and C. Patten. 1984. Metabolism of nitrosamines by cytochrome P-450 isozymes. Pp. 423-428 in N-Nitroso Compounds: Occurrence, Biological Effects and Relevance to Human Cancer. I.K. O'Neill, R.C. Von Borstel, C.T. Miller, J. Long, and H. Bartsch, eds. IARC Scientific Publication No. 57. Lyon, France: IARC.

Yeowell, H.N., P. Linko, E. Hodgson, and J.A. Goldstein. 1985. Induction of specific cytochrome P-450 isozymes by methylenedioxyphenyl compounds and antagonism by 3-methylcholanthrene. Arch. Biochem. Biophys. 243:408-419.

4

Methods for Evaluating Potential Carcinogens and Anticarcinogens

Carcinogenic activity in rodents, following the oral administration of certain dyes, was first demonstrated in the early 1930s. Since then, numerous experimental studies have been conducted to identify carcinogens in the diets of humans. Such studies in the 1930s and 1940s were predominantly experimental and focused on food additives, especially colorants, contaminants, and carcinogens formed during food processing, cooking, and storage. Early experimental studies on the effects of malnutrition on carcinogenicity were also initiated during this period. Relatively few epidemiologic investigations were conducted until the midcentury. Although most investigations concentrated on cancer of the gastrointestinal tract and liver, it soon became clear that cancers at other sites could be induced by ingested chemicals. The oral route became widespread as a convenient method of administering any suspect carcinogen, irrespective of target organ, and a considerable database on chemicals tested for carcinogenicity was developed.

After World War II, results from experimental and epidemiologic studies reinforced the view that dietary patterns were significantly related to geographic variations in cancer incidence. However, in the absence of testable hypotheses and of well-conducted epidemiologic studies, the role of individual dietary components, including potential carcinogens, remained largely unclear for most organ sites, with few exceptions. Nonetheless, while most human studies concentrated on synthetic chemicals or dietary deficiency, the carcinogenic effect of natural carcinogens was not completely ignored. Thus, the senecio alkaloids, cycasin, and aflatoxin were all identified by the early 1960s. By 1970, the possible anticarcinogenic activity of vitamin A was being explored, as were the modifying effects of fruit, fiber, dairy products, and certain vegetables.

In 1969, the International Union Against Cancer (UICC) convened a committee to address issues of cancer testing. The committee held a workshop that focused on the major testing methods and priorities for carcinogenicity testing. In proceedings from the workshop, the committee concluded, "there is general agreement that both (a) the extent to which man is exposed to a substance, and (b) the degree of suspicion with which the substance is regarded, must be considered. In many specific cases (a) or (b) will be clearly dominant. Both natural and synthetic substances must be considered for testing. There is a tendency to consider first substances of the latter category; however, an increasing number of natural products with carcinogenic activity are being found and substances suspected to be in this category deserve more attention." (UICC, 1970).

At about the same time, the National Research Council's Committee on Food Protection conducted a review of naturally occurring toxicants in foods, including carcinogens (NRC 1973), in response to growing public apprehension about the safety of the food supply. The committee's list comprised the major natural carcinogens and toxicants as we know them today, and emphasized that they should be further studied. Neither the UICC committee nor the National Research Council committee suggested that naturally occurring compounds posed any unique problems for testing, nor did they mention any qualitative differences between naturally occurring and synthetic carcinogens.

Most cancers suspected to be diet-related are likely to have a multifactorial origin. The human diet is a complex mixture of nutrients and chemicals that are notoriously difficult to measure in observational studies and many of which might be plausible confounders of the effect under study. Although a single factor might be examined in animals through dietary manipulation, this is rarely possible in humans unless the suspected agent is identifiable, discrete, and present at high levels, such as a mycotoxin. In the past, traditional epidemiologic methods have been effective in identifying exposures to ingested carcinogens, e.g., aflatoxin and arsenic, in the diet at relatively high levels and in raising plausible hypotheses about individual foods and macro- or micronutrients. Modification of one component in a diet is usually associated with a change in others. An increase in calories from fat, for instance, usually reflects a reduced percentage of calories from other sources. However, in studying the role of dietary factors, the problem is even more complex because micro- and macronutrients might behave differently qualitatively and quantitatively between humans and the animals in which they are often studied. Further, experimental diets often compare extreme dietary variations, possibly at toxicologic or pharmacologic levels, leading to inappropriate conclusions in humans, in whom variations are usually within a more modest range. Accordingly, it is necessary to discuss first those limitations that arise from a lack of sensitivity or specificity inherent in the methods used for detecting trivial or minimal exposures and their effects in humans or animals. We must also discuss the issues involved in study of complex mixtures in the presence of multiple plausible confounders.

When adequate human data are not available, it is often necessary to base opinions about human risk on results from experiments in animal models. Animal studies of suspected carcinogens are assumed, with some reservations, to provide qualitative predictions of human risk, especially where there is evidence of common mechanisms and endpoints. However, susceptibility to chemically induced carcinogenesis can show interspecies variability. This discordance results at least in part from differences, either hereditary or induced, among animal species in the steps involved in chemical carcinogenesis, particularly at the level of procarcinogen bioactivation and detoxification. Enzymes involved in bioactivation and detoxification of procarcinogens have now been identified and characterized in multiple animal species, including humans (Gonzalez and Gelboin 1994). There are many instances of interspecies differences in these enzymes, in terms both of catalytic specificity and of regulation (Wright and Stevens 1992). Hence, a given chemical can take divergent metabolic pathways, resulting in different health outcomes, depending on the species exposed.

Furthermore, susceptibility to carcinogenesis can vary significantly within a species. In humans, much of this variability appears to reflect genetic heterogeneity. For example, there are several inherited variations in xenobiotic metabolizing enzymes and in DNA repair enzymes that have been associated with susceptibility to certain malignancies. Genetic predisposition to cancer can also be influenced by inherited mutations in tumor suppressor genes, as illustrated by the Li-Fraumeni syndrome, in which patients inherit mutations in one allele of the *p53* gene, and in hereditary retinoblastoma, which involves the *RB* gene. Interestingly, inherited mutations in either of these tumor suppressor genes increases the susceptibility of individuals to certain radiation-induced tumors (Frebourg and Friend 1992). Inheritance of specific polymorphic alleles of the *ras* oncogene (Weston et al. 1991) and of the *p53* gene (Weston et al. 1992) have been linked to lung cancer risk, but the significance of this association is not known. Recent identification on chromosome 17 of the BRCA1 gene that is associated with familial breast cancer (Miki et al. 1994) might provide a clue as to which genetic factors influence breast cancer risk. In addition, nongenetic factors such as diet and hormones might substantially influence susceptibility to cancer in both humans and inbred laboratory rodents. For example, differences in susceptibility to chemical carcinogenesis have been demonstrated between well-fed and calorie-deprived rodents of the same species, possibly because of calorie-induced differences in the catalytic activities of xenobiotic metabolizing and DNA repair enzymes. Individuals in different age groups might also differ in their susceptibility to chemical carcinogenesis.

Biologic markers are being used to investigate individual susceptibility to various exogenous chemical agents. Cloning genes involved in the activation or detoxification of various xenobiotics and in the fidelity and efficiency of DNA repair, for example, will provide probes that may be used to identify and monitor interindividual variations. Currently used markers relate mainly to DNA-damaging (genotoxic) agents. However, because individuals might vary in their susceptibility to processes not directly involving DNA damage (nongenotoxic effects), markers specific for these changes are needed for routine use in molecular epidemiology studies.

Despite the differences between humans and animals, epidemiologic and experimental models need to be considered as ways to evaluate the potential carcinogenicity of naturally occurring chemicals. For example, epidemiologic data have been crucial in developing the association between cigarette smoking and lung cancer. In addition, such studies have consistently demonstrated the relationship between the consumption of alcoholic beverages and cancer. Further experimental studies in diverse animal species have indicated that alcohol induces cancer by nongenotoxic mechanisms.

In Chapter 4, the following questions are addressed:

· What methods are currently being used to identify and evaluate chemicals as potential carcinogens?
· Should the methods for testing naturally occurring potential carcinogens differ from those used for testing synthetic chemicals?
· Are existing methods adequate?
· How should naturally occurring compounds be prioritized for evaluation of carcinogenic potential?

METHODS FOR EVALUATING CHEMICAL CARCINOGENESIS

Studies in Human Populations

Epidemiology

Epidemiology, a science based on population measurements, can be described as the study of the distribution and determinants of diseases in human populations and the application of the results to disease prevention or control. Epidemiologic approaches to determining cancer risks from chemical constituents of foods require the assessment of exposure (diet) and outcome (disease). Exposure data can be classified as (1) general diet, such as patterns of consumption of macro- and micronutrients, certain non-nutrient constituents, and caloric intake; and (2) the identification, isolation, and biological activity of individual suspected carcinogens and anticarcinogens in the diet. The complexity of the human diet makes it difficult to assess retrospectively. Dietary intake data are often based on the use of food diaries or recall of recent or past diet. These methods have qualitative and quantitative limitations. Over the past 2 decades, laboratory techniques have been developed that attempt to address some of the problems associated with epidemiologic studies of diet and cancer. Biologic markers of intake, either of certain nutrients or of individual chemicals found in foods, might provide a better assessment than has been possible before now of the role of diet in human cancer. Some biologic markers with potential use in epidemiologic studies have recently been reviewed (Riboli et al. 1987), and their use is discussed in more detail in the section on "Molecular Epidemiology." Generally, epidemiologic research follows one of four study designs:

• *Ecologic Studies.* These studies attempt to relate exposures to disease outcomes at a group level. Such studies suffer from several limitations: individual exposure data are not associated with individual outcome; investigators are unable to control for many potential confounders; and measures of exposure are crude. Because of these limitations, the primary value of such studies is in "hypothesis generation" (i.e., suggesting potentially important risk factors for study by methods based on individuals). On the other hand, such studies can often incorporate a broader range of exposures than can studies based on data from individuals. Thus, for weak risk factors, or for risks that occur only at extremes of exposure, this approach might be more useful in identifying or excluding etiologic factors than has traditionally been assumed (Prentice and Sheppard 1990).

A common type of ecologic study in diet and cancer research has been international correlations of per capita food consumption with corresponding incidence or mortality rates from specific cancers (Armstrong and Doll 1975). Other studies have been carried out within national boundaries by the selection of distinctive subpopulations, such as ethnic groups (e.g., in Hawaii and South Africa), religious groups (e.g., Mormons and Seventh Day Adventists), or certain dietary cultures (e.g., vegetarians or abstainers from alcohol) (Lyon and Sorenson 1978, Kolonel et al. 1981). In such studies, the measure of exposure is often a very crude estimate of what individuals might actually be ingesting. Per capita food intakes, for example, use food production and import/export data to determine average exposures for individuals in the population. They do not account for food wastage or food fed to animals, nor for differences in intake by sex and age.

• *Case-Control Studies.* These studies are based on individuals rather than groups, and overcome many of the limitations just cited. In these studies, persons who have the outcome of interest, e.g., breast cancer, are identified, and suitable controls are obtained for comparison. Variables thought to be potential confounders in the relationship can be overcome by matching during control selection or by statistical adjustment at the time of data analysis. Other advantages of this design are that rare diseases (like most cancers) can be studied, results can be obtained rather quickly, and the research is relatively cost-effective. Disadvantages include the fact that exposure data are obtained retrospectively (dietary recall), and that differential misclassification between cases and controls (bias) can occur, despite great care in designing the study and in collecting the data.

Examples of such studies are (1) a comparison of exposure to aflatoxins in foods relative to hepatitis B virus status between persons with liver cancer and controls (Qian et al. 1994); and (2) a study comparing consumption of salted fish by persons with naso-pharyngeal cancer and controls (Ning et al. 1990). Such studies depend on dietary recall methods, primarily on diet histories, in which individuals recall their intake of specific foods at some speci-fied time period in the past. These recall methods are subject to errors in memory. Such errors might be random (nondifferential) or selective (bias). Nondifferential error generally leads to reduced relative risks, so that a true positive finding might be missed. Bias, however, can lead to a false conclusion from the data. Sources of variation in food consumption data are discussed in Chapter 5. Although large sample sizes can help to reduce some of the effects of random misclassification, the effects of bias cannot be dealt with so readily. However, the findings from many case-control studies, such as those on the effects of fruits and vegetables on cancer risk, have been remarkably consistent, attesting to the strength of this approach (Steinmetz and Potter 1991). Nonetheless, there is evi-dence for biased recall in some case-control studies of breast cancer (Giovannucci et al. 1993) and of colorectal cancer (Wilkens et al. 1992).

In some instances, biological specimens (usually serum) have been collected from cases and controls, in an effort to obtain more exact information. Unfortunately, effects of the disease itself on serum levels, variability in serum levels over time, and other factors limit the value of this approach. Newer biologic marker approaches that overcome some of these limitations are discussed below.

• *Cohort Studies.* These studies are generally preferred over case-control studies, because the potential for bias is less. In this design, healthy subjects are classified on exposures of interest prior to disease occurrence. The incidence of disease over time is then compared between the two groups. Since exposure data (e.g., diet histories) are obtained prospectively, recall bias is reduced, but the potential for substantial misclassification is nearly always present. However, prospectively assembled cohort studies are expensive, because very large samples are required, and the subjects must be followed for many years to accrue sufficient numbers of cases for meaningful statistical analysis. Such studies are not generally useful for very rare cancers. An alternative approach is to use pre-existing data sets. However, although this might be less costly, such data might not be ideal.

An example of a cohort study in nutritional epidemiology research is a population of more than 100,000 U.S. nurses being monitored for breast, colon, and other cancers relative to antecedent dietary intakes (e.g., fat and red meat) (Willett et al. 1990, Willett 1994). Other diet-related cohorts in the U.S. include a population of 8,000 Japanese-American men in Hawaii (Heilbrun et al. 1984) and a sample of over 40,000 women in Iowa (Folsom et al. 1990). Cohort studies have often included biochemical measures, such as serum nutrient levels, since data collection occurs prior to the onset of disease. However, because of the lengthy period of follow-up, changes in dietary habits (e.g., fat intake) might occur in the participants, complicating the analyses.

A multicenter, prospective cohort study designed to investigate the relationship of diet, nutritional status, various lifestyles and environmental factors, and the incidence of different forms of cancer is currently being conducted in Europe. The cohort of the European Prospective Investigation Into Cancer and Nutrition (EPIC) study, developed under the auspices of IARC (IARC 1993), will eventually total approximately 350,000 middle-aged men and women. Data on current diet are being collected by means of detailed dietary assessment. A standardized questionnaire is being used to obtain anthropometric measurements, as well as information on physical activity, tobacco smoking, alcohol consumption, occupation, socio-economic status, reproductive history, contraception, use of hormone replacement therapy, previous illness, and current drug use. Blood samples are being collected that will be analyzed at a later date. Samples from subjects who develop cancer will be compared with appropriate disease-free control subjects.

The range of analyses will depend on the type of cancer and availability of techniques.

The EPIC study has several advantages, including the prospective approach, large sample size, and a wide range of dietary exposures. Short-term screening procedures for dietary modulators of cancer risk are also being developed. One problem that needed to be addressed was the necessity of collecting dietary samples from multiple countries in a comparable and standardized manner (Friedenreich et al. 1992).

• *Intervention Studies.* Intervention studies (randomized trials) are theoretically the most desirable of the basic epidemiologic approaches to research. Because they resemble experiments, their results are potentially the most convincing. In intervention studies, individuals are randomly allocated to an experimental or a control group. The experimental arm receives the intervention of interest, while the control arm does not. Because of the randomized design, the potential for bias is minimal, and any differences in outcome between the two groups can be attributed with some confidence to the intervention itself.

Intervention studies that involve dietary manipulation are particularly difficult to perform successfully and to interpret. For example, if the intervention involves decreasing a macronutrient, such as fat, then to maintain weight, protein or carbohydrate must be increased, or energy expenditure decreased. Thus, a change in outcome could be attributable to any of the altered variables, not just to fat. Even an intervention that does not focus on macronutrients could have an effect on total caloric intake. For example, increasing vegetable intake (which adds considerable bulk to the diet) could result in decreased consumption of higher calorie foods, thereby leading to inadvertent weight loss. Even well-designed intervention trials can founder on such obstacles.

Examples of intervention studies related to dietary exposures include a trial of β-carotene supplements to lower risk of skin cancers (Greenberg et al. 1990); a trial of αtocopherol and β-carotene supplements to reduce the incidence of lung and other cancers among male smokers (Alpha-Tocopherol, Beta Carotene Cancer Prevention Study Group 1994); The Carotene and Retinol Efficacy Trial (CARET; Thornquist et al. 1993, Omenn et al. 1994); the Physicians Health Study (PHS; Hennekens et al.); trials of calcium supplements and precursors of colon cancer (Vargas and Alberts 1992); and a trial of low fat intake and breast and colon cancer (the recently begun Women's Health Initiative) (IOM 1993). Under ideal conditions, one would always choose to conduct intervention trials. However, use of trials is limited by several considerations, including the following: (1) excessively large sample size requirements unless very high-risk (and therefore nonrepresentative) populations are selected for the trial; (2) substantial logistical difficulties, such as maintaining compliance to dietary change over extended time periods; (3) the possibility in dietary interventions that the controls might also change their habits on their own initiative, thereby reducing differences between the two groups; (4) very high costs that must be justified; and (5) ethical considerations that often preclude the study (only interventions that are likely to be beneficial and almost certainly not harmful can be tested). Thus, intervention studies can only be justified when substantial supporting evidence from other studies already exists.

Implementation of these four basic designs in epidemiologic research has been expanded in recent years by the incorporation of new discoveries in molecular genetics and advances in molecular biology techniques. This field has been referred to as molecular epidemiology and is discussed in detail below.

Molecular Epidemiology

Research on molecular mechanisms of carcinogenesis will likely provide additional methods for identifying human exposures to potential carcinogens, and mechanistic understanding of value in risk assessment. Conventional approaches in cancer epidemiology have supplied a wealth of information, but, as noted in the previous section, they have several limitations for identifying specific causal factors, particularly for those cancers that result from multifactor interactions. In addition, epidemiologic studies are largely retrospective, and unless very large numbers of individuals are studied, they are quite insensitive to relatively small increases in risk. Molecular epidemiology is an emerging field that combines traditional epidemiologic studies with biochemical, immunologic, and molecular assays of human tissues and biologic fluids. For example, one study in China is measuring DNA or protein-aflatoxin B_1 adducts in individuals at risk for liver cancer. Biologic markers are also being used by NCI to establish efficacy in chemoprevention trials. The usefulness of biologic markers in epidemiologic studies will be determined by their sensitivity, specificity, and predictive value. As noted in the NRC report on Biologic Markers in Immunotoxicology (NRC 1992), the definitions of sensitivity and specificity, as related to epidemiologic studies differ from those used in laboratory studies. While laboratory sensitivity refers to the lowest level that can be reliably analyzed, sensitivity in population studies refers to the proportion of cases that the marker correctly identifies. Similarly, laboratory specificity refers to the ability of the technique to exclude identification of other substances, while specificity in population studies refers to the ability of the marker to identify a true negative correctly. Predictive value is determined by identifying an exposed individual in a population. Laboratory procedures are now available that can be used as biologic markers of factors related to the following: (1) genetic and acquired host susceptibility, (2) metabolism and tissue levels of carcinogens, (3) levels of covalent adducts formed between carcinogens and DNA or other macromolecules, and (4) early cellular responses to carcinogen exposure. Some of these biologic markers are briefly discussed below (for detailed reviews of this subject see Perera and Weinstein 1982,

Harris 1986, Santella 1988, Griffith et al. 1989, Skipper and Tannenbaum 1990, and Weinstein et al. 1995).

Genetic Markers of Susceptibility

As mentioned previously, individual susceptibility to chemical carcinogens is influenced by variation in genes coding for enzymes that activate or detoxify carcinogens, as well as repair damage to DNA. A genetic predisposition to cancer may also be due to mutations in oncogenes and tumor suppressor genes. Once such genes have been identified, an individual's phenotype or genotype can be determined.

Biologic Markers of Internal Dose

Toxicant exposure is often assessed at the level of external source. This approach has limitations with respect to precision, reliability, and the extent to which it reflects internal dose, that is, the amount of compound found within the body following exposure. Highly sensitive analytic procedures and immunoassays now make it possible to measure the amounts of a chemical carcinogen or its metabolites in cells, tissues, or body fluids (saliva, blood, urine, or feces). These biologic markers of internal dose reflect individual differences in absorption or bioaccumulation of the compound in question and indicate the level of the compound within the body and in specific tissues or compartments. Examples of this type of marker include the following chemicals: cotinine in serum or urine resulting from cigarette smoke exposure; urinary 1-hydroxypyrene resulting from exposure to polycyclic aromatic hydrocarbons; aflatoxin in urine from dietary or endogenous sources; and DDT or PCBs in serum or adipose tissue biopsies from environmental contamination. Another example that is not specific to an individual chemical is the Ames *Salmonella typhimurium* mutagenesis assay, which can detect the presence of mutagens in urine that might reflect exposure to cigarette smoke or other genotoxic environmental agents.

Biologic Markers of Biologically Effective Dose

Although markers of internal dose are quite valuable, they do not indicate the extent to which a given compound has interacted with critical cellular targets. In contrast, assays of the biologically effective dose measure the amount of a compound that has reacted with cellular macromolecules, usually DNA, or with a protein such as hemoglobin in the blood (Skipper and Tannenbaum 1990). When DNA from a target tissue is not readily available, sometimes surrogate tissues can be used instead (e.g., placenta or peripheral blood cells). The relationship between the types and levels of adducts in surrogate samples to those in target tissues has not been well characterized in humans, but this relationship has been established for certain carcinogens in laboratory animals. Another limitation is that levels of carcinogen-DNA adducts generally reflect recent exposure rather than cumulative exposure over time and do not indicate if critical targets in DNA such as oncogenes or tumor suppressor genes are affected.

Several methods have been developed for detecting and quantitating carcinogen-DNA adducts in extracts of human peripheral blood cells and tissues. These include physical methods such as fluorescence spectroscopy and gas chromatography/mass spectrometry (GC/MS), the ^{32}P-postlabeling procedure, immunoassays employing antisera to specific carcinogen-DNA adducts, and combinations of these methods (Santella 1988, Weinstein et al. 1995). These methods can detect one carcinogen-DNA adduct per about 10^7 to 10^9 nucleotides, which is equivalent to between 1 and 100

adducts per cell. The enzyme-linked immunoassay (ELISA) procedure has been the most widely used method.

Early Biological Responses and Gene Mutations

The next category of biologic markers in the multistep sequence
of carcinogenesis comprises markers of very early cellular responses
to carcinogen-DNA damage, especially responses thought to play
a role in carcinogenesis. These effects can be measured in target
tissues or more convenient surrogates, such as peripheral white
blood cells. These biologic markers include DNA single- or double-
strand breaks, mutations in various genes, and various cytogenetic
effects, including sister chromatid exchange, micronuclei, and chromosomal aberrations.

Other Types of Biologic Markers

Several nongenotoxic chemicals, including such compounds as
TPA, phenobarbital, TCDD, various PCBS, and hormones (including both natural and synthetic estrogens and androgens) can enhance carcinogenesis without forming covalent adducts with cellular
DNA or proteins (Diamond 1987, Tomatis et al. 1987, Weinstein
et al. 1995). However, there are currently no assays to determine
the biologically effective doses of these agents. One approach
would be to develop assays for biologic markers that assess occu-
pancy rates of high affinity receptors for specific hormones or
TCDD. Because carcinogenesis can involve disturbances in signal
transduction and gene expression, the following assays could be
incorporated into molecular epidemiology studies in the future:
assays to evaluate levels of specific growth factors, growth factor
receptors, second messengers (like cAMP or diacylglycerol) protein

kinases, specific phosphoproteins, and the expression of genes related to cell proliferation and other nongenotoxic endpoints. Other assays that may prove to be useful include immunocytochemical assays of proliferating cell nuclear antigen (PCNA) associated with DNA replication and repair, or of other proteins associated with specific phases of the cell cycle, e.g., cyclins (Weinstein 1991, Weinstein et al. 1995).

Because many epidemiologic studies on diet, nutrition, and cancer have been limited by errors in dietary recall methods (see previous section), it is essential to identify objective biologic markers of exposure to specific dietary constituents. Assays have been used to measure the levels of various vitamins, minerals, and nutrients in human blood, tissues, and urine (Weinstein et al. 1995). It would be useful, in addition, to develop biologic markers that reflect the effects of various dietary factors in the intact individual and the relevance of these factors to the carcinogenic process. Biologic markers related to oxidative damage may prove to be of considerable importance for this purpose. These markers include: urinary levels of oxidized DNA bases; analyses of DNA samples for strand breaks or oxidized bases (thymine glycol, 8-hydroxyguanine, etc.); blood and tissue levels of malonaldehyde, an oxidized product of lipids; and markers of enzymes that detoxify activated forms of oxygen, such as catalase and superoxide dismutase (Teebor et al. 1988, Cerutti and Trump 1991, Pryor 1993).

Although biologic markers can provide useful information for evaluating human risk, molecular epidemiology has some limitations. There can be difficulties in correlating indicators of exposure, effect, or susceptibility with a disease. For example, an Institute of Medicine committee (1993) concluded that there was considerable uncertainty in the use of current TCDD serum levels as indicators of past dioxin exposures of Vietnam veterans. Discrepancies were noted and were attributed to the half-life of the biologic marker, leakage of sequestered material from adipose tissue, and accuracy of the determinations. The widespread use of current biologic markers of exposure is also generally limited to compounds whose structures have been identified. Such a limitation may create problems when the complex mixture of the human diet is investigated. However, as progress is made in understanding the mechanisms of carcinogenesis, additional, biologic markers that can be used in epidemiology will be developed.

Screening Tests in Model Systems

Frequently there are insufficient human data to evaluate the potential carcinogenicity of a chemical. Consequently, human risk must often be assessed using information from experimental models. A number of systems are currently available, including structure-activity analyses, short-term tests, and animal bioassays.

Structure-Activity Analyses

As more potential human and animal carcinogens have been evaluated, it has become apparent that certain structural features of these compounds are associated with the induction of tumors. This observation has led to the development of methods for performing structure-activity analyses to predict carcinogenicity. One approach tests major structural groupings associated with electrophilic carcinogens (Ashby 1985, Ashby and Paton 1993). Because of its reliance on DNA reactivity, this system has been most successful in identifying genotoxic carcinogens. A second approach evaluates the structures of chemicals known to induce tumors in humans or animals to determine functionalities associated with either the presence or the absence of biologic activity (Rosenkranz and Klopman 1990a,b; Rosenkranz 1992).

Using these analyses to evaluate naturally occurring chemicals as carcinogens or anticarcinogens in the diet requires that their structures be determined. It was predicted in one analysis of 98 naturally occurring compounds found in plants that 25% will be carcinogens when evaluated in rodent bioassays (Rosenkranz and Klopman 1990b), but this prediction remains to be confirmed.

A limitation of the structure-activity analyses approach is that it has not been well developed for nongenotoxic agents or agents that inhibit carcinogenesis.

Short-Term Tests

A variety of short-term assays are currently being used to evaluate the carcinogenic potential of chemicals. For the purposes of this discussion, short-term tests include both in vitro systems and in vivo systems that examine the effects of short-term exposures; the end-point is not the induction of cancer, but effects that are likely to be predictive of carcinogenicity. The initial observation that several carcinogens were also mutagens (McCann et al. 1975) provided the basis for developing many short-term tests, the majority of which evaluate genotoxicity. Commonly used endpoints for genotoxicity assays include gene mutation, chromosomal aberration, DNA damage, and mammalian cell transformation. Cell transformation assays can also detect certain nongenotoxic carcinogens. Another assay that can identify nongenotoxic carcinogens involves detecting inhibition of cell-to-cell communication. Generally, a battery of tests based on several endpoints and different cell types is appropriate, although in practice the exact nature of the battery varies. Considerations in choosing tests include the origin of the cells, i.e., bacterial or mammalian, and their capacity for biotransformation, in vivo versus in vitro exposure, as well as sensitivity and selectivity. Only tests that have been standardized should be used.

Several agencies that use short-term test data to evaluate potential carcinogenicity have provided recommendations on the types of assays that they consider appropriate. The U.S. Food and Drug Administration (FDA) suggests three tests, that of gene mutation in *Salmonella typhimurium*, gene mutation in mammalian cells (in vitro), and cytogenetic damage in vivo (FDA 1982). Supplemental tests include an in vitro mammalian cell transformation test and unscheduled DNA synthesis in rat hepatocytes (FDA 1982). The U.S. Environmental Protection Agency (EPA), Office of Pesticide Programs, recommends the same three initial tests as the FDA (Dearfield et al. 1991). The test scheme of the EPA Office of Toxic Substances indicates that a positive result in these assays should be followed by further testing to evaluate germ cell effects (Dearfield et al. 1991). International efforts are currently underway to standardize protocols for the performance of short-term assays and criteria for acceptance of data.

Short-term test data are considered, where relevant, by the International Agency for Research on Cancer (IARC) in evaluating the carcinogenic risk of chemicals to humans (IARC 1987). The endpoints considered are all types of DNA damage, mitotic recombination, gene mutation, sister chromatid exchange, micronuclei, chromosomal aberrations, aneuploidy, cell transformation, and the inhibition of intercellular communication. Particular end points can be detected in prokaryotes, in lower eukaryotes, and in animal or human cells in vitro as well as animal cells in vivo.

Traditionally, short-term tests have been conducted on single chemicals. Aflatoxin B_1, for example, a naturally occurring carcinogen found in the diet, has been positive in a number of genotoxicity assays. However, current methods may pose a problem when investigators try to evaluate foods, which are complex mixtures of potential carcinogens as well as anticarcinogens. One useful approach is to study mixtures via bioassay-directed fractionation (NRC 1988). This method was been used to isolate heterocyclic aromatic amines such as 2-amino-3-methylimidazo [4,5-f] quinoline (IQ) from cooked foods. Organic extracts of the charred surfaces of fish or meat were assayed for mutagenic activity in *Salmonella typhi-*

murium. The mutagenic agents were then characterized chemically, and sufficient quantities were synthesized for animal bioassays. Based on these studies, IQ was judged by the IARC to be an animal carcinogen and a probable human carcinogen (IARC 1993). Brewed coffee and tea have also been evaluated for genotoxicity using a variety of tests (IARC 1993). These examples indicate that short-term tests for naturally occurring dietary carcinogens in mixtures are technically feasible.

While current short-term assays should continue to be used in assessing carcinogenic potential, new assays, particularly those to identify carcinogens that are not DNA-reactive, need to be developed and validated. Short-term assays can provide useful information but, like all experimental models, their limitations need to be considered in evaluating test results. Although positive results in these assays suggest that a chemical may be a carcinogen, they are not sufficient to label a chemical as a human carcinogen, and further testing is often required to confirm these data.

Rodent Carcinogenicity Assays

The evaluation of the carcinogenic potential of chemicals is commonly conducted in rodent bioassays. Medium- and long-term exposures can be used.

Limited or medium-term bioassays provide an opportunity to evaluate the potential carcinogenicity of chemicals by exposing animals in vivo and examining site-specific changes associated with tumorigenesis. The animals generally used have an increased susceptibility to chemical carcinogens. These tests use preneoplastic lesions or benign tumors as markers of a neoplastic response. Preneoplastic lesions are defined as phenotypically altered cells that are not themselves neoplastic but that indicate an increased likelihood that benign or malignant neoplasms will occur (Bannasch 1986). Four main categories of changes have been identified: 1) enzyme content or activity, 2) accumulation of macromolecules, 3) alterations in cellular organelles, and 4) cell proliferation and nuclear changes (Bannasch 1986). A commonly used system is the rat liver foci assay (Pereira 1982, Ito et al. 1992). Assays for the induction of mouse skin papillomas (Slaga 1986) or mouse lung adenomas (Stoner and Shimkin 1982) are also used. Assays to detect tumor induction in specific target organs such as the mammary gland, urinary bladder, or stomach have also been developed in mice and rats (Ito et al. 1992). Some of these assays are based on the multi-stage theory of carcinogenesis, so that agents can be evaluated as affecting different stages. The advantages of these medium-term assays are that they take less time than the standard 2-year rodent bioassays and that they can provide useful mechanistic data. These assays can be performed using single agents as well as complex mixtures. However, these tests have limited sensitivity and tend to evaluate changes in a single tissue.

The long-term rodent bioassay involves exposing animals to the test compound and then determining tumor incidence. Testing is usually performed in male and female rats and mice for 18-24 months.

The U.S. National Toxicology Program (NTP) has defined the following protocol for rodent bioassays (Office of Technology Assessment Task Force 1988). F344 rats and B6C3F$_1$ mice are used as the test strains. Fifty animals of each species and sex are used in the control and exposure groups. Doses are determined from a 90-day exposure study by identifying the highest concentration that causes minimal toxicity and little or no growth suppression. This is done so that animals do not die from non-neoplastic causes during the course of the study, thus ensuring appropriate numbers of control and exposed animals at the end of the study. This estimated maximum tolerated dose (MTD) is used as the highest exposure level. Two or more lower doses are also tested (of NTP tests with positive results, 94% are not MTD only). Animals are exposed to the test agent, beginning at approximately eight weeks of age for up to 104 weeks. Ideally, the route of administration should mimic human exposure; however, the one most commonly used is oral. At the end of the study, each animal is autopsied, gross and microscopic pathologic examinations are performed, and the incidence of tumors in control and experimental groups is compared. Carcinogenicity of a compound is then determined based on the incidence of malignant and benign tumors (Office of Technology Assessment Task Force 1988).

The purpose of the rodent bioassay is to identify compounds that induce tumors in an animal model. It is a qualitative test that alone is not sufficient for human risk assessment (NTP 1992). Consequently, the results should be used in combination with other types of data, to assess the likelihood that the substance in question poses a risk for cancer in humans. While current policy accepts that positive results in rodent bioassays are likely to be predictive of human risk, it has been suggested by the NTP Board of Scientific Counselors that hypothesis-driven mechanistic research be incorporated into the NTP bioassay to place these results in proper perspective (NTP 1992). To do so is particularly important because there are examples (e.g., induction of bladder tumors in rodents by saccharin and renal tumors in male rats by d-limonene) where species-specific responses in rodents can occur that might not be relevant to humans (see Chapter 3).

There are concerns about the design of the long-term rodent bioassay, one of which is the use of the maximum tolerated dose (MTD). The issue of the MTD has been reviewed by a committee convened by the National Research Council, *Committee on Risk Assessment Methodology* (NRC 1993). The reader is referred to that report for a detailed discussion of this issue. The majority of that committee recommended that the MTD should continue to be used as one of the test doses, although a minority suggested that the process of dose selection be modified. It should be noted that MTD/high-dose testing represents not just high-dose exposures, but also can introduce entirely different mechanisms of effect (salt crystals and bladder carcinogenesis; particle overload and lung cancers). In any case, if the compound in question is also positive for carcinogenicity when tested at doses lower than the MTD, then such data might have greater validity.

Although studies spanning the last 60 years have shown that tumor incidence could be altered by dietary modulation, including caloric intake (Kritchevsky 1995), only recently has the concern been raised about the current practice of allowing *ad libitum* feeding in the bioassays. It has been shown that dietary restriction increases survival, decreases the incidence of spontaneous tumors, and may alter susceptibility to chemical carcinogens. Calorie restriction results in a change in the expression of enzymes involved in the biotransformation of xenobiotics that may influence the formation or persistence of toxic products (Manjgaladze et al. 1993). In one instance, caloric restriction resulted in an increase in the formation of benzo(a)pyrene DNA-adducts, while a similar regimen decreased aflatoxin B_1 DNA-adducts (Chou et al. 1993). Cells from animals maintained on a restricted number of calories also showed a reduction in c-H-*ras* oncogene expression compared to animals allowed to feed *ad libitum* (Hass et al. 1993). Dietary restriction has enhanced apoptosis of preneoplastic cells, as well as decreased cell replication; these results suggest that food restriction may provide protection from carcinogens (Grasl-Kraupp et al. 1994). Evaluation of tumor incidence in male and female $B6C3F_1$ mice in 16 NTP bioassays suggests a correlation between tumor incidence and body weight (Turturro et al. 1993). When four chemicals were evaluated under the typical conditions of an NTP bioassay, as well as with dietary restriction protocols, the latter increased survival and decreased tumor incidence in both control and exposed animals (Kari and Abdo 1995). Different rates of tumorigenesis were noted in target organs, suggesting that the sensitivity of the bioassay may be altered by dietary manipulation. With two chemicals, dietary restriction altered the site of tumorigenesis; however, when the *ad libitum* fed animals were compared to weight-matched controls, tumor sites identified under both protocols were detected. Moderate dietary restriction improves the health of animals, thus potentially improving the carcinogenicity bioassay (Keenan and Soper 1995). However, it has been suggested that using dietary restriction will both increase (Keenan and Soper 1995) and decrease (Kari and Abdo 1995) the sensitivity of the bioassay. These and other concerns about the rodent bioassay need to be addressed.

COMPARISON OF METHODS FOR EVALUATING
NATURAL AND SYNTHETIC CARCINOGENS

No evidence to date indicates any consistent, fundamental differences between the known naturally occurring and synthetic carcinogens in terms of mechanisms of action (Chapter 3). Consequently, the potential carcinogenicity of both naturally occurring and synthetic compounds might be evaluated using the same methods, except for essential nutrients, which cannot be tested with a zero control. Either single agents or mixtures can be tested. To test mixtures is particularly relevant, since human exposure to both natural carcinogens and most synthetic carcinogens generally occurs as a result of exposure to mixtures of those agents with other chemicals; however, to evaluate the toxicity of chemical mixtures is problematic and generally avoided. In a 1988 NRC report, *Complex Mixtures* reviewed epidemiologic evidence of effects of exposure to chemical mixtures and proposed strategies for testing mixtures. Much of the epidemiologic evidence was derived from exposures to relatively high doses of substances in the workplace. This report concluded that detecting the effects of mixtures at low doses will require better methods for documenting relevant exposures and better ways to avoid misclassification of both exposures and outcomes. This problem is certainly germane to evaluating the potential effects of chemicals that occur in low concentrations in foods. *Complex Mixtures* concluded that although testing such mixtures in the laboratory presents a formidable scientific problem, "reasonably standardized techniques that were developed for the testing of single chemicals can usually be adapted to study complex mixtures" (NRC 1988). In addition, when complex mixtures are tested, problems such as interspecies and high-to-low dose extrapolation are no different from those encountered when testing single agents.

One of the central issues associated with testing mixtures, whether synthetic or naturally occurring, is identifying the causative agents. If a dietary component is suspected to increase or decrease cancer risk, bioassay-directed fractionation might identify the responsible agent. Complete chemical characterization of complex and diverse mixtures is unlikely to be "prudent or possible" (NRC 1988); however, when individual chemicals and their biologic effects are known, such information should be utilized. The activity of a specific chemical component of a food or other mixture, suspected to increase or decrease cancer risk when administered alone, might be altered when exposure occurs to the mixture. Alterations might result from interactions with the other components of the mixture that, for example, might change the component's structure, activity, dose-response relationship, bioavailability, metabolism, or biologic effects.

CRITERIA FOR SELECTING AND TESTING

Carcinogens

In 1984, the IARC identified general criteria for selecting agents for carcinogenicity evaluation (see Table 4-1). Although they were developed primarily to set priorities for testing synthetic compounds, these criteria are also appropriate, with minor modifications, for testing naturally occurring compounds (Table 4-1). For

Table 4-1 Criteria for Selecting Agents for Evaluating Carcinogenic or Anticarcinogenic Potential

Synthetic[a]	Naturally Occurring
Environmental occurrence and human exposure	Occurrence in diet and extent of exposure
Population at risk	Population at risk
Extent of occurrence and use patterns	Usual dietary concentrations; use patterns in children versus adults; regional and ethnic or racial differences in consumption
Stability and persistence in the environment	Stability and persistence in dietary constituents
Structure-activity relationship with known carcinogens and/or mutagens	Structural comparison with known synthetic or naturally occurring carcinogens
Results from short-term tests for genetic and nongenetic end points	Results from short-term tests for genetic and nongenetic end points
Known human carcinogenicity, but no animal data	Suspected human carcinogenicity, but no animal data
Availability for testing	Availability for testing

[a]Adapted from IARC 1984.

these compounds, the presence of an agent in the food and the amount consumed should be considered and might influence the ranking of priorities. For example, constituents present in food in low concentrations, particularly if the foods are consumed in small quantities, might rate a lower priority than those that are relatively abundant in foods and are eaten by a large segment of the population. Exceptions would be chemicals known to be highly potent in other assays, for example mutagenicity assays.

Dietary consumption patterns should also be considered since they are known to differ between children and adults. Geographic, racial, and ethnic patterns of food use also exist. In addition, important information can be gained by comparing the structure of the compound of interest, if known, with other naturally occurring and synthetic chemicals. Higher priority should be given to naturally occurring compounds that fall in the same chemical class as known carcinogens, that contain the same chemical groups, that are likely to form reactive intermediates, or are likely to be persistent. Short-term tests can play a role in prioritizing chemicals for long-term rodent bioassays, and the latter assays can help prioritize chemicals for epidemiologic studies. In turn, epidemiologic and molecular epidemiology studies might highlight dietary constituents that warrant further examination in short-term tests and rodent bioassays, thus providing further verification of their carcinogenic potential.

As noted earlier in this chapter, current methods for evaluating chemicals as carcinogens and anticarcinogens have limitations. Consequently, only agents that substantially meet these criteria should be considered for testing.

Anticarcinogens

Two general approaches have been used to identify a chemical's potential to prevent cancer. The first involves assessing properties that have been associated with cancer prevention, e.g., antioxidant activity, induction of detoxification systems such as glutathione and superoxide dismutase, or the ability to block interaction of reactive species with cellular constituents. Such studies are often used as screening systems that help to identify components for further study. The second approach involves treatment with the potential cancer prevention agent before or after treatment with a carcinogenic agent. This approach is used in short-term, in vitro systems and in long-term, in vivo systems. Examples of this approach include adding of cancer prevention agents to mutagenesis assay systems before or after treatment with carcinogens or mutagens; treating animals with agents before or after treatment with a carcinogen; or measuring the impact of the agent on the metabolism of the carcinogen or on enzyme systems that are induced by the carcinogen. It should be noted that the problems associated with extrapolating results from rodent carcinogenicity studies to humans are also inherent in the experiments designed to assess anticarcinogenicity. The use of a high-dose carcinogen, high-dose treatment with the agent under study, and short-term observation periods all limit the application of these results to humans.

Studying the effect of anticarcinogenic agents on specific stages of cancer development has identified whether the agents modify genotoxic or nongenotoxic processes. For example, studies have evaluated the ability of cancer prevention agents to inhibit nongenotoxic effects such as cell proliferation, by applying these agents before or after treatment with the phorbol ester TPA following exposure to a genotoxic agent. A recent approach to assessing cancer prevention is the use of intermediate markers for tumor formation, such as aberrant crypts and hyperplasia. This approach permits the study of potential cancer prevention agents in humans.

In selecting agents to be evaluated as anticarcinogens, the criteria shown in Table 4-1 for establishing testing priorities can be applied to both synthetic and naturally occurring agents.

SUMMARY AND CONCLUSIONS

To limit the human risk of cancer, it is necessary to evaluate the carcinogenic potential of chemicals, whether they are synthetic or naturally occurring. Current strategies for identifying and evaluating potential naturally occurring carcinogens and anticarcinogens can be grouped into epidemiologic studies and those using experimental animal and cell models. The methods to assess carcinoge-

nicity have been presented in this chapter and the following conclusions derived.

• As stated in Chapter 3, there is no reason to assume that the
mechanisms involved in the process of carcinogenesis differ between naturally occurring and synthetic carcinogens. Consequently, they can be evaluated by the same methods.
• Current methods to identify potential human carcinogens,
whether naturally occurring or synthetic, have limitations. Existing
tests should be modified and coupled with new methods developed
that reflect current understanding of the mechanisms of chemical
carcinogenesis.
• The value of traditional epidemiologic approaches to identifying dietary carcinogens would be expanded by incorporating into
their research designs new biochemical, immunologic, and molecular assays based on human tissues and biologic fluids.
• Despite their limitations, experimental models serve as important screening tests to identify potential human carcinogens. However, there are concerns about extrapolating the results from these
models to humans, both with respect to carcinogenic risks and to
risks at levels of human exposure. With respect to risk extrapolating, data from screening tests should be used in combination with
mechanistic and other available information to predict more reliably the potential human carcinogenicity of a given substance. This
is true for both synthetic and naturally occurring compounds.

REFERENCES

Alpha-Tocopherol, Beta Carotene Cancer Prevention Study
    Group. 1994. The effect of vitamin E and beta carotene on
    the incidence of lung cancer and other cancers in male
    smokers. N. Engl. J. Med. 330:1029-1035.
Armstrong, B. and R. Doll. 1975. Environmental factors and

cancer incidence and mortality in different countries, with special reference to dietary practices. Int. J. Cancer 15:617-631.

Ashby, J. 1985. Fundamental structural alerts to potential carcinogenicity or noncarcinogenicity. Environ. Mutagen. 7:919-921.

Ashby, J. and D. Paton. 1993. The influence of chemical structure on the extent and sites of carcinogenesis for 522 rodent carcinogens and 55 different human carcinogen exposures. Mutat. Res. 286:3-74.

Bannasch, P. 1986. Preneoplastic lesions as end points in carcinogenicity testing. I. Hepatic preneoplasia. Carcinogenesis 7:689-695

Cerutti, P.A. and B.F. Trump. 1991. Inflammation and oxidative stress in carcinogenesis. Cancer Cells 3:1-7.

Chou, M.W., J. Kong, K.T. Chung, and R.W. Hart. 1993. Effect of caloric restriction on the metabolic activation of xenobiotics. Mutation Research 295:223-235.

Dearfield, K.L., A.E. Auletta, M.C. Cimino, and M.M. Moore. 1991. Considerations in the U.S. Environmental Protection Agency's testing approach for mutagenicity. Mutat. Res. 258:259-283.

Diamond, L. 1987. Tumor promoters and cell transformation. Pp. 731-734 in Mechanisms of Cellular Transformation by Carcinogenic Agents. Grunberger, D. and S. Goff, eds. Elmsford: Pergamon Press.

FDA (U.S. Food and Drug Administration). 1982. Toxicological Principles for the Safety Assessment of Direct Food Additives and Color Additives used in Food. U.S. Food and Drug Administration, Bureau of Foods.

Folsom, A.R., S.A. Kaye, R.J. Prineas, J.D. Potter, S.M. Gapstur, and R.B. Wallace. 1990. Increased incidence of carcinoma of the breast associated with abdominal adiposity in postmenopausal women. Am. J. Epidemiol. 131:794-803.

Frebourg, T. and S. H. Friend. 1992. Cancer risks from germline p53 mutations. J. Clin. Invest. 90:1637-1641.

Friedenreich, C.M., N. Slimani, and E. Riboli. 1992. Measurement of past diet: review of previous and proposed methods. Epidemiol. Rev. 14:177-196.

Giovannucci, E., M. J. Stampfer, G. A. Colditz, J. E. Manson, B. A. Rosner, M. Longnecker, F. E. Speizer, and W. C. Willett. 1993. A comparison of prospective and retrospective assessments of diet in the study of breast cancer. Am. J. Epidemiol. 137:502-511.

Gonzalez, F.J., and H.V. Gelboin. 1994. Role of human cytochromes P450 in the metabolic activation of chemical carcinogens and toxins. Drug Metab. Rev. 26(1-2):165-183.

Grasl-Kraupp, B., W. Bursch, B. Ruttkay-Nedecky, A. Wagner, B. Lauer, and R. Shulte-Hermann. 1995. Food restriction eliminates preneoplastic cells through apoptosis and antagonizes carcinogenesis in rat liver. Proc. Natl. Acad. Sci. U.S.A. 91:9995-9999.

Greenberg, E. R., J. A. Baron, T.A. Stukel, M. M. Stevens, J. S. Mandel, S. K. Spencer, P. M. Elias, N. Lowe, D. W. Nierenberg, G. Bayrd, J. C. Vance, D. H. Freeman, Jr., W. E. Clendenning, T. Kwan, and the Skin Cancer Prevention Study Group. 1990. A clinical trial of beta carotene to prevent basal-cell and squamous-cell cancers of the skin. N. Engl. J. Med. 323:789-795.

Griffith, J., R.C. Duncan, and B.S. Hulka. 1989. Biochemical and biological markers: Implications for epidemiologic studies. Arch. Environ. Health 44:375-381.

Hass, B.S., R.W. Hart, M.H. Lu, and B.D. Lyn-Cook. 1993. Effects of caloric restriction in animals on cellular function, oncogene expression and DNA methylation in vitro. Mutation Research 295:281-289.

Harris, C.C., ed. 1986. Biochemical and Molecular Epidemiology of Cancer. New York: Alan R. Liss. 473 p.

Heilbrun, L.K., A.M. Nomura, and G.N. Stemmermann. 1984. Dietary cholesterol and lung cancer risk among Japanese men in Hawaii. Am. J. Clin. Nutr. 39:375-379.

IARC (International Agency for Research on Cancer). 1984. Chemicals and Exposures to Complex Mixtures Recommended for Evaluation in IARC Monographs and Chemicals and Complex Mixtures Recommended for Long Term Carcinogenicity Testing. IARC Intern. Tech. Rep. No. 84/002. Lyon, France: IARC.

IARC (International Agency for Research on Cancer). 1987. IARC monographs on the evaluation of carcinogenic risks to humans. Genetic and related effects: an updating of selected IARC monographs from volumes 1-42. Supplement 6.

IARC (International Agency for Research on Cancer). 1993. Biennial Report, 1992-1993. For the period 1 July 1991 to 30 June 1993. Lyon, France: IARC. Pages 44-49.

IARC (International Agency for Research on Cancer). 1993. IARC monographs on the evaluation of carcinogenic risks to humans. Vol. 56.

IOM (Institute of Medicine). 1993. An Assessment of the NIH Women's Health Initiative. Thaul, S. and D. Hoftra, eds. National Academy of Sciences. Washington, DC: National Academy Press. 142 pp.

IOM (Institute of Medicine). 1993. Veterans and Agent Orange: health effects of herbicides used in Vietnam. National Academy of Sciences. Washington, DC: National Academy Press.

Ito, N., T. Shirai, and R. Hasegawa. 1992. Medium-term bioassays for carcinogens. Pp. 353-388 in Mechanisms of Carcinogenesis and Risk Identification. Vainio, H., P. N. Magee, D. B. McGregor, and A. J. McMichael, eds. IARC Scientific Publications 116.

Kari, F.W., and K.A. Abdo. 1995. The sensitivity of the NTP bioassay for carcinogen hazard evaluation can be modulated by dietary restriction. Pp. 63-78 in Dietary Restriction: Implications for the Design and Interpretation of Toxicity and Carcinogenicity Studies. R.W. Hart, D.A. Neumann, and R.T. Robertson, eds. Washington, D.C.: ILSI Press.

Keenan, K.P., and K.A. Soper. 1995. The effects of *ad libitum* overfeeding and moderate dietary restriction on Sprague-Dawley rat survival, spontaneous carcinogenesis, chronic disease and the toxicologic response to pharmaceuticals. Pp. 99-126 in Dietary Restriction: Implications for the Design and Interpretation of Toxicity and Carcinogenicity Studies. R.W. Hart, D.A. Neumann, and R.T. Robertson, eds. Washington, D.C.: ILSI Press.

Kolonel, L.N., J.H. Hankin, J. Lee, S.Y. Chu, A.M.Y. Nomura, and M.W. Hinds. 1981. Nutrient intakes in relation to cancer incidence in Hawaii. Br. J. Cancer 44:332-339.

Kritchevsky, D. 1995. Fat, calories, and cancer. Pp. 155-165 in Dietary REstriction: Implications for the Design and Interpretation of Toxicity and Carcinogenicity Studies. R.W. Hart, D.A. Neumann, and R.T. Robertson, eds. Washington, D.C.: ILSI Press.

Lyon, J.L. and A.W. Sorenson. 1978. Colon cancer in a low-risk population. Am. J. Clin. Nutr. 31:S227-S230.

Manjgaladze, M., S. Chen, L.T. Frame, J.E. Seng, P.H. Duffy, R.J. Feurers, R.W. Hart, and J.E.A. Leakey. 1993. Effects of caloric restriction on rodent drug and carcinogen metabolizing enzymes: implications for mutagenesis and cancer. Mutat. Res. 295:201-222.

McCann, J., E. Choi, E. Yamasaki, and B. N. Ames. 1975. Detection of carcinogens as mutagens in the *Salmonella*/microsome test: assay of 300 chemicals. Proc.Natl. Acad. Sci. (USA) 72:5135-5139.

Miki, Y., J. Swensen, D. Shattuck-Eidens, P.A. Futreal, K. Harshman, S. Tavtigian, Q. Liu, C. Cochran, L.M. Bennett, W. Ding, R. Bell, J. Rosenthal, C. Hussey, T. Tran, M.

McClure, C. Frye, T. Hattier, R. Phelps, A. Haugen-Strano, H. Katcher, K. Yakumo, Z. Gholami, D. Shaffer. S. Stone, S. Bayer, Christian Wray, R. Bogden, P. Dayananth, J. Ward, P. Tonin, S. Narod, P.K. Bristow, F.H. Norris, L. Helvering, P. Morrison, P. Rosteck, M. Lai, J.C. Barrett, C. Lewis, S. Neuhausen, L. Cannon-Albright, D. Goldgar, R. Wiseman, A. Kamb, M.H. Skolnick. 1994. A strong candidate for the breast and ovarian cancer susceptibility gene BRCA1. Science 266(5182):66-71.

NRC (National Research Council). 1973. Toxicants occurring naturally in foods, 1st edition, 1966; 2nd edition, 1973. Committee on Food Protection. Washington, DC: National Academy Press.

NRC (National Research Council). 1988. Complex Mixtures. Washington, DC: National Academy Press.

NRC (National Research Council). 1992. Biologic Markers in Immunotoxicology. Washington, DC: National Academy Press.

NRC (National Research Council). 1993. Issues in Risk Assessment. Washington, DC: National Academy Press.

NTP (National Toxicology Program). 1992. Final Report of the Advisory Review by the NTP Board of Scientific Counselors; Request for Comments. Federal Register 57:312721-31730.

Ning, J.-P., M. C. Yu, Q.-S. Wang, and B. E. Henderson. 1990. Consumption of salted fish and other risk factors for nasopharyngeal carcinoma (NPC) in Tianjin, a low-risk region for NPC in the People's Republic of China. J. Natl. Cancer Inst. 82:291-296.

Office of Technology Assessment Task Force. 1988. Identifying and regulating Carcinogens. Michigan: Lewis Publishers.

Pereira, M. A. 1982. Rat liver foci bioassay. J. Amer. Coll. Toxicol. 1:101-117.

Perera F.P. and I. B. Weinstein. 1982. Molecular epidemiology and carcinogen-DNA adduct detection: new approaches to studies of human cancer causation. J. Chronic Dis. 35:581-600.

Prentice, R. L. and L. Sheppard. 1990. Dietary fat and cancer: Consistency of the epidemiologic dats, and disease prevention that may follow from a practical reduction in fat consumption. Cancer Causes and Control 1:81-97.

Pryor, W. A. 1993. Measurement of oxidative stress status in humans. Cancer Epidemiol. Biomarkers Prev. 2:289-292.

Qian, G.S., R.K. Ross, M.C. Yu, J.-M. Yuan, Y.-T. Gao, B.E. Henderson, G.N. Wogan, and J.D. Groopman. 1994. A follow-up study of urinary markers of aflatoxin exposure and liver cancer risk in Shanghai, People's Republic of China. Cancer Epidemiol. Biomarkers and Prevention 3:3-10.

Riboli, E., H. Ronnholm, and R. Saracci. 1987. Biological markers of diet. Cancer Surveys 6:685-718.

Rosenkranz, H. S. 1992. Structure-activity relationships for carcinogens with different modes of action. Pp. 271-277 in Mechanisms of Carcinogenesis and Risk Identification. Vainio, H., P. Magee, D. B. McGregor, and A. J. McMichael, eds. IARC Scientific Publication 116.

Rosenkranz, H. S. and G. Klopman. 1990a. Structural basis of carcinogenicity in rodents of genotoxicants and non-genotoxicants. Mutat. Res. 228:105-124.

Rosenkranz, H. S. and G. Klopman. 1990b. Natural pesticides present in edible plants are predicted to be carcinogenic. Carcinogenesis 11:349-353.

Santella, R. M. 1988. Application of new techniques for the detection of carcinogen adducts to human population monitoring. Mutat. Res. 205:271-282.

Skipper, P. L. and S. R. Tannenbaum. 1990. Protein adducts in the molecular dosimetry of chemical carcinogens. Carcinogenesis 11:507-518.

Slaga, T. J. 1986. SENCAR mouse skin tumorigenesis model versus other strains and stocks of mice. Environ. Health

Persp. 68:27-32.

Steinmetz, K. A. and J. D. Potter. 1991. Vegetables, fruit, and cancer. I. Epidemiology (Review). Cancer Causes Control 2:325-357.

Stoner, G. D. and M. B. Shimkin. 1982. Strain A mouse lung tumor bioassay. J. Amer. Coll. Toxicol. 1:145-169.

Teebor, G. W., R. J. Boorstein, and J. Cadet. 1988. The repairability of oxidative free radical mediated damage to DNA: a review. Int. J. Radiat. Biol. 54:131-150.

Tomatis, L., A. Aitio, J. Wilbourn, and L. Shuker. 1987. Human carcinogens so far identified. Jpn J. Cancer Res. 80:795-807.

Turturro, A., P.H. Duffy, and R.W. Hart. 1993. Modulation of toxicity by diet and dietary macronutrient restriction. Mutat. Res. 295:151-164.

Vargas, P. A. and D. S. Alberts. 1992. Primary prevention of colorectal cancer through dietary modification. Cancer (Suppl) 70:1229-1235.

Weinstein, I. B. 1988. The origins of human cancer: molecular mechanisms of carcinogenesis and their implications for cancer prevention and treatment. Cancer research 48:4135-4143.

Weinstein, I. B. 1991. Cancer Prevention: recent progress and future opportunities. Cancer Res. (suppl.) 51:5080S-5085S.

Weinstein, I.B., R.M. Santella, and F. Perera. 1995. Molecular Biology and Epidemiology of Cancer. Pp. 83-110 in Cancer Prevention and Control, P. Greenwald, B.S. Kramer, and D.L. Weed, ed. New York: Marcel Dekker, Inc.

Weston, A., L.S. Perrin, K. Forrester, R. N. Hoover, B. F. Trump, C. C. Harris, and N. E. Caporaso. 1992. Allelic frequency of a p53 polymorphism in human lung cancer. Cancer Epidemiol. Biomarkers Prev. 1:481-483.

Weston, A., P. Vineis, N. E. Caporaso, T. G. Krontiris, J. A. Lovergaw, and H. Sugimura. 1991. Racial variation in the distribution of H-*ras*-1 alleles. Mol. Carcinog. 4:265-268.

Wilkens, L. R., J. H. Hankin, C. N. Yoshizawa, L. N. Kolonel, and J. Lee. 1992. Comparison of long-term dietary recall between cancer cases and noncases. Am. J. Epidemiol. 136:825-835.

Willett, W.C. 1994. Diet and health: What should we eat? Science 264:532-537.

Willett, W.C., M.J. Stampfer, G.A. Colditz, B.A. Rosner, and F.E. Speizer. 1990. Relation of meat, fat, and fiber intake to the risk of colon cancer in a prospective study among women. N. Engl. J. Med. 323:1664-1672.

Wright, S.A., and J.C. Stevens. 1992. The human hepatic cytochromes P450 involved in drug metabolism. Crit. Rev. Toxicol. 22(1):1-21.

5

Risk Comparisons

Previous chapters of this report have discussed the ways in which dietary carcinogens are identified and documented the presence in the human diet of both naturally occurring and synthetic substances that may possess carcinogenic potential. In this chapter, we discuss the relative risks posed by natural and synthetic dietary carcinogens.

Throughout this report, the term *diet* is used to refer to foods and beverages consumed intentionally and customarily in the U.S., not as a result of accident or deprivation. As in previous chapters, it is convenient to differentiate among constitutive, derived, acquired, pass-through, and added naturally occurring food chemicals. The definition of a carcinogen adopted in this report is that used by the International Agency for Research on Cancer, namely any agent capable of increasing the incidence of malignant neoplasia. Operationally, the committee treats as carcinogens those agents classified in certain IARC categories (i.e., 1, 2A, and 2B) and in the National Toxicology Program's (1994) Annual Report as known to be or reasonably anticipated to be carcinogenic.

The level of risk associated with a carcinogenic agent depends on both the potency of the agent and on the level of exposure to that agent. Carcinogenic potency can be estimated using clinical and epidemiologic data on humans or toxicologic data derived from animal bioassays. Exposure to carcinogenic agents present in the diet depends on both food consumption patterns and the concentration of those agents in foods consumed. Food consumption data can be collected through the use of food diaries, or by using questionnaires designed to gauge the frequency with which specific foods are consumed or to identify by recall those foods recently consumed. Concentrations of carcinogenic agents in the food supply can be determined by analytic techniques, such as chemical analyses for pesticide residues present on foods.

Inferences about dietary cancer risks are complicated by several factors. Diet is a complex mixture containing a large number of micro- and macroingredients. Components of the diet may interact with one another in a synergistic or antagonistic way. Some dietary components, such as aflatoxin, might increase cancer risks, whereas others, such as fruits and vegetables rich in antioxidants, might reduce cancer risk.

Food-consumption patterns can be highly variable even among individuals in the same population subgroup. Food consumption varies depending on availability, ethnic customs, age, economics, and other factors. Chemical contaminants, extraneous matter, and pesticide residues can be present in food at variable concentrations. Food composition and products derived from preparation and processing of food are also variable. In addition to variability in dietary intakes, individuals may also vary with respect to their susceptibility to food components with carcinogenic potential. Each of these sources of dietary variability can effect individual exposures to food chemicals, as well any associated risks.

Estimates of potential dietary cancer risks are subject to considerable uncertainty; for example, epidemiological studies have failed to provide unambiguous evidence of the effects of dietary fat on cancer risk. Estimates of potential cancer risks associated with low levels of individual food chemicals derived on the basis of laboratory results are highly uncertain. The application of animal cancer test data to humans requires extrapolation from the high doses used in laboratory studies to much lower doses corresponding to concentrations in the human diet, and extrapolation from animals to humans. The joint effects of ingestion of multiple agents in the form of complex dietary mixtures are also difficult to define. Consequently, in evaluating dietary cancer risks, it is important that both uncertainty and variability be recognized and, if possible, characterized.

Recognizing that estimates of cancer risk are uncertain, this chapter focuses on the following questions:

• Does diet contribute to an appreciable proportion of human cancer?
• What are the relative contributions of naturally occurring and synthetic agents to dietary cancer risk?
• Are there significant interactions between either synthetic or naturally occurring carcinogens and anticarcinogens in the diet?

To determine whether synthetic or natural chemicals classified as carcinogens pose the greater risk, it is necessary to know 1) the identity of the carcinogens present in the diet; 2) levels of ingestion of specific dietary carcinogens, both natural and synthetic; and, 3) the carcinogenic potency of these chemicals. Although this information might be used to evaluate the potential risks associated with individual food chemicals, it is more difficult to evaluate the overall risk posed by carcinogens present in the diet as a whole. The human diet is a complex mixture of food chemicals that interact in ways that are not generally well understood. Consequently, much of the discussion in this chapter of the comparative risks of naturally occurring and synthetic carcinogens present in the diet will focus on individual substances rather than mixtures.

The levels of exposure to dietary carcinogens vary widely, depending on food-consumption patterns and dietary concentrations of carcinogenic substances. Because consumption patterns vary among individuals, it is important to consider the range of exposures within the population of interest, particularly those persons with high dietary intakes of naturally occurring or synthetic carcinogens.

For purposes of risk comparison, a quantitative measure of the potency of naturally occurring and synthetic carcinogens is required. A widely used measure of carcinogenic potency is the TD_{50}, defined as the level of exposure resulting in an excess lifetime cancer risk of 50% (Peto et al. 1984, Sawyer et al. 1984). The TD_{50} can be derived from either epidemiologic or toxicologic investigations. Because the TD_{50} is often derived from high-dose experimental data, it does not necessarily provide an appropriate basis for making inferences about cancer risks at low levels of exposure. To obtain a measure of carcinogenic potency that is closer to human exposure levels, the committee also used the TD_{01} as an index of carcinogenic potency. Because risk is a function of exposure and potency, the ratio of exposure to potency has been proposed as a means of comparing the relative risk of exposure to different carcinogens (Ames and Gold 1987).

This chapter reviews existing data on the comparative potency of naturally occurring and synthetic carcinogens. Specifically, the committee compiled a database on the carcinogenic potencies of 37 natural and 70 synthetic carcinogens known to occur in the diet. These substances were identified as being carcinogenic in animals or humans by either the U.S. National Toxicology Program or the International Agency for Research on Cancer. All of these chemicals were classified by the NTP as known or reasonably anticipated to be carcinogens or by IARC as known (Group 1), probable (Group 2A), or possible (Group 2B) human carcinogens. Although the potency of naturally occurring dietary carcinogens as a group was on average greater than that of the synthetic carcinogens, the potencies of both types vary widely with considerable overlap. As discussed above, they are also subject to considerable uncertainty. Based on this limited number of chemicals, which might not represent the universe of naturally occurring and synthetic dietary carcinogens, it appears difficult to distinguish between the potencies of the two classes.

The overall contribution of diet to the human cancer burden is also considered. Although tobacco and diet are thought to account for the large majority of human cancer, the contribution of the diet is less well understood than that of tobacco and is subject to far greater uncertainty as to the attributable risk fraction. Recent reviews of the causes of human cancer have suggested that synthetic carcinogens present in the diet might be responsible for a very small fraction of the human cancer burden (Ames et al. 1995, Higginson 1988), due in part to regulations that have limited the use of pesticides, including those with carcinogenic potential, and preclude the use of carcinogenic substances as direct food additives. In terms of risk from food substances, calories and fat may represent the most important naturally occurring dietary constituents. Food chemicals produced naturally by plants for self-defense have not been investigated to the same extent, and therefore the degree to which they contribute to human cancer is less clear.

MONITORING FOOD CONSUMPTION

Sources of Information

Pesticides in the Diets of Infants and Children (NRC 1993a) addresses issues of food and water consumption in the U.S. population. Directed primarily at the pediatric population, the report discusses approaches to quantifying food and water consumption in the population at large, and the limitations of methods for food consumption monitoring.

National food surveys are conducted by the U.S. Department of Agriculture (USDA) and the Department of Health and Human Services. The USDA's Human Nutrition Information Service (HNIS) conducts a comprehensive Nationwide Food Consumption (NFC) Survey about every ten years. In the interim, the service conducts Continuing Surveys of Food Intakes of Individuals (CSFII). Both the 1977-1978 and the 1987-1988 NFC Surveys were reviewed in *Pesticides in the Diets of Infants and Children*. However, the 1987-1988 survey was considered less reliable for estimating dietary exposures because of the low response rate (34%). Other limitations of the 1987-1988 USDA survey are discussed by the Government Accounting Office (1991).

Although subject to serious limitations, the USDA surveys provide the only comprehensive data currently and publicly available on food consumption by people of all ages. Some surveys focus on segments of the U.S. population: for example, the 1985-1986 CSFII emphasized women 19-50 years old and their children ages 1-5, a sample of low-income women and their children, and in 1985 only, men ages 19-50 years. In the CSFII 1989, 1990, and 1991 surveys, data were collected on individuals of both sexes in all age classes, with response rates higher than those of the 1987-1988 NFC Survey (over 50%). The results of the 1989 and 1990 surveys are available commercially (Technical Assessment Systems 1995a,b) and on computer media from the National Technical Information Service.

There is substantial uncertainty in such food consumption data due to a variety of factors, including recall bias, measurement error, and recording errors. The fact that the numbers of people surveyed are relatively small and response rates poor makes generalization to the U.S. population at large difficult. The optimal system for collecting and validating data on food consumption has yet to be developed. Ideally, complete and accurate records of the types and quantities of food consumed by the survey respondents could be used as a reference against which different surveys providing estimates of consumption could be compared. Because of the problems in measuring actual food intake, however, validation studies have in the past focused on the comparisons of results obtained from different surveys using different data collection methods.

Another series of food consumption surveys that provides nationwide data is conducted by DHHS's National Center for Health Statistics (NCHS). Since 1960, the center has conducted seven health examination surveys of the U.S. population. The National Health and Nutrition Examination Surveys (NHANES), including the recently completed NHANES III, were designed to obtain representative information on the health and nutritional status for the U.S. population through health and medical histories, dietary interviews, direct physical examinations, and laboratory measurements. NFC and NHANES surveys deal primarily with nutritional considerations and are less useful for evaluating ingestion of naturally occurring chemicals and food additives.

NHANES I (1971-1974) and NHANES II (1976-1980) sought data on medical conditions, especially nutrition-related disorders (obesity, growth retardation, anemia, diabetes, atherosclerotic cardiovascular diseases, hypertension, and deficiencies of vitamins or minerals). Both were directed at the civilian, noninstitutional population. (Excluded were the homeless, residents of hotels, rooming houses, dormitories, Native American reservations, military posts, prisons, hospitals, and residential treatment centers for drug addiction, alcoholism, and obesity.) Both surveys covered the 48 contiguous states, although Alaska and Hawaii were included in NHANES II. These surveys are discussed in detail in the NRC report *Diet and Health* (NRC 1989a). NHANES II data have been used to evaluate the proportion of the population at risk for deficiencies of vitamin A, vitamin C, folate, iron, zinc, and protein.

The target population for NHANES III was the U.S. civilian, noninstitutional population aged 2 months or older. The survey design called for a stratified sample of counties, blocks, and persons randomly selected from households. National samples were drawn during 1988-1991 and 1991-1994. Eighty-one counties were selected from 26 states; from these, approximately 40,000 persons of all races were selected, and about 30,000 agreed to participate in the medical examination. Precise estimates of health characteristics were needed for relatively small population subgroups (children, older persons, black, and Mexican Americans), which were subject to oversampling.

Some of the 30 topics investigated in NHANES III were high blood pressure, high blood cholesterol, obesity, passive smoking, lung disease, osteoporosis, HIV, hepatitis, helicobacter pylori, immunization status, diabetes, allergies, growth and development, blood lead, anemia, food sufficiency, and dietary intake, including fats, antioxidants, and nutritional blood measures. Results from NHANES III are being analyzed by NCHS and are not yet available.

Although NHANES data are extensive and derive from a broad range of measurements, the data are of limited use in the study of chronic diseases, in part because of the sample size, response rates, and recall bias. NHANES provides only cross-sectional data on a periodic basis. *Diet and Health* provides an in-depth discussion of the limitations of NHANES data.

A number of factors need to be considered when using food composition and consumption data in estimating dietary cancer risks. For example, food composition databases do not contain data on the concentration of many of the potential carcinogenic constituents found in foods (USDA 1992). Information on macronutrients and on certain micronutrients with carcinogenic or anticarcinogenic potential is available for a large variety of foods. However, data on many other microconstituents, naturally occurring and synthetic, are lacking. For example, little information is available on plant biocides, non-nutritive plant products with anticarcinogenic potential, or compounds generated by cooking. Furthermore, databases frequently do not take into consideration variability among food samples, population groups, and individuals, or consumption patterns that vary over time.

Sources of Variation in
Food Composition and Consumption

Individuals vary in their dietary habits, people of different ages have different dietary requirements, and the concentration of food constituents can differ substantially. This section addresses some of the sources of variation in exposure to carcinogens in the diet.

Dietary risk assessments should take into consideration that food samples can vary greatly in composition (see Chapter 2). For example, plants may produce natural chemicals for purposes of self-defense when they come in contact with certain pests (Harborne 1993). The concentrations of these substances in a particular food can vary considerably among samples, depending on the extent of the stress to the plant prior to harvesting. Factors such as storage, cooking, and pesticide application rates also have effects on food composition. This variability could result in substantial seasonal, geographic, and individual variation among food samples and, consequently, among human exposure levels. Similarly, cultivars of fruits and vegetables may differ in the content of naturally occurring constituents. For example, a cultivar of Idaho potatoes had to be taken off the market when it was found to contain toxic levels of the neurotoxin solanine (IFBC 1990).

Dietary assessments should also allow for consumption patterns that may vary among population subgroups (defined in terms of sex, ethnicity, income, and other characteristics) (Kolonel et al. 1983, USDA 1987). Using data from the 1977-1978 USDA survey, *Pesticides in the Diets of Infants and Children* concluded that infants and children consume more calories relative to body weight than adults, eat far less-varied diets, and consume far greater amounts of milk in some form. Because of the lack of diversity of infant diets, infants can consume much greater quantities of certain foods than adults: the average 1-year-old consumes approximately 40-fold more apple juice relative to body weight than the average adult (Murdoch et al. 1992). Other population subgroups whose dietary habits differ from those of the general population include vegetarians and religious groups with special dietary restrictions. However, such groups may also exhibit nondietary differences from the general population, with respect to other factors such as socioeconomic status and smoking habits (Lyon et al. 1980).

Water is a major component of food (see Chapter 2) containing trace levels of a number of chemicals and should be considered in any analysis of dietary risk. This fact is particularly important when estimating the risks to children from dietary exposures. *Pesticides in the Diets of Infants and Children* considered three types of water in its analysis of dietary risks: water intrinsic to food, tap water added to food during preparation, and the direct consumption of tap water. The report indicates that dietary sources of water represented by fruits, liquids (especially fruit juices and milk), and vegetables are greater for infants than for older children or adults, and should be considered in estimating the risk from dietary exposure to potential human carcinogens. Such age-dependent differences in dietary patterns need to considered when evaluating lifetime cancer risks (Goddard et al. 1995).

Dietary patterns can change markedly over time with changes in food preferences and the introduction of new foods. For example, artificial sweeteners were unknown until the discovery of saccharin in 1879 (cf. Arnold et al. 1983); however, since its approval for widespread use as an artificial sweetener, aspartame has become a common constituent of the diets of many Americans. In addition, fabricated and genetically engineered foods introduced in recent years have also afforded consumers with new dietary choices.

Finally, food consumption data and survey methods need to be standardized to make them more useful in estimating exposures and determining risk. Currently, there is no simple, uniform method for conversion of a food, as consumed, to its components in terms of raw agricultural constituents. In addition, surveys should be coordinated among concerned organizations and carried out in a timely manner in order to identify trends in food and water consumption.

Factors Affecting Susceptibility

Individuals within a subgroup may vary with respect to their susceptibility to the toxic effects of those agents. Most carcinogens, whether naturally occurring or synthetic, will be metabolized in the body to a greater or lesser degree by different individuals. Some of these substances may be activated to their carcinogenic derivatives, while others are detoxified. Some of the enzymes involved in these reactions, such as certain of the cytochrome P450 mixed function oxidases, are not only inducible but also encoded by polymorphic genes (Idle et al. 1992). As a result, individuals vary in their susceptibility to carcinogens (Omenn et al. 1990).

Prescription and over-the-counter drugs may affect specific constituents of food, such as cholesterol and fat. Several million people take cholesterol-lowering agents, and new drugs are being developed to block lipid absorption. Information on the use of pharmaceutical products that may affect dietary cancer risks is therefore of interest.

DIETARY EXPOSURE TO POTENTIAL CARCINOGENS AND ANTICARCINOGENS

Despite a substantial degree of measurement error in assessing food intakes, as well as limitations in the current food composition and consumption databases, useful estimates of human exposure to some naturally occurring constituents of foods can often be derived. Estimating exposures to synthetic agents is more problematic. Residues of pesticides, chemicals added in processing, and carcinogens produced during cooking can be extremely variable in foods and are usually present in microquantities. In addition, exposure estimates based on dietary intakes (as opposed to serum or tissue measurements) do not account for the bioavailability of food constituents, which depends on many factors, such as other foods consumed at the same time, and the manner in which constituents are structurally bound in food.

In the sections that follow, dietary exposure levels to naturally occurring and synthetic carcinogens and anticarcinogens are discussed. Major food sources and concentrations found in those foods are discussed in detail in Chapter 2.

Naturally Occurring Carcinogens

Table 5-1 classifies chemicals identified as naturally occurring carcinogens that may be present in the diet into five categories: constitutive, derived, acquired, pass-through, and added. The chemicals listed in each category have been classified by IARC or NTP as carcinogens. The remainder of this section discusses potential exposure to these substances and focuses on a few agents in each class for which relatively high intakes are expected.

Constitutive Exposures

Included in this group are the sex hormones (e.g., estradiol 17β, estrone, acetate, progesterone, testosterone), metabolic intermediates in plants (e.g., acetaldehyde), caffeic acid, and natural furocoumarins (5-methoxy and 8-methoxypsoralen). The sex hormones are present in fairly low quantities in consumed meats, although exposure to some can be increased above natural levels through their legal and illegal use as growth promoters in meat production.

Acetaldehyde is a metabolic intermediate in the formation of ethanol during anaerobic respiration, a process which plant tissues can only tolerate for brief periods. Acetaldehyde has been identified as a volatile component of essential oils from a variety of fruit and spice plants, and as a natural constituent of numerous edible berries and other fruits. Acetaldehyde is also formed in animals, during the intracellular oxidation of ethanol, and is present at relatively low concentrations in meat. However, the extent that low levels of acetaldehyde in foods poses a carcinogenic risk is unclear.

Table 5-1   Naturally Occurring Animal and Human Carcinogens[a] That
Might Be Present in U.S. Diets

Constitutive:
  Acetaldehyde[b], benzene, caffeic acid, cobalt[c], estradiol 17β, estrone, ethyl
  acrylate, (with UV light exposure), 8-methoxypsoralen (xanthotoxin) (with
  UV light exposure), progesterone, safrole, styrene, testosterone
Derived:
  A-alpha-C, acetaldehyde[b], benz(a)anthracene, benzene, benzo(a)pyrene,
  benzo(b)fluoranthene, benzo(j)fluoranthene, benzo(k)fluorathene,
  dibenz(a,h)acridine, dibenz(a,j)acridine, dibenz(a,h)anthracene, formalde-
  hyde[b], glu-P-1, glu-P-2, glycidaldehyde, IQ, Me-A-alpha-C, MeIQ, MeIQx,
  methylmercury compounds, N-methyl-N'-nitro-nitrosoquanidine, N-nitroso-
  N-dibutylamine, N-nitrosodiethylamine, N-nitrosodimethylamine, N-
  nitrosodi-N-propylamine, N-nitrosomethylethylamine, N-nitrosopiperidine,
  N-nitrosopyrrolidine, N-nitrososarcosine, PhIP, Trp-P-1, Trp-P-2, urethane
Acquired:
  Aflatoxin B, aflatoxin M$_1$, ochratoxin A, sterigmatocystin, toxins derived
  from *Fusarium moniliforme*
Pass through:
  Arsenic, benz(a)anthracene, benzo(a)pyrene, beryllium[b], cadmium[b], chromi-
  um[b], cobalt, indeno(1,2,3)pyrene, lead, nickel[b]
Added:
  Contaminant introduced through tap water: arsenic, asbestos[b], benzene,
    beryillium[b], cadmium[b], hexavalent chromium[b], dibenzo(a,l)pyrene,
    indeno(1,2,3,-cd)pyrene, radon
  Indirect through use as drug or in packaging: i) veterinary drugs— estradiol
    17β, progesterone, reserpine, testosterone, ii) food-packaging material—
    benzene, cobalt, ethyl acrylate, formaldehyde[b], nickel[b]
  Direct food additives: acetaldehyde[b], ethyl acrylate, formaldehyde[b]
  Traditional foods and beverages: alcoholic beverages, betel quid, bracken
    fern, hot maté, pickled vegetables, salted fish (Chinese style)

[a]Chemicals classified by IARC as Group 1, 2A, or 2B carcinogens or by NTP
as known or reasonably anticipated to be carcinogens.
[b]Carcinogenicity established by, for example, inhalation, injection, or dermal
routes. The degree to which these agents should be considered carcinogenic
via dietary exposures is uncertain.

The risk for oral exposure appears to be substantially less than for inhalation exposures (ILSI, 1993). For this reason, estimates of the amount of exposure to acetaldehyde via the diet are not made.

Caffeic acid, a metabolic precursor of lignin, a structural polymer found in all land plants, is ubiquitous in the food supply. It accumulates primarily in conjugated forms, which can be hydrolyzed to free caffeic acid in the digestive tract (see Chapter 2). In the conjugated form, it is widely distributed in fruits and vegetables. Concentrations of these conjugates and free caffeic acid have been measured in a variety of food plants by Herrmann (1989) and colleagues. The most recently reported values for caffeic acid in these food sources are assumed to be the most reliable, because of the use of improved analytical techniques involving gas and high performance liquid chromatography. Using the concentrations reported by Herrmann and colleagues and USDA food consumption data, rough estimates of human intake are obtained and presented in Table 5-2.

Table 5-2 reports ranges rather than single values for caffeic acid intake, to reflect both the uncertainty and variability in caffeic acid exposure. Caffeic acid exists primarily as conjugates (esters and glucosides) in unprocessed food plants (see Chapter 2); while these conjugates may be converted to free caffeic acid during food processing and after ingestion, the extent of the conversion is unknown. Human ingestion of chlorogenic acids gave rise to urinary metabolites of caffeic acid in one study, but the amount of the conversion was not measured (Booth et al. 1957). Although other work has indicated that chlorogenic acids are hydrolyzed in the digestive tract of the rat before caffeic acid appears in the bloodstream, the amount of hydrolysis was not reported (Czok et al. 1974). A more recent study of the metabolism of caffeic acid by humans concluded that the phenolic acid is extensively and rapidly metabolized (i.e., within 4 hours), but accounted for only 11% of the acid administered (Jacobson et al. 1983). In calculating average intakes of caffeic acid for the general population, 100% hydrolysis of caffeic acid

Table 5-2   Concentrations of Caffeic Acid, Selected Foods, and Predicted Intake of Caffeic Acid from These Foods in the General Population

Fresh and Prepared Food	Concentration[a] (mg/kg)	Average Intake[b] (mg/kg-day)
Apples	71 (33-203)	0.008 - 0.08
Carrots	33 (12-62)	0.0006-0.006
Celery	80-130[c]	0.0006-0.006
Citrus	0-5[d]	0.001-0.01
Lettuce	64 (43-84)[e]	0.001-0.01
Peaches	139 (39-478)	0.002-0.02
Pears	68 (33-143)	0.0005-0.005
Plums	318 (53-478)	0.002-0.02
Potatoes	30 (15-51)	0.003-0.03
Seed of pea, bush bean, broad bean	None detected	—
Spinach	None detected	--
Tomatoes	33 (14-67)	0.006-0.06
Total from food	--	0.02-0.2[f]
Coffee[g]	492	0.9-9

[a]Concentration as caffeic acid. Unless otherwise noted, calculated from concentrations of caffeic acid conjugates provided by Herrmann (1989). Range reflects values obtained for different varieties.
[b]Intake values calculated using consumption data from the USDA's Continuing Food Consumption Surveys for years 1987-1992, with the software programs EXPOSURE 1® and 4® and databases provided by Technical Assessment Systems (TAS, 1995a). Similar values were obtained using the USDA 1977-78 survey data. The upper bound indicates results assuming complete hydrolysis of caffeic acid conjugates, and the lower bound assumes only 10% hydrolysis.
[c]From Herrmann (1978).

Table 5-2 Continued

[d]Risch and Herrmann (1988) report that caffeic acid esters are minor components in citrus. A range of 0-5 mg/kg (caffeic acid equivalents) can be calculated from concentrations of esters cited.
[e]Mean value of measured levels of outer leaves (56 and 84 ppm) and inner
leaves (43 and 71 ppm) of field grown, head lettuce (Winter and Herrmann
1986).
[f]Estimates for young children, aged 1-6, are roughly a factor of 2 higher and for
non-nursing infants under age 1, roughly a factor of 5 higher.
[g]Concentration of caffeic acid (in mg per liter of liquid) using data of Clinton
(1985), who reports 190 mg chlorogenic acid (97 mg caffeic acid equivalent) per
cup of drip-brewed 6.7 ounce (197 ml) cup of coffee and a national average
consumption of 3.58 cups per day for coffee drinkers. To estimate intake for
the general population, it was assumed that 41% were coffee drinkers (USDA
Continuing Food Consumption Survey for 1989-1991). Lower intake value
assumes 10% hydrolysis of chlorogenic acid in the digestive tract; upper value
assumes complete hydrolysis.

conjugates was assumed in deriving the upper bound and 10%
hydrolysis in deriving the lower bound. Estimates of average daily
intake of caffeic acid from food for the general population were
0.02-0.2 mg/kg. Daily intakes for high consumers of produce can
be considerably greater (e.g., the 95th percentile estimates for children aged 1-6 are 0.2-3 mg/kg). Estimates of caffeic acid intake
from coffee for moderately high consumers are also considerably
higher: 0.9-9 mg/kg for the general population.

Most exposure to natural furocoumarins is derived from limes
and other citrus and umbelliferous plants, with *per capita* exposure
estimated to be 1.3 mg per day (Wegstaff 1991).

Derived

Included in this group are compounds generated by cooking (e.g.,
polycyclic aromatic hydrocarbons [PAHs], heterocyclic amines,

benzene, and glycidaldehyde), and those compounds that appear in preserved or cured foods (e.g., nitrosamines) and in technologically altered foods.

PAHs are present in a variety of prepared foods. They can be endogenously produced, or enter food through environmental contamination from both natural (e.g., forest fires) and anthropogenic sources (IARC 1983). The potential for high exposures to benzo(a)-pyrene, one of the most potent carcinogenic PAHs, is greatest with consumption of charred meats, smoked fish, vegetable oils, tea, roasted coffee, and some fruits and vegetables.

The formation of heterocyclic amines during the cooking of proteinaceous foods was discussed earlier. Data are limited concerning the intake of these substances. Layton et al. (1995) analyzed the consumption of foods containing five of the principal heterocyclic amines by 3,563 persons who provided 3-day dietary records in a USDA-sponsored survey conducted in 1989. They calculated average intakes (ng/kg per day) of the five principal heterocyclic amines as follows: PhIP, 16.64; AαC, 5.17; MeIQx, 2.61; DiMeIQx, 0.81; and IQ, 0.28. One of the study authors indicates that these calculated intake levels are probably (within a factor of 5) those consumed by the average person, but that the intake for high consumers of meats cooked "well-done" (95th percentile) could be considerably greater than the average value (J.S. Felton, Lawrence Livermore National Laboratory, personal communication).

Preformed *N*-nitroso compounds may be present in the diet, mainly in foods cured with nitrate or nitrite. Cured meats and beer are the most important sources of nitrosamines. In 1981, the National Research Council (NRC 1981) estimated the daily intake of nitrosamines from dietary sources to be 1.1 µg; the same estimate was obtained for 1979 for *N*-nitrosodimethylamine intake by males in Germany (Preussmann 1984). Estimates of *N*-nitrosodimethylamine intake from food have recently been published for European countries, and U.S. intake levels are expected to be similar. Daily intakes of *N*-nitrosodimethylamine from food were estimated to be roughly 0.1 µg (≈ 0.0014 µg/kg-bw) in eastern France (Biaudet et al. 1994), 0.2 µg (≈0.003 µg/kg-bw in West Germany; Tricker et al. 1991), and, for all volatile nitrosamines, less than 0.1 µg in the Netherlands (Ellen et al. 1990).

N-nitrosodimethylamine levels in beer of 1-5 ppb were common in the early 1980's (Scanlan 1983), and in 1981 a National Research Council (NRC 1981) committee estimated a daily consumption of 0.9 µg (≈0.027 µg/kg-bw) from a level of 2.8 µg/l in beer (Scanlan and Barbour 1991). A recent analysis of nearly 200 U.S. and Canadian beers by Scanlan and Barbour (1991) found a mean concentration level of 0.074 µg/kg; current daily consumption (apparently for beer consumers) of *N*-nitrosodimethylamine from beer was estimated to be around 0.026 µg (≈0.00037 µg/kg-bw), or about 3% of the value a decade ago. The decrease in exposure from the 1981 NRC value was due to measures taken to reduce the formation of *N*-nitrosodimethylamine in malt. Concentrations of roughly 0.5 µg/kg were observed for a few types of beer, and thus high consumers of those beers would be exposed to relatively high levels of *N*-nitrosodimethylamine. Concentrations roughly double those observed by Scanlan and Barbour (1991) were reported for analyses of 170 retail samples of beer by Massey et al. (1990) (range <0.1 to 1.2 µg/kg, with mean of 0.2 µg/kg).

In addition to preformed *N*-nitroso compounds, humans are exposed to a wide range of nitrogen-containing compounds and nitrosating agents that can react in vivo to form *N*-nitroso compounds (Bartsch 1991), including *N*-nitrosodimethylamine (Pignatelli et al. 1991). Residual nitrites in cured meats and fish are an important source of nitrosating agents in the stomach (NRC 1989a). Potentially endogenous formation can lead to exposures substantially higher than from direct ingestion of preformed compounds. The above calculations do not account for endogenous formation of *N*-nitroso compounds.

Urethane is formed naturally in fermented beverages and foods, such as alcoholic beverages, leavened bread, soy sauce, yogurt, and olives, and has also been measured in milk (Battaglia et al. 1990, Zimmerli and Schlatter 1990, Dunn et al. 1991). High levels in beverages have been associated with the use of urea as a yeast food and the use of the antimicrobial agent diethylpyrocarbonate. Both of these uses are now prohibited in the U.S. Tabulations of reported measured levels in most fermented foods are in the low parts per billion, with the mean values falling below 1 ppb for cheese, milk, and yogurt, and below 10 ppb for bread (Battaglia et al. 1990, Dunn et al. 1991). Somewhat higher levels have been observed for soy sauce, with mean values reported ranging from 4.4 to 18 ppb. Single samples of other fermented foods also indicate possible levels in the low ppb range: olives (1.1 ppb), sauerkraut (0.3 ppb), orange juice (1.5 ppb), apple vinegar (3.3 ppb). Assuming that a level of 1 ppb occurs in milk products, taking mean levels reported in the literature for the other food items, and using the results from the USDA Continuing Survey of Food Intakes by Individuals (as codified by TAS 1995a,b), estimates for daily intake of urethane in food were obtained: 1.4×10^{-5} mg/kg for the general population, and 4.4×10^{-5} mg/kg for children aged 1-6, with an upper 95th percentile for this group of 9.5×10^{-5}. The greatest contribution was from milk products, for which data are scanty and an upper bound concentration estimate was used; thus, the intake results should be seen as upper bound estimates. The estimate for the general population is in the range of that for the Swiss population published by Zimmerli and Schlatter (1991; 10-20 ng/kg-bw, i.e., 10 to 20×10^{-5} mg/kg). Zimmerli and Schlatter report intakes moderately higher than those received from food are associated with consumption of wine and spirits; moderate consumption of wine (95th percentile for general population) was associated with approximately a 5-fold increase over the mean population level. However, moderate daily consumption of stone fruit distillates (30 ml/day) can increase exposure by roughly 60 fold (Zimmerli and Schlatter 1991) to roughly 0.01 mg/kg.

Acquired

Included in this group are naturally occurring chemicals absorbed by food organisms from the environment (e.g., lead) and mycotoxins (e.g., aflatoxin, ochratoxin, sterigmatocystin, and toxins derived from *Fusarium moniliforme*). Of the agents in this group studied for carcinogenicity and found to be carcinogenic, mycotoxins are predominant and have the greatest human exposure potential. Exposures to the mycotoxins aflatoxin, fumonisin B1, and sterigmatocystin are described below:

• *Aflatoxin.* Levels of aflatoxin in crops vary geographically and over time, with the southeastern United States frequently referred to as an area where high levels in corn can occur. Field corn, which is primarily used for animal feed and milling, has been the primary concern. Sweet corn is considered to be of no major consequence as a source of dietary exposure to aflatoxin. Human consumption of peanuts and peanut products are the other major source of aflatoxin exposure. FDA routinely samples aflatoxin in corn and peanuts for human consumption and the American Peanut Product Manufacturers, Inc. has established a surveillance system for peanuts destined for human consumption. Using the results of the FDA surveillance for 1984-1989, and of a USDA survey (year not specified), the FDA recently estimated for a 60 kilogram person an average intake for aflatoxin B_1 of 17 ng/day from corn and peanut products. The upper 90th percentile estimate was 40 ng/day (Springer 1994). Subgroups who regularly consume large amounts of certain corn products (e.g., grits, corn tortillas), in areas where aflatoxin contamination is frequent, may be exposed to larger quantities.

• *Fumonisin B_1.* Data on fumonisin occurrence are being developed and at present are limited. In a recent tabulation by Pohland (1994), fumonisin B1 was present in a majority of samples of field corn products, with levels as follows: corn meal, average approximately 1 ppm (47/48 positive); corn flour, 0.12-0.25 (2/2); grits, average 0.2 (5/5); corn bran cereals, 0.06 - 0.33 (5/5); corn flakes 0.01 - 0.055 (4/19); fiber cereal 0.06-0.13 (2/2 positive); hominy, 0.06 (1/1); masa 0.017 (1/1); popcorn (0.01 - 0.06 (6/8); puffed corn, 0.79-6.1 (6/6); torilllas 0.06-0.12 (2/4); tortilla chips 0.03 - 0.32 (4/6). With respect to whole corn, fumonisin B_1 occurred in 9 of 27 frozen corn samples (0.08 - 0.35 ppm), 33 of 73 canned (0.03- 0.34 ppm), and 2 of 16 sweet corn samples (0.07 and 0.79 ppm). From the USDA 1978 survey data and the above concentrations, crude estimates of average daily exposures to fumonisin B1 were calculated to fall between 2×10^{-6} to 4×10^{-5} mg/kg-day. Subgroups consuming corn in areas subject to high contamination may be exposed to substantially greater levels.

• *Sterigmatocystin and ochratoxin A.* Data on sterigmatocystin occurrence and exposure are difficult to locate. IARC (1976) notes that sterigmatocystin has been found as a natural contaminant of green coffee beans (1.1 ppm) and wheat (0.3 ppm), and that it can be identified in salami inoculated with *Aspergillus versicolor.* It can also be isolated from cultures of *A. versicolor* found on country hams. Calculation of exposure estimates thus awaits better and more complete data. Ochratoxin A is a contaminant of stored grain. It appears to be relatively uncommon in the U.S., because the winter storage climates are fairly cold (Miller 1994). However, occasional outbreaks occur. IARC (1993) notes that pork products, contaminated via feed grains, can be a significant human dietary source of ochratoxin A.

Pass-Through

Inorganic metals and organic contaminants, such as polycyclic aromatic hydrocarbons (PAHs), can enter the food supply following uptake by plants and animals from the environment. Levels of some PAHs in vegetables decrease, for example, with increased distance from industrial centers and highways (Shibamato and Bjeldanes 1993). In fact, environmental contamination is seen as a major source of relatively high PAH levels observed in vegetable oil (Shibamoto and Bjeldanes 1993), fresh vegetables, meats, seafoods, oils, grains, and fruits (IARC 1983). Vegetation, especially that with a high lipid content, can be a major vehicle for removing PAHs from the atmosphere (Simonich and Hites 1994). Examples of benzo(a)pyrene levels due to uptake include: cereal (0.2-4 ppb), grain (0.7-2.3 ppb), flour (dried, 4 ppb), lettuce (2.8-12.8 ppb), margarine (0.9-36 ppb), coconut fat (0.9-43 ppb), and sunflower oil (different reports: 0.2; 5; 29-62 ppb).

Intentional Food Additives and Constituents of Spices

Intentional food additives are plotted in Figure 5-1 in decreasing order of annual per capita disappearance, which reflects usage in food. Disappearance exceeds actual human intake because of wastage and losses due, for example, to volatilization and leaching during processing, storage, distribution, and final preparation. The data were compiled in 1980 from NAS surveys, supplemented and checked against independently acquired information. Dietary patterns change only slowly; e.g., sucrose, the dominant caloric sweetener in 1980, has been replaced in part by low-fructose corn syrup, but this has not altered the overall pattern of ingredient usage.

In this figure (5-1), section 1 of the curve contains the caloric sweeteners, major functional ingredients such as acidifiers, but no spices or flavors. Section 2 contains pH-adjusting agents, processing aids, and a few major spices and flavors, such as vanilla extract, the synthetic flavor vanillin, and black pepper. Section 3 consists largely of minor spices and herbs, essential oils, and the major synthetic flavors. Section 4 of the curve, below a few milligrams per year, contains most of the flavors added to foods and a few of the

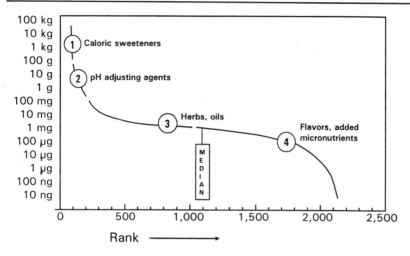

Figure 5-1 Rank ordering of food ingredients by per capita annual disappearance.

smaller-volume, intentionally added micronutrients. The median intake of the entire group is approximately 1 mg per person per year.

Some substances, such as nitrate and nitrite, occur as natural components and as intentional additives. Nitrate is reduced endogenously to nitrite. Although there is no evidence that either nitrate or nitrite alone is carcinogenic, nitrite consumed with nitrosatable amines results in the endogenous formation of carcinogenic nitrosamines.

Dietary nitrate intake is estimated to vary from about 75 to 270 mg (NRC 1981). The extent to which nitrate is reduced endogenously to nitrite depends on gastric acidity and the nature and number of bacteria present. Dietary nitrite intakes are much lower than those of nitrate.

Vegetables are the primary source of nitrate and nitrite in food, although cured meat and dairy products also contribute to overall exposure. Concentrations of nitrate in vegetables depend on agricultural practices, the temperature and light in which they are grown, the concentrations of nitrate in the soil, fertilizers, and water used to grow the vegetables, and on storage conditions (NRC 1981).

The concentrations of nitrate and nitrite in cured-meat products depend on the curing process and on the amounts added as preservatives. Concentrations of nitrite in bacon, for example, can be as high as 120 ppm, the maximum allowed by law (9CFR 318.7B). Nitrate and nitrite are used as preservatives because of their ability to inhibit the growth of *Clostridium botulinum* (NRC 1981). However, improved manufacturing processes have led to a steady decline in the concentrations of nitrate and nitrite in preserved meats; in fact, nitrate is now used only rarely.

Dairy products contain low concentrations of nitrate and nitrite in general, rarely exceeding 5 mg/kg in milk (NRC 1981).

Approximately 100 spices and herbs are used for dietary purposes in the United States, most in very small quantities. A majority of these are available commercially and are regulated under the Food, Drug and Cosmetic Act. Some are grown in home herb gardens, and others are gathered wild. Teas made from herbs gathered by amateurs are a well-recognized cause of human poisonings. The carcinogenic properties of most of these spices have not been evaluated. Most are generally recognized as safe by the U.S. Food and Drug Administration.

The animal carcinogens so far identified in spices and flavors are listed with their plant sources and levels of occurrence in Appendix A. The appendix notes only that there has been some degree of carcinogenicity testing with some positive results reported. Among the plant constituents, those associated with spices include benzaldehyde, capsaicin, estragole, eugenol (also reported to be anticarcinogenic), and safrole. Constitutive substances reported to be inhibitors of carcinogenesis are listed in Appendix B. The comparative carcinogenic potency of constitutive and nonconstitutive substances is addressed later in this chapter.

Traditional Foods

The International Agency for Research on Cancer has identified more than 69 agents capable of causing cancer in humans, including the following whole foods and beverages: bracken fern (or fiddleheads), Chinese salted fish (Cantonese style), hot maté, betel quid (with tobacco leaves), and alcoholic beverages. The carcinogenicity of these agents was established through epidemiologic studies. With the exception of alcoholic beverages, risks of these agents are confined to relatively small groups in the United States. (For example, Chinese salted fish is used in some communities to wean infants.) However, alcoholic beverages are consumed by a relatively large subpopulation at moderate to high levels.

Recent advances in genetic engineering are expected to lead to the development of new technologically altered foods in the future. Very limited quantities of the first such technologically altered food, the Flavr/Savr™ tomato, were released for public consumption in 1994. The introduction of such novel foods may affect overall food consumption patterns by augmenting or displacing consumption of traditional foods.

Synthetic Carcinogens

Table 5-3 classifies synthetic carcinogens found in the diet into six categories: pesticide residues, potential animal drug residues, packaging or storage container migrants, residues from food processing, colors, and direct food additives. The chemicals listed under each category have been classified by IARC or NTP as carcinogens. In the remainder of this section, potential exposures to these categories of chemicals will be discussed.

Table 5-3   Synthetic Animal and Human Carcinogens[a] That Might Be Present in the Diet

Pesticide residues

Acrylonitrile, amitrole, aramite, atrazine, benzotrichloride, 1,3-butadiene, captafol, carbon tetrachloride, chlordane, chlordecone (Kepone), chloroform, 3-chloro-2-methylpropene, p-chloro-o-toluidine (impurity), chlorophenoxy herbicides, creosotes, DDD, DDE, DDT, DDVP (Dichlorvos), 1,2-dibromo-3-chloropropane, p-dichlorobenzene, 1,2-dichloroethane (ethylene dichloride), 2-dichloroethane, dichloromethane, 1,3-dichloropropene (telone), dimethylcarbamoyl chloride, 1,1-dimethylhydrazine (UDMH) (as a breakdown product and contaminant of alar), ethylene dibromide, ethylene thiourea, heptachlor, hexachlorobenzene, hexachlorocyclohexane), mirex, nitrofen (technical grade), N-nitrosodiethanolamine (atrazine contaminant), pentachlorophenol, o-phenylphenate sodium, 1,3-propane sulfone, propylene oxide, styrene oxide, sulfallate, tetrachlorodibenzo-p-dioxin (as a contaminant of chlorophenoxy herbicides), thiourea (past), toxaphene, 2,4,6-trichlorophenol

Potential animal drug residues

Diethylstilbesterol (now banned), ethinyl estradiol, medroxyprogesterone acetate, methylthiouracil, 5-(morpholinomethyl)-3-[(5-nitrofurfurylidene)-amino]-2-oxalolidione, N-[4-(5-nitro-2-furyl)-2-thiazolyl]acetamide, nortestosterone, propylthiouracil

Packaging or storage container migrants

Acrylamide[b], acrylonitrile[b], 2-aminoanthraquinone, BHA[b], 1,3-butadiene[b], chlorinated paraffins, carbon tetrachloride[b], chloroform[b], 2-diaminotoluene[b], di(2-ethylhexyl)phthalate[b], dimethylformamide[b], diethyl sulfate[b], dimethyl sulfate[b], 1,4-dioxane[b], (synthesized ethyl acrylate[b]), epichlorohydrin[b], ethylene oxide[b], ethylene thiourea, 2-methylaziridine, 4,4'-methylenedianiline, 4,4'-methylene bis(2-chloroaniline) (now prohibited), 2-nitropropane[b], 1-nitropyrene, phenyl glycidyl ether, propylene oxide[b], sodium phenyl phenate[b], sodium saccharin[b], styrene[b], styrene oxide[b], tetrachloroethylene[b], toluene diisocyanate[b], vinyl chloride[b]

Residues from food processing

Dichloromethane(as a solvent), epichlorohydrin (to crosslink starch, not now practiced), NTA trisodium salt monohydrate

Table 5-3 Continued

Residues from environmental contamination (partial list)
Tap water: acylamide, benzene, benzotrichloride, bromodichloromethane, carbon tetrachloride, chloroform, 1,2-dibromo-3-chloropropane, 1,2-dichloroethane, dichloromethane, p-dichlorobenzene, tetrachloroethylene, vinyl chloride

Particle deposition onto foods: 1,6-dinitropyrene, 1,8-dinitropyrene, 2-nitrofluorene, 1-nitropyrene, 4-nitropyrene, soots

Persistent environmental contaminants: chlordecone, hexachlorocyclohexane, DDT, DDD, DDE, polybrominated biphenyls, polychlorinated biphenyls, tetrachlorodibenzo-p-dioxin

Direct food additives[c]
BHA, potassium bromate, saccharin

---

[a]Chemicals classified by IARC as Group 1, 2A, or 2B carcinogens or by NTP as known or reasonably anticipated to be carcinogens.
[b]Agents listed in the FDA priority-based Assessment of Food Additives data base as indirect food additives (Benz 1994).
[c]Although carcinogenic agents cannot be used as food additives because of the Delaney Clause, saccharin had a congressional over-ride, and BHA appears to operate by mechanisms where low-level exposures are unlikely to pose a risk.

Pesticide Residues in Foods

Pesticide residue data can be obtained from a variety of sources, including the FDA, state regulatory agencies, the food-processing industry, retail distributors, the agricultural chemical industry, and food commodity associations. Although all these sources of information are useful, no one source is necessarily preferable to another for purposes of assessing exposure. Residue analyses are complex, difficult to perform, and expensive. All data should be judged in this context.

Residue levels depend on several factors, the most important of which are the percentage of crop acreage treated with the pesticide, the sampling design of the survey, and the analytical limit of detection for the pesticide in that food. Other factors include the stability of the chemical; the time between pesticide application, harvest, and sampling; and the degree of postharvest processing.

Processing may increase, decrease, or have no effect on the concentration levels of pesticide residues in foods. Washing the raw foods tends to reduce residues, blanching reduces them further, and canning reduces them even further (Elkins 1989). For example, malathion levels in tomatoes were reduced 99% when subjected to all three processes. However, ethylene thiourea (ETU) levels in frozen turnips increased 94.5% as a result of maneb degradation during cooking in a saucepan. Similarly, when the plant-growth regulator Alar was used in apple production, the concentration of unsymmetric dimethyl hydrazine was several-fold greater in apple juice and apple sauce than in fresh apples, because of the breakdown of Alar.

In 1993, the NRC Committee on Pesticides in the Diets of Infants and Children determined that FDA's market basket sampling and analysis provided the most comprehensive residue data at this time. More than 100 different pesticides were reviewed by the NRC using the FDA surveillance data. Pesticides were detected most frequently in fresh fruits and vegetables, such as apples, peaches, pears, bananas, peas, green beans, and carrots. Detectable levels were found in less than 10% of the samples for most crop-pesticide combinations with 2-year samples larger than 25. The percentage of positive detections ranged from 0.3% for captan on carrots and peas to 50% for benomyl on peaches. Of those residues that were detected, most were well below the EPA tolerance levels. Only six crop-pesticide combinations had maximum residues exceeding EPA tolerance levels, with all mean concentrations of detected residues well below these levels.

Veterinary Drug Residues

The U.S. FDA (1985) regulates the concentrations of veterinary drugs that are known to be carcinogenic. Specifically, it requires analytical methods capable of detecting drug residues in edible meat at concentrations in the human diet that have estimated lifetime cancer risks of less than 10^{-6}. For some of the hormone residues, FDA prohibits detectable levels in edible tissues. Scheuplein (1990) estimates the total daily dose of these animal drug residues to be less than 100 ppb.

Packaging Materials

Humans may be exposed to trace quantities of chemicals that migrate into food from packaging materials. Regulations governing packaging components and their constituents are based primarily on the characteristics and uses of these materials. These characteristics and uses are very different from those of direct additives, and also from those of the indirect additives (e.g., pesticidal residues). The primary purpose of packaging is to protect the food it contains from air, moisture, light, contamination, attack by pests, tampering, quality loss, and physical damage. Packaging also can carry information and advertising, and it may aid in dispensing the food. Serving these functions requires materials that typically are insoluble, inert, and specifically intended not to enter the food or to affect it in any way other than to protect it. Moreover, the packaging regulations provide a list of thousands of options. There is no way of knowing which particular sets of options, employed in packaging each of many tens of thousands of foods, are in use across the entire food supply at any particular time. As a result, human exposures to such agents are difficult to estimate.

The most common restrictions on packaging components and their constituents are the following: good manufacturing practices

(GMP); a provision that they may be used "in an amount not to exceed that required to accomplish the desired technical effect"; and provisions that confine usage to particular technical effects (e.g., preservatives or emulsifiers). In a few instances, such as some monomers used in fabricating plastic resins, the regulation will limit the amount used or the level remaining in the packaging component or constituent to below a particular quantity. This limitation is usually based on extraction tests using specified methods. It is intended to ensure that when humans consume food that has been in contact with a component that might contain a questionable substance, such exposure cannot exceed a value that will provide a reasonable assurance of safety. The U.S. Food and Drug Administration has proposed to set a threshold for regulation to correspond to a toxicologically insignificant exposure level for food-contact substances, as described later in this chapter.

Residues from Food Processing

Carcinogenic residues can sometimes form as a result of processing. For example, cooking can increase the level of ethylene thiourea, a degradation product of maneb and related pesticides, and was observed to dramatically increase the levels of unsymmetric dimethyl hydrazine in apple products due to the degradation of Alar. Methylene chloride residues introduced during the production of decaffeinated coffee were the subject of considerable concern.

Direct Food Additives

A variety of additives are allowed into the final food product to assure its safety in the package. It is important to note that this vast array of substances are strictly regulated by the FDA. Among these additives are antioxidants.

One of these direct food additives is the antioxidant butylated hydroxyanisole (BHA), which is generally recognized as safe by the FDA at levels less than 0.02% of the fat content of food. It is also codified as a prior-sanctioned ingredient for use in food-packaging materials. Products that may contain BHA include breakfast cereals, potato flakes, poultry and meat products, sausage, shortenings, oils, food packaging materials, dessert and beverage mixes, glazed fruits, chewing gum, and flavoring agents. Based on the NRC (1979) report, *Use and Intake of Food and Color Additives*, estimates of mean BHA intakes for various age groups ranged from 0.12 to 0.35 mg/kg day. At the 90th percentile, intakes ranged from 0.27 to 0.76 mg/kg-day It should be noted that an ad hoc expert panel of the Federation of American Societies for Experimental Biology excluded the most recent NRC estimates of BHA intake data from consideration because it was felt that the estimates (which were about 25% the previous NRC values) were tempered by lack of survey compliance data.

Anticarcinogens

Fiber

There is a paucity of data on the amounts and kinds of dietary fiber in foods. Although data for crude fiber are available in food-composition tables, this is an inadequate indicator of dietary fiber because the method of analysis for crude fiber involves treatment of foods with acids and alkalies that destroy many of the components of dietary fiber (NRC 1989). The first surveys to include an estimate of dietary fiber were the 1985 and 1986 CSFIIs (USDA 1987). In these surveys, dietary fiber included the insoluble fraction (neutral detergent fiber) and soluble fraction (such as gums in cereal grains and pectin in fruits and vegetables). Foods highest in dietary fiber include whole (unrefined) grains and breads made from them, legumes, vegetables, fruits, nuts, and seeds. According to the 1985

CSFII Survey, average intake of dietary fiber per day for women 19 to 50 years of age was 10.9g; for children 1 to 5 years old, 9.8g (both based on 4 days of intake); and for men 19 to 50 years old, 18g (based on a 1-day intake).

The 1986 CSFII (USDA 1987) indicated that women in the west and midwest sections of the U.S. had higher intakes of dietary fiber than those in the south or northeast.

Micronutrients

Several nutrients, including vitamins A, C, D, E, folic acid, calcium, selenium, and iron, have been extensively studied in cancer chemoprevention. Intake of these agents, particularly vitamins A, C, calcium, and iron, has been estimated in food consumption surveys. Data on the intake of vitamins D, E (alpha-tocopherol or alpha-TE), selenium, and folic acids in foods are less complete.

A previous NRC report (1989a) reviewed the intake of vitamins A, C, D, E, folic acid, calcium, and iron from major food sources in relation to the recommended daily allowances (RDAs) for these substances. The RDA of vitamin A ranges from 400 to 1,000 µg depending on age, with additional supplements recommended for pregnant and lactating women. Although this RDA is not achieved by all individuals, the 1985 CSFII indicated that the majority of the population appeared to consume the recommended levels. Intakes tended to be lower among low-income groups and higher in the western United States. RDAs for vitamin C range from 35 to 60 mg, again with supplements for pregnant and lactating women. Both the 1985 CSFII and the 1977 NFCS indicated average intakes of this vitamin exceeding the RDA, with intakes positively correlated with economic status. RDAs for vitamin D range from 5 to 10 µg; however, its intake is only estimated in national surveys monitoring food consumption, because little information is available on vitamin D in foods. The RDAs for vitamin E range from

3 to 4 mg for children to 11 mg for lactating women. Vitamin E intakes were first reported in the 1985 CSFII, with average intake levels near or above the RDA.

The RDAs for folic acid range from 35 to 40 μg for infants to 800 μg for pregnant women. Data from the 1985 CSFII indicate average intakes of 305 μ/day and 189 μg/day for men and women 19 to 50 years of age, respectively. Results for folic acid are limited by the inherent variability in laboratory methods of analysis of folacin in foods, and by the high percentage of folacin concentrations in foods that were imputed rather than measured.

Calcium RDAs range from 360 mg to 1,200 mg in children 11 to 18 years of age and in pregnant or lactating women. Mean intakes of calcium were less than the RDA in most population subgroups, although men 19 to 50 years of age consumed an average of 115% of the RDA in the 1985 CSFII.

RDAs for iron range from 10 to 18 mg. While the mean intake among children 1 to 5 years old was 78% of the RDA, only 4% of women met or exceeded the RDA.

Estimates of selenium intake for the U.S. population range from 0.071 to 0.152 mg selenium/day (Schrauzer and White 1978, Welsh et al. 1981, FDA 1982, Levander 1987, Schubert et al. 1987, Pennington et al. 1989).

Non-Nutritive Constituents

Several investigations suggest that non-nutrient components of plants consumed in the diet contribute significantly to cancer prevention. Of particular interest are members of the flavonoid class, such as quercetin and kaempferol glycosides, which are widely distributed in foods. Others include isoflavonoids and phytoestrogens. However, unlike the nutrients, intakes of non-nutritive constituents have not been extensively studied. No quantitative exposure information is available on the anticarcinogenic non-nutritive constituents. Their numerous conjugated forms in plants have not been investigated, and estimates of exposure are further complicated because these constituents are hydrolyzed in the gut to other products.

Comparisons of Exposure Predictions for Naturally Occurring and Synthetic Carcinogens

Predicted exposure levels to some of the naturally occurring and synthetic carcinogens in the diet are provided in Tables 5-4 and 5-5. These estimates are subject to considerable uncertainty, and should be considered ballpark figures, accurate to at most an order of magnitude.

MEASURES OF CARCINOGENIC POTENCY

To estimate cancer risks, information is required on the carcinogenic potency of the agent of interest, in addition to the level of exposure to the agent. Recent developments in measuring carcinogenic potency are related to the TD_{50} index introduced by Peto et al. (1984a) and Sawyer et al. (1984). Formally, the TD_{50} is defined as the dose that reduces the proportion of tumor-free animals by 50% at a specified point in time. Letting P(d) denote the probability of a tumor occurring at dose d, the TD_{50} is that dose d that satisfies the equation

$$R(d) = [P(d)-P(0)]/[1-P(0)] = 0.5, \tag{1}$$

where R(d) is the extra risk over background at dose d. Note that the TD_{50} is inversely related to potency, in the sense that the more potent the carcinogen, the lower the TD_{50}. Thus, once the dose-

Table 5-4 Predicted Daily Intake Levels of Selected Naturally Occurring Carcinogens in the Diet

	Daily Intake (μg/kg-bw/day)	
	U.S. Population Average	High Consumers
Constitutive		
Caffeic acid		
Food	20-200	60-600 (upper 95 percentile estimate for children ages 1-6)
Coffee[a]	200-2,000	900-9,000 (upper 95 percentile adult)
8-methoxypsoralen(xanthotoxin)	0.5	2 (children ages 1-6)
Derived		
PhIP[b]	0.017 (0.003-0.085)	0.2 (high consumers of well-done meats)
Urethane		
Food[c]	<0.02	<0.1 (children)
Alcohol[d]	0.001-0.003	0.014 (average per day when consumed) 1 (moderate consumption of imported fruit brandy (1 dl/day))
N-nitrosodimethylamine		
Food[e]	0.001-0.003	0.002 (average on days consumed)
Beer[f] 1990	0.00005-0.0001	0.07
1980	0.002	
Acquired		
Aflatoxin[g]	0.0003	0.0007 (90th percentile consumer)

[a]See Table 5-2 and accompanying text for details.

Table 5-4 Continued

[b]Estimate derived by Layton et al. (1995). Values in parenthesis indicate the judgment of one of the study authors regarding the plausible range for the actual average. See text for details. USDA CSFII and the ranges of concentrations of PhIP observed in foods cooked at different temperatures for different periods of time suggests that high consumers of well-done meats could consume at least 10 times that of the average individual.

[c]Calculated on the basis of USDA CSFII using Exposure 1® and 4® (TAS 1995a) and concentration levels reported in the literature. The results should be considered upper bounds. The greatest contributions were calculated to occur from milk products, for which the upper estimate for urethane concentration of 1 ppb was used.

[d]Population averages and the value for moderate wine drinkers were derived from U.S. average concentrations from the sampling effort of the Bureau of Alcohol, Tobacco, and Firearms (BATF 1987, 1988) as reported by Dunn et al. (1991) and USDA survey data using the Exposure 1® and 4® (TAS 1995a) to model beer and wine consumption. Similar figures were derived from the per capita consumption data of the National Institute on Alcohol Abuse and Alcoholism (1988).

[e]Derived from food intake levels reported by Biaudet et al. (1994) and Tricker et al. (1991) for eastern France and West Germany, respectively. Based on earlier reports (Preussman 1984, NRC 1981) U.S. values are expected to be similar.

[f]U.S. beer consumption assumed to follow 1989-1991 USDA CFSII, as modeled by Exposures 1® and 4® (TAS 1995a). For 1990 average population estimates, lower bound corresponds to the average concentration of 0.074 µg/kg reported by Scanlan and Barbour (1991); upper bound estimates to that by Massey et al. (1990). For high consumer estimates, the lower bound is for contamination of average levels, and the upper bound represents consumers of highly contaminated beer (by today's standards). For the 1980 estimate, an average concentration of 2.8 µg/kg (Scanlan and Barbour 1991) was assumed.

[g]Derived from average and upper bound estimates presented by the US FDA (Springer 1994); see text for details.

response relationship P(d) has been determined, the TD_{50} may be estimated from equation (1).

More generally, the TD_{100p} is the dose corresponding to an excess risk of 0<p<1. In this chapter, the TD_{01} will also be considered as the basis for comparing the potency of naturally occurring and synthetic carcinogens. The TD_{01} is closer to human exposure levels,

Table 5-5 Predicted Daily Exposure Levels of Selected Synthetic Carcinogens in the Diet

	Daily Intake ($\mu g/kg\text{-}bw/day$)	
	U.S. Population Average	High Consumers[a]
Pesticide Residues		
DDD, DDE, and DDT 1954 (DDE and DDT)[a]	4	
1965 (DDT)[a]	0.57	28
Ethylene thiourea[b]	0.2; 0.6	
Unsymmetrical dimethyl-hydrazine (UDMH) - 1989[b]	0.05	0.4 (average non-nursing infant)
Packaging Migrants		
Diethylhexylphthalate		
1982 report[c]	83	
1991 report[d]	4	29
Environmental Contaminants		
TCDD equivalents from PCDDs and PCDFs[e]	$1 - 3 \times 10^{-6}$	7×10^{-5} (average nursing infant, to age 6 months)
Polychlorinated biphenyls[f]	0.2	4.2 (average nursing infant, to age 6 months)
γ-Hexachloro-cyclohexane[g]		
1964-1969	0.05	
1980	0.003	
1988	0.001	

	Daily Intake (µg/kg-bw/day)	
	U.S. Population Average	High Consumers[a]
Intentional Food Additives		
Butylated hydroxyanisole[h]	120-350	270-760 (90th percentile intakes for different age groups)
Potassium bromate[i]	--	0.08 (high consumer of bread with relatively high residues)
Saccharin - 1977[j]	120	650; 2,200 (upper 95th and 99th percentile for the general population)

[a]From WHO 1979.

[b]Larger value from US EPA (1989a), lower value corresponds to more recent residue data and account for discontinued uses subsequent to the 1989 analysis (EPA 1992).

[c]DHHS (1982).

[d]DHHS (1991).

[e]Average intake estimated by Fürst et al. (1991) for industrialized countries. WHO (1988) estimated average intake via breast milk for nursing infants aged 0 to 6 months.

[f]From WHO (1988, 1993). A somewhat lower estimate (1.9 µg/kg-d) can be calculated from the figures of Rogan et al. (1991) for infants nursing for 9 months on breast milk contaminated at the 90th percentile level (2.97 ppm).

[g]From US FDA total diet study, as summarized by WHO (1991).

[h]Taken from NRC (1979a). Comparable levels were found more recently by Kirkpatrick and Lauer (1986) for intake in Canada, which imposes similar constraints on BHA concentration in fats (mean intakes of 0.13-0.39 mg/kg-bw/day, depending on age group).

[i]Potassium bromate was used widely, but usage is declining (Ranum 1992, Jackel 1994). Analytical techniques to reliably detect concentrations less than 1 ppm in bread have not been available until recently (Ranum 1992). NRC (1979a) reported an average value of 1.8 µg/kg-bw-day, but indicated that it was an overestimate. The figure for the high consumer in the table corresponds to an upper bound consumer of bread (at 100 grams/day) with 50 µg/kg potassium bromate (see, e.g., Dennis et al., 1994).

Table 5-5 Continued

[j]From the NRC (1979b). These were similar to the results from a study by Market Research Corporation of America for the NRC (1978) Committee for a Study on Saccharin and Food Safety, but averages for teenage consumption (not reported in the table) were lower by factors of 2-3 for surveys done during the same period (see Morgan et al. 1982).

yet still not sufficiently low that it depends strongly on the dose-response model chosen to represent P(d).

Sawyer et al. (1984) used a hazard function of the form

$$\lambda(t;d) = (1+\beta d)\lambda_0(t), \qquad (2)$$

where $\lambda_0(t)$ denotes the baseline hazard at time t in the absence of exposure. Use of this function leads to an essentially linear dose-response relationship

$$P(d;T) = 1\text{-exp}\{-[\lambda_0(T)+\beta d]T\} \qquad (3)$$

at a fixed time T, in the absence of mortality from causes other than tumor occurrence. Other hazard functions based on either the empirical or biologically based dose-response models could be used to accommodate nonlinear dose-response relationships (Krewski et al. 1992).

Ideally, the time of tumor occurrence would be used as the basis for statistical inference about the hazard function for tumor induction. Unfortunately, because most tumors in laboratory animals are unobservable before sacrifice, the tumor onset time is generally unknown. Sawyer et al. (1984) avoided this problem by using the time of death of those animals with tumors as a proxy for the time of tumor onset. Although this assumption is appropriate for tumors that are rapidly lethal, Portier and Hoel (1987) found that estimates of the TD_{50} are quite sensitive to assumptions about tumor lethality.

Finkelstein and Ryan (1987) addressed this problem by using the methods of Peto et al. (1980) for combining tumor mortality and prevalence data to estimate the TD_{50}. Bailar and Portier (1993) used survival-adjusted quantal response data as described by Bailar and Portier (1988) to estimate the TD_{50}. Dewanji et al. (1993) used Weibull models for the time of tumor onset, the time to death due to tumor occurrence, and the time to death from competing risks to estimate the TD_{50}. This latter approach can be applied to rapidly lethal or incidental tumors, or to those of unknown lethality.

Gold et al. (1984, 1986, 1987, 1990, 1993, 1995) have tabulated the TD_{50} values for a large number of chemical carcinogens in their Carcinogenic Potency Database (CPDB). The TD_{50} values in the CPDB were calculated using the statistical methods developed by Sawyer et al. (1984). All TD_{50} values are expressed in common units of mg/kg body weight/day, and corrected for intercurrent mortality whenever individual animal survival times are available. The CPDB currently includes data on over 4,000 experiments on more than 1,000 different chemicals. The carcinogenic potency of these chemicals expressed in terms of the TD_{50} varies by more than 10 million fold.

Although the TD_{50} represents a useful measure of carcinogenic potency, it is based on experimental observation at doses generally well above those to which humans may be exposed. Another measure of potency, which has been used by the U.S. Environmental Protection Agency (1986a), is the estimate of the linear term q_1 in the multistage model

$$P(d) = 1 - \exp\{-(q_0 + q_1 d + \ldots + q_k d^k)\},$$

where $P(d)$ denotes the probability of tumor occurrence at dose d. Because the extra risk $P(d) - P(0)$ is approximated by $R(d) = q_1 d$ at low doses, the value of q_1 may be used to estimate the risk associated with environmental exposures to a dose d of a carcinogen. In practice, an upper confidence limit q_1^* on the value of q_1 is used, because of the instability of the maximum likelihood estimate of the linear term in the multistage model (Crump 1984). This application is commonly referred to as the linearized multistage (LMS) model and represents an upper bound on risk. This procedure was used to estimate the TD_{01}, later in this report, for comparing the carcinogenic potencies of naturally occurring and synthetic carcinogens.

Another approach for estimating low-dose risks is the model-free extrapolation (MFX) method proposed by Krewski et al. (1991). This procedure assumes that the dose-response curve is linear only at low doses and is based on a series of secant approximations to the low-dose region. Upper confidence limits on the slope of the dose-response curve based on MFX are generally close to the values of q_1^* obtained from the LMS model.

Although the preceding measures of carcinogenic potency are useful, they are subject to certain limitations. The TD_{50} is based on data obtained at high doses and may not reflect potency at low doses. Krewski et al. (1990) noted that the TD_{50} will exceed the highest dose used in animal cancer tests in some cases and thus require extrapolation outside the range of the experimental data. Because the TD_{50} can vary appreciably with the period of exposure (Dewanji et al. 1993), it is important that $TD_{50}s$ used for comparative purposes be standardized. When data on the dependency of cancer risk on age and exposure time are not available, standardization of TD_{50} values in the Carcinogenic Potency Database is done under the assumption that risk increases in proportion to time to the second power. Inferences about carcinogenic potency at low doses require extrapolation of animal bioassay data to low doses outside of the experimentally observable range. In the absence of information to the contrary, extrapolation is generally performed under the assumption that the dose-response relationship is linear at low doses.

To avoid low-dose and high-dose extrapolation, an intermediate measure of potency such as the TD_{05} or TD_{10} is preferred. The TD_{01} represents perhaps the lowest indicator of carcinogenic potency that remains near the experimentally observable response range and is used in the comparison of potencies of naturally occurring and synthetic carcinogens presented in a later section of this chapter. Van Ryzin (1980), Farmer et al. (1982), and Gaylor et al. (1994) used the TD_{01} as the basis for linear extrabolation to lower doses. Krewski et al. (1993) showed that the TD_{50}s of rodent carcinogens, based on either the one-stage or multistage models, are tightly clustered around their MTDs. For the one-stage model, $TD_{01} = TD_{50}/69$.

Correlation Between Cancer Potency and Other Measures of Toxicity

Several investigators have noted a strong correlation between the TD_{50} and the MTD (Bernstein et al. 1985, Gaylor, 1989, Krewski et al. 1989, Reith and Starr 1989, Freedman et al. 1993). This correlation (r=0.924) is illustrated in Figure 5-2 using a sample of 191 carcinogens selected from the CPDB (Krewski et al. 1993). Although the TD_{50} values used in this analysis are based on an essentially linear dose-response model, the correlation is equally high when it is obtained with TD_{50}s estimated using the Armitage-Doll multistage model. Bernstein et al. (1985) attributed this high correlation to the limited range of possible TD_{50} values relative to the MTD, and to the large variation among MTDs for different chemicals. Subsequent analytical results by Kodell et al. (1990) and Krewski et al. (1993) support this argument.

Krewski et al. (1989) noted that the values of q_1^* derived from the linearized multistage model fitted to 263 data sets were also highly correlated with the maximum doses. As with the TD_{50}, this association between q_1^* and the MTD occurs as a result of the limited range of values that q_1^* can assume once the MTD is

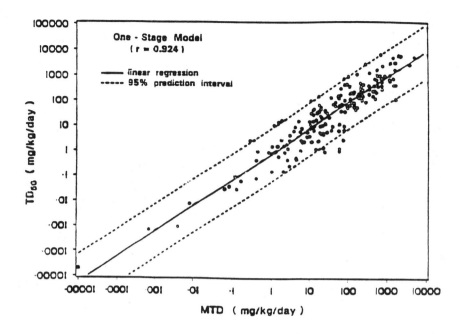

Figure 5-2 Association between carcinogenic potency and MTD. Source: NRC 1993b.

established. This correlation is illustrated in Figure 5-3 using the same data presented in Figure 5-2. As indicated in Figure 5-3, there is a strong negative correlation between q_1^* and the MTD. Thus, the MTD has a strong influence on measures of carcinogenic potency at both high and low doses.

The absence of points in the upper lefthand triangular region in Figure 5-2 is due to the lower limit on the number of tumors required for statistical significance observed in the exposed groups. This limit implies that highly toxic chemicals of weak carcinogenic potency would likely go undetected in a standard bioassay, because such agents would not yield a measurable excess of tumors at the MTD (NRC 1993b). Crouch et al. (1987) attribute the absence of points in the lower right hand triangular region (Figure 5-2) to a

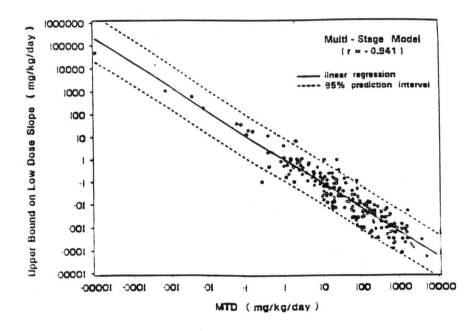

Figure 5-3 Association between upper bounds on low-dose slope and MTD.
Source: NRC 1993b.

lack of chemicals with extremely high potencies relative to their MTDs. An informal search for such "supercarcinogens" conducted by the National Research Council (1993b) failed to reveal any points clearly embedded in this region.

The relationship between acute toxicity and carcinogenic potency has been the subject of several investigations. Parodi et al. (1982) found a significant correlation (r = 0.49) between carcinogenic potency and acute toxicity. Zeise et al. (1982, 1984, 1986) reported a high correlation between acute toxicity, as measured by the LD_{50}, and carcinogenic potency. Metzger et al. (1989) reported somewhat lower correlations (r = 0.6) between the LD_{50} and TD_{50} for 264 carcinogens selected from the CPDB. McGregor (1992) calculated the correlation between the TD_{50} and LD_{50} for different classes of carcinogens considered by IARC. The highest correlations were observed in IARC Group 1 carcinogens (i.e., known human carcinogens) with $r = 0.72$ for mice and $r = 0.91$ for rats, based on samples of size 9 and 8, respectively. Goodman and Wilson (1992) calculated the correlation between the TD_{50} and LD_{50} for 217 chemicals that they classified as being either genotoxic or nongenotoxic. The correlation coefficient for genotoxic chemicals was approximately $r = 0.4$ regardless of whether rats or mice were used, whereas the correlation coefficient for nongenotoxic chemicals was approximately $r = 0.7$. Haseman and Seilkop (1992) showed that chemicals with low MTDs (i.e., high toxicity) were somewhat more likely to be rodent carcinogens than chemicals with high MTDs, but this association was limited primarily to gavage studies.

Travis et al. (1990a,b, 1991) investigated the correlation between the TD_{50} and composite indices based on mutation, toxicity, reproductive anomalies, and tumorigenicity data derived from the Registry of Toxic Effects of Chemical Substances (RTECS) (Sweet, 1987). This analysis confirmed the previously reported correlation of $r = 0.4$ between mutagenic potency in the Ames assay and the TD_{50} estimated from rodent carcinogenicity studies (McCann et al. 1988, Piegorsch and Hoel 1988); the correlation of $r = 0.7$ between LD_{50} and TD_{50} was also somewhat greater than that reported by Metzger et al. (1989). Using all of the RTECS assays, the correlation of the composite potency index with the TD_{50} was $r = 0.80$, 0.87, or 0.79, depending on whether data for rats, mice, or the most sensitive species were used.

Hoel et al. (1988) explored the relationships between toxicity and carcinogenicity for 99 chronic studies conducted in rodents. Only seven of the 53 carcinogenicity studies reporting positive results exhibited target organ toxicity that could have been the cause of observed carcinogenic effects. Those findings suggested that only a small number of chemical carcinogens that induce tumors in rodents solely by indirect mechanisms may be limited.

Tennant et al. (1991) examined 31 chemicals, of which 22 were classified as rodent carcinogens. Regardless of their mutagenic potential, chronic toxicity was not always sufficient to produce neoplasia. This suggests that effects other than mutagenicity or toxicity may be responsible for the carcinogenicity of some chemicals.

Gaylor and Gold (1995) used the correlation between the MTD and cancer potency to obtain preliminary estimates of cancer risk based on the 90-day MTD and not on 2-year bioassays in rodents. Using results from studies conducted by the National Toxicology Program, estimates of the regulatory virtually safe dose (VSD), corresponding to an estimated maximum lifetime cancer risk of less than one per million, were obtained by linear low-dose extrapolation for 139 rodent carcinogens. Based on these cases, the geometric mean ratio of the MTD to the VSD was 740,000. Of the 139 cases examined, only five ratios differed from the mean ratio by more than a factor of 10. Here, the VSD is roughly a small fraction of the rodent test doses. A similar result can be obtained using the acute toxicity measure the LD_{50}, compared with a dose corresponding to an estimated risk of less than one per million (Zeise et al. 1984). Hence, it may not be worthwhile to conduct a chronic bioassay when levels of human exposure are so low as to suggest negligible risk (see the section below on toxicologically insignificant exposures).

Interpretation of Carcinogenic Potency

Little information is currently available on the relative potencies of various carcinogens and anticarcinogens in the human diet. Although reasonable estimates may be determined for a few substances, such as aflatoxin, most of the data are sparse. Although precise potency data for humans on each substance of interest would be ideal, an absolute measure is not essential for comparative purposes, and a relative measure could serve.

Nondietary exposures may influence the degree of toxicity of dietary carcinogens and anticarcinogens. For example, cigarette smoking induces aryl hydrocarbon hydroxylase, one of the cytochrome P450 isozymes, which in turn may affect the metabolism of substances in the diet.

As noted earlier in the section, most information on the potencies of carcinogens in humans is inferred from animal experiments. In fact, the U.S. EPA *Guidelines for Carcinogen Risk Assessment* (1986a) specify that if there are adequate data demonstrating an agent's carcinogenicity in laboratory animals, it should be regulated as a human carcinogen. However, the issue of extrapolating the results of animal bioassays to humans for regulatory purposes is controversial. The current animal bioassay was designed as a qualitative screen for carcinogenicity; it was not designed to provide information on an agent's biologic mechanisms of action or on its dose-response characteristics at low doses. Most cancer bioassays use the MTD, which is generally much higher than environmental exposure levels likely to be encountered by humans. The MTD is used in cancer studies to increase the likelihood of detecting any potential carcinogenic effects of a chemical in experiments involving small numbers of laboratory animals. The problem with using such high doses is that they may cause other effects that could influence the likelihood of tumor formation; for example, high doses can lead to changes in food consumption, recurrent cytotoxicity in specific organs, hormonal imbalance, or combinations of these and other effects (NRC 1993b). Such effects have been associated with both increases and decreases in tumor incidence in laboratory animals (Reitz et al. 1980, 1990; Turnbull et al. 1985; Roe 1988). Thus, dose-response data from high dose studies can be of limited value for low-dose risk prediction (NRC 1993b). In addition, testing at high doses that result in lower body weights may reduce the incidence of some types of tumors (Turturro et al. 1993).

When quantitative estimates of human cancer risk must be made on the basis of animal data, an interspecies scaling factor may be employed. Gaylor and Chen (1986) have shown that estimates of cancer potency in rats and mice are correlated, although potencies can differ by a factor of 100-fold or more in some cases. Although quantitative interspecies extrapolation has been done on the basis of body weight or surface area in the past, Travis and White (1988) have suggested that an intermediate scaling based on body weight to the 3/4 power may be more appropriate. Watanabe et al. (1992) note that the available data do not permit one to distinguish between surface area or 3/4 scaling and that different chemicals may warrant different scaling procedures. Physiologic pharmaco-kinetic models offer a more sophisticated approach to interspecies extrapolation through the use of predicted tissue doses in the species of interest (NRC 1987). However, whenever human risks are inferred from animal test data, considerable uncertainty may remain about the magnitude of the risk.

ESTIMATING HUMAN CANCER RISKS

Risk-Estimation Methods

Estimates of human cancer risks are based primarily on findings from human epidemiologic studies or results from laboratory tests involving experimental animals. Epidemiologic studies have the advantage of providing information on carcinogenic risks directly in humans. However, the results of such studies may be subject to biases due to confounding factors or errors in exposure and disease ascertainment. Nonetheless, these studies have been used to identify 69 agents capable of causing cancer in humans. Of these, only a few (including salted fish, alcoholic beverages, and aflatoxin B_1) are present in the U.S. diet. Epidemiologic studies may not be sufficiently sensitive to detect the hazards to humans from expo-sures to low levels of carcinogens in the environment. In contrast, toxicologic studies can achieve greater sensitivity through the use of high doses and because they can be designed to control for potential sources of bias. These gains are offset to a certain extent, however, when extrapolating from high to low doses and from animals to humans. Nonetheless, about 600 chemicals have been shown to demonstrate carcinogenic potential in animal cancer tests (Gold et al. 1995).

Quantitative predictions of human cancer risk are generally obtained by fitting a suitable dose-response model to either toxicologic or epidemiologic data. Many epidemiologic studies provide little information on dose-response relationships, making it difficult to estimate risks at exposure levels different from those observed in the original study. When dose-response data are available, a linear model is often sufficient to describe the observed dose-response relationship.

Toxicologic experiments involving only two or three relatively high doses also provide limited information on dose-response. Important questions have been raised about the relevance to humans of results observed at the high doses used in laboratory studies. Ames and Gold (1990a) argue that cancer risks may be increased at high doses through the induction of mitogenic effects that would not be expected to occur at low doses. After reviewing the use of the MTD in animal cancer tests, a committee of the National Research Council (1993b) concluded that results obtained at the MTD need to be interpreted with care, although a majority of that committee saw no clear alternative at the time.

Attempts have been made to strengthen cancer risk-assessment methods through the use of biologically based risk assessment models (Goddard and Krewski 1995). Biologically based models are appealing because the model parameters have a direct biological interpretation. Such models can also lead to a greater understanding of cancer mechanisms when they fail to fit the data. In such cases, different mechanistic assumptions must be made to obtain a parsimonious description of the data.

As noted previously, the linearized multistage procedure does not enable one to account for tissue growth and cell kinetics. These features can be incorporated into multistage modeling at the expense of achieving a somewhat over-parametrized model. For this reason, simpler biologically based models, such as the two-stage clonal expansion model described by Moolgavkar and Luebeck (1990) are of value. This model is based on the assumption that two mutations are required to transform a normal cell into a cancer cell; provision is made both for natural growth of normal tissues, and for selective clonal expansion of initiated cells that have sustained the first mutation. This model has recently been used in a biologically based reanalysis of data on lung cancer in Colorado uranium miners exposed to radon and cigarette smoke (Moolgavkar et al. 1993). Other biologically based models incorporating data on metabolic activation (Krewski et al. 1994) and receptor binding (Kohn and Portier 1993) have been proposed in an attempt to build a comprehensive pharmacokinetic/pharmacodynamic risk assessment model (Andersen et al. 1993).

A clear understanding of the process of carcinogenesis and considerable data are required if the results of biologically based approaches are to be viewed with confidence. Lacking that data necessary to develop biologically based models, empirical approaches to cancer risk estimation are often invoked. If the dose-response curve is assumed to be linear in the low-dose region, estimates of human cancer risk at low doses can be obtained using the linearized multistage model described by Crump (1984), or the model-free approach to linear low-dose extrapolation discussed by Krewski et al. (1991). In practice, these two methods yield similar results. Linear extrapolation from the TD_{50} also yields similar predictions when estimating cancer risk at low doses (Krewski 1990).

Uncertainty Analysis

In the past, methods for quantitative cancer risk assessment focused on a single estimate of risk—either a best estimate or an upper-bound estimate derived from the most likely model of carcinogenesis and for the expected exposure conditions. However, such estimates are subject to variability and uncertainty. For example, both food consumption patterns and concentrations of carcinogenic substances present in the diet can vary widely, leading to appreciable variation in individual intake of dietary chemicals. Uncertainty about the mechanisms of carcinogenic action and the relative sensitivity of animals and humans leads to uncertainty about the risk associated with a given level of exposure.

Recently, attempts have been made to evaluate both variability and uncertainty in cancer risk assessment. *Pesticides in the Diets of Infants and Children* (NRC 1993a) proposed methods to describe the variation in food-consumption levels and in pesticide residues found in foods. This analysis was accomplished by combining consumption and residue distributions to arrive at a single intake distribution of pesticide residue in the diet, reflecting both sources of variation.

Using existing databases, Gaylor et al. (1993) examined the uncertainties in cancer potency estimates resulting from experiment, strain, and species variability. They concluded that estimates of potency for human carcinogens, based upon animal data, are likely to be within a factor of 110 for most cases. Cancer rates in humans are commonly estimated by basing cancer risk estimates on the most sensitive rodent species, strain, and sex, and using an interspecies dose scaling factor based on body surface area. However, this practice appears to overestimate cancer rates in humans by about an order of magnitude (Gaylor et al. 1993). Hence, for chemicals where the dose-response relationship is nearly linear at doses below the experimental range, cancer risk estimates based on animal data are not necessarily conservative. Sources of underestimation not fully addressed by these comparisons include saturable pharmacokinetics (as seen, for example, with vinyl chloride and tetrachloroethylene (Bois et al. 1994)); less-than-lifetime animal bioassay (e.g., diethylnitrosamine (Peto et al. 1984b); human occupational data (e.g., benzidine (IARC 1982)); and human heterogeneity (e.g., 4-aminobiphenyl (Bois et al. 1995)). For a more complete discussion of underestimation, see Portier and Kaplan (1989), Finkel (1995), and Zeise (1989).

Portier and Kaplan (1989) analyzed the uncertainty surrounding the values of model parameters and its impact on model-based predictions of metabolites reaching target tissues. This analysis was conducted on model parameters in physiologically based pharmacokinetic models for methylene chloride. They demonstrated that uncertainty surrounding the values of the model parameters implied considerable uncertainty in tissue doses of the proximate carcinogen. Similar analyses have been conducted by Farrar et al. (1989), Bois et al. (1990), and Hetrick et al. (1991). Methods for uncertainty analysis are described in a recent text by Morgan and Henrion (1990).

Krewski et al. (1995) proposed a general methodology for analyzing uncertainty, variability, and sensitivity in physiologically based pharmacokinetic models. This approach takes into account a number of natural constraints on the model parameters, such as the upper limit on the sum of tissue volumes imposed by total body volume. Using this approach, it is possible to evaluate the uncertainty in model-based predictions of tissue dose attributable to the uncertainty associated with individual model parameters, as well as the total uncertainty conferred by all model parameters. The impact of interindividual variability in model parameters is assessed, including physiological parameters that are related to body weight, which varies considerably among individuals. Methods are also proposed for identifying sensitive parameters that play a critical role in model-based predictions concerning metabolites. These analyses may guide efforts to improve the reliability of estimates derived for the most critical model parameters.

Finkel (1995) analyzed the uncertainties associated with the cancer risks of aflatoxin and alar (a synthetic organic growth regulator formerly used on apples). Although single estimates of risk suggested aflatoxin to be 18 times more potent than Alar, the risks of these two substances could not be distinguished when all of the relevant uncertainties were taken into account.

Mechanistic Considerations

Methods currently used to calculate cancer potencies generally do not incorporate mechanistic considerations. The methods are based on the assumption that if a chemical increases tumor rates at high doses in animal bioassays, it may increase cancer risk among human populations exposed to lower levels found in the environment or the diet. This is an important consideration because chemicals that increase tumor rates at high doses by increasing cell proliferation as a result of tissue damage may not be carcinogenic at low doses. Some chemicals in the diet that test positive in cancer bioassays using high doses may not necessarily be carcinogenic at doses likely to be encountered by humans in the environment. Therefore, studies of the carcinogenicity of some chemicals at high doses are of limited value in assessing the dose-response relationships occurring at low exposure levels that are likely to be encountered in the human diet (Cohen and Ellwein 1990, Cohen et al. 1991).

In addition, some chemicals induce cancer in rodents by mechanisms that are likely not to be operative in humans (Cohen and Ellwein 1990, Boorman et al. 1994). An example is the induction of urinary bladder cancer in male rats as a consequence of microcrystal formation after ingestion of high doses of sodium salts. Although these chemicals demonstrate carcinogenic activity in rats, they may pose little or no carcinogenic risk to humans.

The International Agency for Research on Cancer (IARC 1992) has provided guidelines on the use of mechanistic information in carcinogenic risk assessment. These guidelines allow for the possibility that certain animal carcinogens are unlikely to be human carcinogens, and are hence considered unclassifiable (Group 3) with respect to human carcinogenicity. The guidelines also allow for the classification of an agent as a human carcinogen (Group I) in the absence of positive epidemiologic evidence. Such classification could occur in the presence of strong animal evidence for carcinogenicity and molecular evidence that the agent is likely to be effective in humans.

Toxicologically Insignificant Exposure Levels

The concept of toxicologically insignificant exposures (TIE) in the regulation of certain chemical substances found in food is currently receiving considerable attention (Rulis 1986, 1989, 1992; FDA 1993), particularly indirect food additives that migrate into food from packaging materials. Under the assumption that a new chemical in a particular class is no more toxic than the most toxic chemicals previously in that class, an upper bound on the potency of the new substance can be inferred. In turn, this upper bound on potency can be used to establish a toxicologically insignificant exposure for that chemical, below which only trivial risks are assumed to arise. This concept is discussed in more detail by Munro (1990).

The concept of toxicological insignificance has advantages and disadvantages in safety assessment. Because inferences on the potential toxicity of the substance in question are made in relation to the toxicity of other chemicals, the need to perform extensive toxicity studies is eliminated. However, the assumption that a new chemical is as potent as the more potent substances in the selected reference class of chemicals may impart a high degree of conservatism in evaluating its safety, especially when this assumption is applied to all new chemicals. In addition, the possibility that the new chemical of interest may be more potent than any in the reference class cannot be ruled out.

After analyzing approximately 220 chronic toxicity studies collected from the literature, Frawley (1967) proposed a toxicologically insignificant level of exposure of 0.1 ppm for food additives and other ingredients of the human diet. Since then, several hundred chemicals have been tested for tumorigenicity in rodents. With the increasing emphasis on tumorigenicity as an endpoint in chemical regulation, and the recognition that tumorigens are more stringently regulated than other chemicals, additional studies have examined the possibility of establishing a TIE level for potentially tumorigenic indirect additives. One such attempt is that of Rulis (1992), who proposed a threshold of regulation for indirect additives (packaging materials) of 500 ppt, based on his analysis of the Carcinogenic Potency Database described earlier. However, contamination by some agents with moderately high carcinogenic activity could be a concern at this level.

Risks of Joint Exposures and Mixtures

Risk assessment methods for joint exposures and mixtures have been examined in detail by the National Research Council (1988) and the International Agency for Research on Cancer (Vainio et al. 1990). The effects of a specific dietary constitutent may be influenced by the concentrations of other carcinogens or anticarcinogens in the diet. This fact complicates the task of estimating cancer risk for a complex mixture such as food. That is, substances may not act independently, and dietary constituents may interact. Examples of such interaction are provided by the recent studies by the National Toxicology Program (NTP 1995) designed to evaluate the effect of diet restriction on chemical-induced carcinogenicity. Chronic exposure studies conducted by the NTP usually involve administration of the test chemical to rodents maintained on the basal diet ad libitum for a period of about two years. Animals maintained under these conditions typically develop obesity; in contrast, diet restriction results in leaner animals that live longer.

In the series of studies conducted by the NTP, groups of 50-60 rats and mice per dosage group were fed diet either ad libitum or in amounts that restricted mean body weights to approximately 85% of the ad libitum bodyweight. After adjusting for intercurrent mortality, the effect of butyl benzyl phthalate on the incidence of pancreatic tumors was substantially higher in animals allowed to feed ad libitum and killed after 2 years, as compared with those on restricted feed. Specifically, pancreatic tumors were not observed in animals exposed to the compound but on restricted feed and killed after 2 years, and were only observed in exposed animals on restricted feed and killed at 30 months. Salicylazosulfapyridine caused an increased incidence of liver neoplasms in male mice fed ad libitum relative to the ad libitum-fed and weight-matched controls. This increase did not occur in the restricted feed protocols; in fact, decreases in combined hepatocellular carcinomas and adenomas were observed in salicylazosulfapyridine-exposed animals on restricted feed and sacrificed after 2 years, and decreases in hepatocellular carcinomas in those sacrificed after 3 years.

A further example is the interaction of aflatoxin and hepatitis B in the induction of liver cancer, as observed in epidemiologic investigations of humans exposed to both agents. Liver cancer incidence rises more rapidly for those individuals exposed to aflatoxin and testing positive for the hepatitis B virus than for those exposed to aflatoxin but testing negative for hepatitis. Cancer potency estimates differ by approximately a factor of 10 for the two groups (Wu-Williams et al. 1992). These findings are consistent with results from molecular studies (Bressae et al. 1991, Hsu et al. 1991).

Vainio et al. (1990) note that interactions among chemicals may occur during absorption, distribution, metabolism, and excretion. Compounds may interact chemically to create new toxic components or to change the bioavailability of mixture components. The matrix in which mixture components exist, such as soil, also may alter the carcinogenicity of a mixture. Evidence from animal and human studies indicates that interactive effects may cause deviations from simple additivity of risks, although these deviations are usually much less than one order of magnitude. Vainio et al. (1990) conclude that the most relevant quantitative data for making risk estimates for complex mixtures comes from epidemiologic studies of populations exposed to the complete mixture, not from studies of individual components.

Similarly, the EPA *Guidelines for the Health Risk Assessment of Chemical Mixtures* (1986b) state that the carcinogenic effects of a mixture can best be examined by testing the mixture. In the absence of such information, test results from a similar mixture may be adequate. Estimates of carcinogenic potencies for mixtures are not usually available, whereas estimates of potencies for the primary components of a mixture may be obtained in a number of cases. Thus, the EPA guidelines further state that if estimates of the effects of interactions among the components are available, the cancer risk for the mixture can be predicted. If it can be assumed that such interactions are negligible, the cancer risk for the mixture is generally estimated from the sum of the risks of the individual components. This practice does not imply that response additivity should be considered a universal phenomenon that occurs without exception, but that it should be a default position in the absence of evidence to the contrary (Krewski and Thomas 1992). Where a series of related chemicals causes cancer by the same mechanism, and the relative potency of such chemicals is known, estimates of cancer risk associated with a mixture of such chemicals may be based on the sum of the effective doses of each component.

The presence of a chemical in a mixture may increase or decrease the carcinogenic potency of other components through the induction of detoxification enzymes or DNA repair, competition for receptors, or saturation of metabolic pathways. Experimental studies involving simultaneous exposure to high doses of two carcinogens have demonstrated both synergistic and antagonistic effects with respect to cancer risk. Interaction among components at low doses, on the other hand, may be minimal, due in part to the lack of competition for reactive agents. However, it is possible that two innocuous chemicals can combine to form a toxic compound, even at low doses.

Increased cell proliferation provides an increased opportunity for genetic events that lead to cancer. The concentration of an individual component of a mixture may not be adequate to cause mitogenesis by itself. However, the cumulative concentration of several components that increase mitogenesis by the same process may result in an increase in cell division. Hence, the cancer risk for a mixture could exceed the sum of the cancer risks of its components.

The occurrence of spontaneous tumors indicates that there are sufficient background levels of exogenous carcinogens, endogenous factors, and spontaneous tumorigenic events to produce tumors. The addition of a chemical that augments the background carcinogenic process will increase cancer risk to an extent that is proportional (linearly related) to the chemical dose at low doses. In this case, the use of a response-additive model is inappropriate, and a dose-additive model should be used (NRC 1989b). Krewski et al. (1995) reviewed this issue of additivity to background doses and low-dose linearity of risk. As the number of carcinogenic components increases in a mixture, the chance of augmenting a carcinogenic process increases; this process, in turn, increases the probability that the relationship between cancer risk and dose of the mixture is linear at low doses. Where the dose-response relationship is nearly linear at low doses, a response-additive and a dose-additive approach will give essentially the same result (NRC 1989b).

Apart from any chemical or biological interactions, the cancer risk from two chemicals acting on the same stage of a multistage process is the sum of the risks of the individual chemicals (Gibb and Chen 1986). Continuous, lifetime exposure of two chemicals acting on different stages of a multistage process results in multiplicative relative risks (Gibb and Chen 1986). For less than lifetime exposure, Brown and Chu (1989) show that the effect of two chemicals acting on the first and penultimate stages of a multistage process depends upon the age of the exposed animal and duration of the exposure. Nearly additive relative risks result when the two exposure periods occur simultaneously and are of short duration, while multiplicative relative risks result from lifetime exposure.

Kodell et al. (1991) describe the nature of interactions possible under the commonly used (approximate) form of the Moolgavkar-Venzon-Knudson two-stage clonal expansion model of carcinogenesis. In this analysis, interaction among initiators (agents that increase the first-stage mutation rate), promoters (agents that increase the rate of proliferation of initiated cells that have sustained the first mutation), and completers (agents that increase the second-stage mutation rate) was evaluated in terms of age-specific relative risk. It was found that joint exposure to two initiators or to two completers resulted in additivity of the age-specific relative risks, whereas joint exposure to an initiator and a completer or to an initiator and a promoter led to a multiplicative relative risk relationship. Supramultiplicative relative risk can occur with simultaneous exposure to two promoters. These results assume that there are no chemical or biological interactions between the two agents involved.

Kodell and Gaylor (1989) discuss the difficulties of distinguishing between additive and multiplicative relative risks for carcinogens. For the small, relative risks that would be expected at low doses, estimates of cancer risk for a mixture are approximately additive (NRC 1988). This is readily seen by a simple example. Suppose the relative risks for three components of a mixture are 1.01, 1.02, and 1.03. Using a multiplicative relative risk model, the relative risk for the mixture is 1.01 x 1.02 x 1.03 = 1.061. The additional risk of 0.061 is approximately the sum of the additional risk from each component 0.01 + 0.02 + 0.03 = 0.060. For most low-dose situations, there is no need to distinguish between additive and multiplicative risks. Thus, at low doses, the risk for a mixture generally can be approximated by the sum of the risks of the components.

For chemicals that can be grouped according to structural properties, such as polycyclic aromatic hydrocarbons, dibenzo-*p*-dioxins, and dibenzofurans, the combined carcinogenicity of a mixture can be estimated on the basis of a potency-equivalence approach based on a representative chemical of the class (NRC 1989b).

The combined effect of eating fruits and vegetables results in a reduction in some types of cancer. Both carcinogens and anticarcinogens may occur in a single food (e.g., citrus fruits contain vitamin C, which has anticarcinogenic properties, but also quercetin, a mutagen and possible carcinogen), and certainly both types of substances can be consumed in a single meal (NRC 1989b). Accordingly, individuals are exposed not only to mixtures of carcinogens, but also to mixtures of carcinogens and anticarcinogens. The net effect of such complex exposures is difficult to predict and is best determined empirically. Thus, although fruits and vegetables contain substances that may be carcinogenic in humans (Stolz et al. 1984), they also contain protective substances, and epidemiologic data strongly suggest that the risk of cancer is significantly reduced among individuals who consume higher amounts of these foods (Steinmetz and Potter 1991). It is not known whether the net beneficial effect of these foods results from interactions between the carcinogens and the anticarcinogens, or whether the combined beneficial effect simply exceeds the carcinogenic effect. However, from a public health perspective, people are encouraged to consume these foods because of the anticarcinogenic effects, which outweigh any carcinogenic risks posed by naturally occurring constituents.

DIETARY CANCER RISKS

Overall Impact of Diet on Cancer

The NRC Committee on Diet and Health (NRC 1989a) systematically examined the evidence relating dietary components to the occurrence of cancer. That committee found suggestive evidence linking specific cancers to the diet (e.g., alcoholic beverage intake and increases in esophageal and colorectal cancers), but the committee did not estimate the overall effect of diet on cancer mortality and incidence rates. Doll and Peto (1981) gave as a best estimate that 35% of all cancer mortality reported in the U.S. is related to diet, with an uncertainty range of 10-70%. Doll (1992) recently asserted that "the estimate that the risk of fatal cancer might be reducible by dietary modification by 35 percent remains a reasonable estimate." In discussing these and other estimates, the Committee on Diet and Health noted that "because few relationships between specific dietary components and cancer risk are well-established, it is not possible to quantify the contribution of diet to individual cancers (and thus to total cancer rates) more precisely." Similarly, the earlier NRC Committee on Diet, Nutrition, and Cancer (1982) found that cancers of most major sites are influenced by dietary patterns, but concluded that "the data are not sufficient to quantitate the contribution of diet to the overall cancer risk or to determine the percent reduction in risk that might be achieved by dietary modification."

After reviewing all the evidence available to date, Ames et al. (1995) conclude that 1) reduction of smoking, 2) avoidance of intense sun exposure and high levels of alcohol consumption, 3) control of infections, and 4) increased consumption of fruits and vegetables, as well as increases in physical activity are likely to reduce the risks of specific cancers. The authors also suggest that reduced consumption of red meat may decrease the incidence of colon and prostate cancer and that modification of sex hormone levels might have some effect on breast cancer incidence.

Impact of Dietary Constituents on Human Cancer

Although only a few individual carcinogens in the diet have been identified through epidemiologic studies (e.g., aflatoxin and arsen-

ic), these studies have identified dietary components as either contributing to or reducing cancer risk. Carcinogenic and anticarcinogenic dietary components strongly supported by epidemiologic
studies at the time of the NRC Committee's report on Diet and
Health in 1989, are shown in Table 5-6.

Many commonly consumed foods also contain chemical substances that have both carcinogenic and anticarcinogenic potential.
Cooked beef steak contains a number of derived pyrolysis products
such as benz(a)anthracene that have been shown to be carcinogenic
in animals (cf. IARC 3:45, 32:135). Heterocyclic amines formed
during cooking of beef steak, such as 2-amino-3-methylimidazo[4,5-
f]quinoline (IQ), are also in low concentrations ranging up to 20
ng/g (IARC 40:261, 56:165). Beef steak may also contain traces of
naturally occurring carcinogens acquired from the environment,
including arsenic and ochratoxin A, a mycotoxin resulting from
feed contamination (IARC 10:191, 31:191, 42:262, 56:489). Synthetic carcinogens such as 2,3,7,8-tetrachlorodibenzo-*p*-dioxin and
other chlorinated polycylic hydrocarbons may also be present in
beef steak as a consequence of contamination of packaging materials (IARC 15:41). In addition to trace levels of these carcinogenic
substances, beef steak contains anticarcinogenic substances such as
conjugated linoleic acid and selenium.

Many other foods contain carcinogenic and anticarcinogenic
constituents. For example, broccoli may contain trace levels of
arsenic, a widely distributed natural contaminant. Broccoli also
contains chlorogenic and neochlorogenic acids; both are metabolized to caffeic acid, which is found in broccoli at concentrations up
to 10 mg/kg. Anticarcinogenic substances found in broccoli include ascorbic acid, indole and other isothiocyanates, and sulfora-
phane.

Assessing dietary cancer risks requires consideration of both
these types of agents, carcinogenic and anticarcinogenic. Ames et
al. (1993b) have suggested that antioxidants such as ascorbate, tocopherol, and carotenoids found in fruits and vegetables may re-

Table 5-6 NRC Committee on Diet and Health[a]: Findings on Diet and Cancer

Cancer-Causing Dietary Components	Tumor Sites
Alcoholic beverages[b]	Oral cavity, pharynx, esophagus, larynx, colon and rectum, (possibly) liver, (maybe) breast
High salt intake and frequent consumption of salt-cured and salt-preserved foods	Stomach
Aflatoxin[c]	Liver
Obesity	Endometrium, (maybe) post menopausal breast
Dietary fat[d]	Possibly breast, prostate, and colorectal[c]

Cancer-Preventing Dietary Components	Tumor Sites
Fresh fruits	Stomach, lung
Vegetables	Stomach, colorectal
High intake of green and yellow vegetables (possibly due to β-carotene and other carotenoids)	Colorectal, lung

[a]NRC 1989b.

[b]The committee associated heavy, sustained intake with cancers of the oral cavity, pharynx, larynx, and esophagus (especially in combination with cigarette smoking). The committee noted that there was some epidemiologic evidence that alcohol consumption is associated with primary liver cancer and moderate beer drinking with colorectal cancer, and found the association between alcohol consumption and breast cancer less clear.

[c]The committee noted that there was no evidence that aflatoxin, as an individual substance, makes a major contribution to cancer in the United States.

[d]The committee found the evidence between high fat intake and cancers of the breast, prostate, and colon suggestive, but not definitive.

duce cancer risk. Calorie restriction may also be effective in reducing cancer risk (Pariza and Boutwell 1987, Youngman et al. 1992).

Role of Calories and Fat

Excess Calories

Although animal models have shown effects of caloric intake on tumor incidence, especially a protective effect of reduced energy intake (Pariza and Boutwell 1987), in human beings the relationship of caloric intake to cancer risk has not yet been clarified. Because caloric intake and the intake of macronutrients (especially fat) are highly correlated in individuals, an effect of calories needs to be distinguished from one of fat or other macronutrients. Unfortunately, many early epidemiologic studies of diet and cancer did not assess total caloric intake, and others did not adjust for calories when examining the effects of fat or other macronutrients (NRC 1989a). Moreover, recent studies that examined total energy intake have not been consistent in their findings. For example, studies have shown both positive associations (West et al. 1989) and no association (Goldbohm et al. 1994) for total energy intake and colon cancer. Others have found independent effects of fat (or other macronutrients) on cancer risk after adjusting for caloric intake (Van't Veer et al. 1990, Willett et al. 1990, Giovannucci et al. 1993).

Epidemiologic evidence suggests that energy expenditure is also related to cancer risk, particularly inverse associations between physical activity and cancers of the colon, breast, and prostate (Peters et al. 1989, Whittemore et al. 1990, Lee et al. 1991, Lee et al. 1992, Friedenreich and Rohan 1995). The association of both caloric intake and physical activity with cancer of the colon suggests that net energy balance may be an important determinant of risk for some cancers. Moreover, positive associations have been found between obesity and the risk of cancer of the endometrium, colon, and breast (Henderson et al. 1983, Hunter and Willett 1993, Potter et al. 1993). Although the determinants of obesity are not fully understood (Berry et al. 1987), this association offers additional support to the hypothesis that net energy balance is related to cancer risk. In general, epidemiologic studies suggest that high caloric intake, low levels of physical activity, and obesity cause a moderate (i.e., 2- or 3-fold) increase in cancer risk.

Estimates of per capita caloric intake in the U.S. show relatively little change over the period 1909-1985, because increases in fat intake were largely offset by decreases in carbohydrate levels, while protein intake remained relatively constant (NRC 1989a). Data from food consumption surveys in recent years show variation in energy intake between sexes and among age groups. For example, in the 1977-1978 Nationwide Food Consumption Survey (see earlier section of this chapter on Sources of Information), men 75 years and older averaged 1,866 kcal per day, whereas women in the same age group consumed 1,417 kcal per day. Men in the age group 15-18 years of age, in contrast, consumed an average of 2,568 kcal per day.

Fat

Many epidemiologic studies have found a positive association between dietary fat intake and cancer at certain sites, such as the colon, prostate, and breast (NRC 1989a). Ecological studies, for example, have shown a positive relationship between per capita fat intake level by country and corresponding incidence or mortality rates for several cancers. In some instances, the associations were stronger for animal fat than for vegetable fat consumption (Rose et al. 1986, Prentice and Shephard 1990).

The findings from these ecological analyses have not been confirmed in analytical epidemiologic studies based on data collected directly from individuals. Thus, whereas a combined analysis of 12 case-control studies found a weak positive association between fat intake and breast cancer risk (Howe et al. 1990), 6 large cohort studies found no significant elevation in the risk of breast cancer among women with the highest levels of fat intake (Hunter and Willett 1993). Epidemiologic data on diet and prostate cancer are less abundant but suggest overall a positive association between dietary fat, especially animal or saturated fat, and risk of this cancer (Nomura and Kolonel 1991). Colon cancer has also been associated with saturated or animal fat, in both case-control and cohort studies (Whittemore et al. 1990, Willett et al. 1990). Cancers at other sites, such as the ovary and lung (Goodman et al. 1988, Risch et al. 1994), have also been associated with dietary fat, but the evidence at present is very limited.

In some populations, fat intake is highly correlated with the consumption of meat, a major source of saturated fats in the diet. Furthermore, some recent studies found strong positive associations between the intake of meat, especially red meat, and the risk of cancers of the prostate and colon (Giovannucci et al. 1993, Le Marchand et al. 1994). Meat may contain carcinogens other than fat, because cooking such foods at high temperatures (as in broiling or frying) can generate potentially carcinogenic polycyclic hydrocarbons and heterocyclic amines (Sugimura 1985). Thus, a causal relationship between dietary fat and cancer in humans has not yet been conclusively established.

Animal studies also show a relationship of dietary fat to cancer, although the only fatty acid that has been shown unequivocally to enhance carcinogenesis in animal models is linoleic acid (see Chapter 2). Although dietary fat and calories appear to interact in modifying cancer risk in animals (Welsch et al. 1990, see Chapter 2), an independent effect of fat has also been demonstrated (Birt et al. 1993).

Per capita intake of fat in the U.S. appears to have increased throughout the period 1909-1913 to 1985. During this time, estimated saturated fat intake rose from about 50 g/day to 65 g/day.

As a percent of total calories, fat has remained relatively constant (approximately 40%) during the past twenty years (NRC 1989a). However, the data for these apparent trends are difficult to interpret, because survey methods have varied over time.

Risk Estimates Derived from Epidemiologic Studies

In only a few cases can dietary risks be estimated from human data. The example of aflatoxin shows the difficulties in risk estimation, even for a well-studied case with human data. Several investigators have estimated the cancer risk associated with aflatoxin B_1 exposure of individuals living in southern China. The range of estimates varies considerably, depending upon whether additive or multiplicative models were chosen and whether the exposed individuals also tested positive for the hepatitis B virus. Using a relative risk model, Hoseyni (1992) calculated a lifetime risk for liver cancer of 2.5 per million per ng/kg body weight/day for aflatoxin B_1 in hepatitis-negative individuals and 62 per million per ng/kg body weight/day in hepatitis-positive individuals. Wu-Williams et al. (1992) calculated a lifetime risk of primary hepatocellular carcinoma for males of 5.6 per million per ng/kg body weight/day using a multiplicative relative risk model, and 46 per million per ng/kg body weight/day using an interactive risk model. Risk levels were at least an order of magnitude higher for hepatitis B-positive individuals. Bowers et al. (1993) estimated a lifetime cancer risk of 9 per million per ng/kg body weight/day and 230 per million per ng/kg body weight/day for hepatitis B-negative and -positive individuals, respectively. Aflatoxin B_1 exposure levels are generally on the order of a few ng/kg body weight/day. Thus, primary hepatocellular carcinoma risks from aflatoxin appear to be on the order of one per 10,000, which would account for a fraction of the liver cancer in the U.S. However, those infected with hepatitis B (which, for example, is endemic to the Asian immigrant community) could face liver cancer risks on the order of 10^{-3} to 10^{-2}.

Data from rats, the species most sensitive to aflatoxin, shows carcinoma potency estimates from aflatoxin is considerably greater than that derived from epidemiologic data (i.e., cancer potency estimates of 5,000 to 20,000 (mg/kg-day)$^{-1}$ for the rat *versus* 5 to 50 (mg/kg-day)$^{-1}$ for the hepatitis B negative humans).

Risk Estimates Derived from Toxicological Studies

Cancer risk estimates can also be derived from toxicological studies, although such estimates are uncertain due to the need to extrapolate from high to low doses, and from animals to humans. An example of risk estimation relying on toxicological information for the cancer potency estimate is given here for illustrative purposes. Gaylor and Kadlubar (1991) investigated the cancer risk to humans exposed to (polycyclic) heterocyclic amines formed during the cooking of food. Cancer potency estimates were derived from rodent data. With one exception, the animal bioassays consisted of only one dose level and controls. Hence, the potency estimates were based on the one-hit model. Cancer potency estimates for several of the heterocyclic amines were as high as one in a 100,000 per ppb in the total diet. Data on exposures in the human diet were sketchy, with ranges from 0.02 to 83 ppb in the total diet. Based on these data, it was estimated that the upper limit on cancer risk in the total average diet due to heterocyclic amines formed during cooking is on the order of one per 10,000.

Recently, Layton et al. (1995) examined the cancer risk of heterocyclic amines in cooked foods, establishing concentrations of heterocyclic amines from published literature. Average consumption of foods containing heterocyclic amines were obtained from 3-day dietary records of a random survey of 3563 individuals conducted by the USDA in 1989. Cancer potencies were taken from Bogen (1994), which accounted for the induction of tumors at multiple tissue sites. An upper bound estimate at the incremental cancer risk of heterocyclic amines produced by cooking is 1.1×10^{-4} using cancer potencies based on body surface area. Nearly half of the risk was due to the ingestion of 2-amino-1-methyl-6-phenylimidazo[4,5-6] pyridine (PhIP). Consumption of beef and fish products accounted for about 80% of the total risk. The authors calculated that the ingestion of these dietary heterocyclic amines might account for at most a small fraction (0.25%) of colorectal cancers in the United States.

Apportionment of Dietary Cancer Risk

Lutz and Schlatter (1992) recently estimated cancer risks to humans from known animal and human carcinogens present in the diet. Human exposure estimates were based on average daily intake estimates for dietary carcinogens in Switzerland. The total cancer risk was compared with the number of cancer cases attributed by epidemiologists to dietary factors, about 80,000 cases per 1 million people. The investigators state that, "Except for alcohol, the known dietary carcinogens could not account for more than a few hundred cancer cases." This estimate is only a small fraction of the risk estimate provided by Doll (less than 0.01%). In deriving these estimates, Lutz and Schlatter did not consider potential interactions among the known human carcinogens, the unspecified (and unknown) carcinogens, and dietary macronutrients, nor did they consider the multifactorial nature of cancer causation in humans. Consideration of these factors could result in substantially greater risk estimates than those provided.

Because their estimate proved to be negligible, Lutz and Schlatter (1992) searched for other possible contributors to risk and concluded that the vast majority of dietary cancers may be due to overnutrition. As already discussed, epidemiologic studies have demonstrated an association between excess calories and the occurrence of breast, colon, and prostate cancer. Furthermore, studies in animals have shown that dietary restriction results in significant reductions in spontaneous and induced cancer incidence, as well as increases in tumor incidence in animals fed ad libitum when compared to dietary-restricted control animals. These studies suggest that the increased tumor incidence may be attributed to the excess food intake.

To test this assumption, Lutz and Schlatter determined that the average calorie intake in Switzerland between 1985 and 1987 for the age group 20-39 was 2315 kcal/person/day (excluding alcohol). Basal requirements for this age group are 1963 kcal/person/day. Thus, the investigators concluded that the average Swiss adult is overnourished by about 5.5 kcal/kg/day, or 1.9 g food/kg body weight/day. Using a TD_{50} of 16g/kg/d for excess feed in rats, the authors estimate that 60,000 cancer cases in a population of one million could be attributed to excess food intake in Switzerland, noting that "this value is provocatively close to the number of cancer cases not explained by the human dietary chemical carcinogens."

Scheuplein (1990) examined the contribution of various food categories to overall human cancer risk. His estimates of daily intakes of selected food categories are shown in Table 5-7. The intake of a food category that is calculated to be carcinogenic is also shown. This intake was calculated by multiplying the food intake by the proportion estimated to be carcinogenic, yielding "unverified estimates that seem reasonable." Assuming equal potencies (i.e., equal risk per mg of carcinogen) across food categories, the naturally occurring carcinogens account for 99.8% of human dietary cancer. Assuming that the potencies of traditional food, spices and flavors, charred protein, and mycotoxins are 0.01, 0.1, 100, and 1000 times the potencies of synthetic chemicals, respectively,

Table 5-7 Daily Intakes of Dietary Carcinogens in Selected Food Categories[a]

Food Category	Daily Intake	Assumed Proportion Carcinogenic	Predicted Intake of Carcinogenic Substances (mg)
Traditional foods	1,000 g	0.001	1,000
Spices and flavors	1 g	0.01	10
Indirects	20 mg	0.1	2
Pesticides and contaminants	200 µg	0.5	0.1
Animal drugs	1 mg	0.1	0.1
Charred protein	1 g	0.0001	0.1
Mycotoxins	10 µg	0.1	0.001

[a]Adapted from Scheuplein (1990).

Scheuplein estimated that naturally occurring carcinogens account for approximately 91% of the cancers attributable to the human diet.

Scheuplein's attempt to quantitate the contribution of dietary risk factors to human cancers demonstrates the gaps in our present knowledge. There is a need to systematically investigate the role of dietary modulation of malignant neoplasia. Using available data, plausible assumptions, and mathematics, he effectively challenges the scientific community to prove or disprove his hypotheses. Although the Surgeon General's Report on Nutrition and Health (1988) concludes that many food factors are involved, it cites in particular the "disproportionate consumption of food high in fats, often at the expense of food high in complex carbohydrates and fiber—such as vegetables, fruits, and whole grain products that may be more conducive to health."

Risks of Naturally Occurring
Versus Synthetic Carcinogens in the Diet

Potency of Naturally Occurring and Synthetic Carcinogens

Distribution of Potency

Only a small fraction of chemicals, natural or synthetic, has been adequately tested for carcinogenicity. Over 13 million chemicals have been assigned CAS numbers by the Chemical Abstracts Service. Testing has been undertaken for less than 0.01% of those, a number of these because of suspicions regarding their potential carcinogenicity.

Both naturally occurring and synthetic agents currently found in the U.S. diet have been identified as carcinogens by the International Agency for Research on Cancer (IARC) or the National Toxicology Program (NTP). Appendix B lists all agents identified by IARC as group 1, 2A, or 2B carcinogens or by the NTP as known or reasonably anticipated to be carcinogens. This list of carcinogens is divided into four tables: agents that may be encountered in U.S. diets (Table B-1), agents formerly encountered in U.S. diets but no longer (Table B-2) agents rarely or accidentally encountered in U.S. diets (Table B-3), and agents unlikely to be present in U.S. diets (Table B-4). When available, TD_{01} values are provided for these agents. The committee also attempted to determine whether an agent listed in the appendix should be considered as synthetic or naturally occurring as defined in Chapter 1. Naturally occurring agents are further subclassified as constitutive, derived, acquired, or added. The subclassification of naturally occurring agents was sometimes arbitrary, with some agents belonging in more than one category.

Table 5-8 compares the geometric means of the TD_{01} values for various synthetic versus naturally occurring carcinogens found in

U.S. diets. As depicted in Figure 5-4, TD_{01} values for the constitutive agents are higher than the TD_{01} values for the nonconstitutive agents, indicating that the constitutive agents are less carcinogenic. This may be an artifact of selection bias, however, since few constitutive agents have been identified and TD_{01} values are available on even fewer of these. In addition, because of the uncertainty in the TD_{01} estimates, the differences are not considered to be of practical significance. As shown in Figure 5-4, a comparison of TD_{01} values for synthetic versus naturally occurring agents indicates that the latter appear to be somewhat more potent, with lower TD_{01} values. Because the selection of the agents for testing is not random, and the number of naturally occurring and synthetic dietary agents tested is relatively small, the extent to which these results can be generalized is not known.

Table 5-8 Comparison of TD_{01} Values for Selected Synthetic and Naturally Occurring Carcinogens[a] in the Diet

Occurrence in the Diet	Number of Agents	TD_{01} Geometric Mean (mg/ kg/day)	Geometric Standard Deviation
Naturally occurring	37	0.002	11
Constitutive	4	0.03	27
Derived	27	0.001	7
Acquired or pass-through	6	0.001	17
Synthetic	60	0.02	25
Total	97	0.007	23

[a]Chemicals classified by IARC as Group 1, 2A, or 2B carcinogens, or by NTP as known or reasonably anticipated to be carcinogens.

Interpretation of Results

Figure 5-4 supports the conclusion that, quantitatively, the carcinogenic activities of naturally occurring and synthetic dietary agents

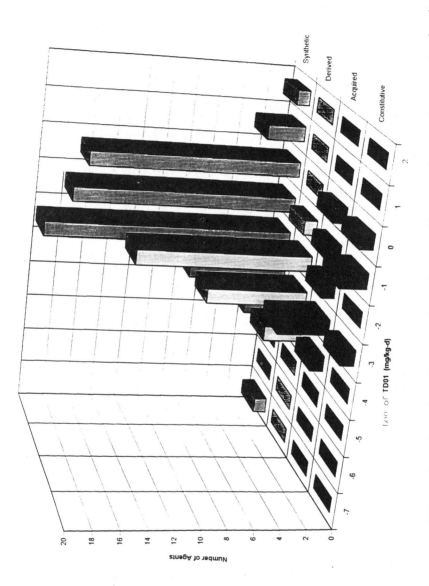

Figure 5-4 TD$_{01}$ values for selected synthetic and naturally occurring carcinogens in the diet.

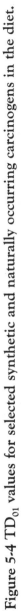

do not appear to differ substantially. Although the considerations involved in making this inference have been mentioned, a more extensive discussion of issues arising in the comparative carcinogenicity of dietary naturally occurring and synthetic carcinogens is now given.

Route of Exposure. Several naturally occurring carcinogens inherent in commonly eaten foods were identified as carcinogenic on the basis of findings reported in occupational studies, in which workers were exposed to high concentrations, or from inhalation bioassays conducted in animals. Cancer potencies may differ, depending on the route of exposure. This appears to be the case for several of these agents. For example, the cancer activity associated with oral exposure appears to be considerably less than that for inhalation exposures for asbestos, crystalline silica, hexavalent chromium, cadmium, nickel, formaldehyde, and acetaldehyde; furthermore, the degree to which oral exposures to these agents poses a cancer risk is currently the subject of debate. Cancer potencies for these naturally occurring agents as a result of inhalation are not representative of the cancer potencies associated with dietary intake and thus were not used in the comparisons. The fact that the FDA has permitted the addition of acetaldehyde to various foods and formaldehyde to milk (as a vitamin D carrier) underscores the fact that carcinogenic activity associated with the two routes is understood to be substantially different. Any of the above-mentioned agents, if active by the oral route, would have oral TD_{01} values considerably higher than the inhalation values.

Definition of Naturally Occurring. The distinction made here is between those agents not known to occur in nature (as noted by IARC) and the rest of the chemical world. Thus, benzo(a)pyrene and a number of other pyrolytic products are classified as naturally occurring dietary carcinogens, even though relatively large dietary contributions can result from plant uptake of fossil fuel combustion byproducts.

Selection Bias. The agents for which cancer potency estimates are available do not represent a random sample of the universe of synthetic and naturally occurring agents. For the most part, cancer testing has been guided by suspicions of carcinogenicity from noted similarities to other compounds recognized as carcinogens, structure-activity considerations, mechanistic data, and indications from epidemiologic studies (Rosenkranz 1992). Finding one bad actor typically leads to the identification of other bad actors. For example, the finding that mutagenic products are formed during cooking has stimulated considerable research, including the conduct of cancer bioassays. As a result, this class of agents is relatively well identified (see Table 5-1). Similarly, observations of an increased incidence of bladder cancer among workers exposed to synthetic dyes and dye intermediates led to the discovery of the carcinogenicity of benzidine and related dyes; consequently, cancer potency estimates are available for a number of these agents. In contrast, only a few constitutive agents, normally present in U.S. diets, have been well studied by the oral route and identified as carcinogenic. The extent to which these are representative of all carcinogenic constituents is unknown. There may be literally millions of constitutive agents. Caffeic acid is one of the prevalent constitutive carcinogens, but as Lutz and Schlatter (1992) point out, the compound may be carcinogenic only at high doses (see, for example, Ito et al. 1991); thus it is improbable that the risks derived from animal bioassay data using standard techniques are representative of actual risks for human beings. The estimated carcinogenic potency of caffeic acid is therefore unlikely to be indicative of its activity under conditions of most human exposures. Further, whether caffeic acid actually poses a human cancer risk is unclear.

Uncertainty in Potency Estimates. The risks predicted using cancer potency values such as the reciprocal of the TD_{01} are often described as upper bound estimates. It is widely recognized that these risk predictions are not precise and that the uncertainty inherent in risk calculations is usually large. Ratios of cancer poten-cies for dissimilar agents can be subject to larger uncertainty. Statistical techniques can be applied to estimate the error in deriving potency parameters from bioassay data (e.g., the error in deriving the β parameter). Areas that are uncertain and not as amenable to quantification include interspecies extrapolation, estimation of lifetime risks from experiments conducted for less than a lifetime, and the application of potency parameters to exposure levels and patterns considerably different from those in the bioassay that has served as the basis for calculating the potency. In addition, comparisons of potencies for multiple agents in a mixture carry even greater uncertainty, as was discussed previously.

HERP Approach

A number of recent papers by Ames and colleagues have discussed the relative importance of naturally occurring and synthetic carcinogens with respect to dietary cancer risk (Ames et al. 1987, 1990a,b; Ames and Gold 1990a,b,c, 1995; Gold et al. 1992, 1993b, 1994). In these papers, the investigators compare the ratios of human exposure to animal cancer potency for different agents, noting that the result serves as a guide to priority setting (Ames et al. 1987). One of these ratios, the Human Exposure/Rodent Potency index (HERP), is constructed by dividing an estimate of human exposure by the TD_{50}. The larger the value of the HERP index, the closer the level of human exposure is to the dose estimated to cause a 50% excess cancer risk in animals (Gold et al. 1990, 1992). Based on a tabulation of HERP indices for various carcinogens using data from the Carcinogenic Potency Database, these investigators assert that the risks associated with exposure to natural carcinogens is greater than many synthetic agents. For example, the HERP index for 8-methoxypsoralen in a quarter of a parsnip (0.06) is larger than the HERP index for chloroform in one liter of tap water (0.001). However, Ames and Gold (1990b) offer assurances that the exposure to individual natural and synthetic carcinogens is low, and there is no cause for alarm for those who eat a balanced diet.

Ames and his associates investigated agents they identified as naturally occurring and synthetic pesticides to determine their role in the induction of cancer in humans (Ames et al. 1990a,b; Gold et al. 1993a). They calculated "that 99.99% (by weight) of the pesticides in the American diet are chemicals that plants produce to defend themselves" (Ames et al. 1990b). In another study Ames et al. (1993) compared the HERP indices for agents they identified as natural plant pesticides to the indices of synthetic organic pesticides used to enhance agricultural productivity. On the basis of these results, they concluded that dietary exposure to naturally occurring pesticides, weighted by carcinogenic potency, is greater than dietary exposure to synthetic pesticides. They further noted that a high proportion of "natural pesticides" were positive in animal cancer tests and concluded that naturally occurring and synthetic chemicals present in the diet are equally likely to test positive in animal cancer tests, and that the potential risks of dietary residues of synthetic organic compounds are insignificant.

Comparisons of HERP indices among different types of naturally occurring carcinogens have also been made (Gold et al. 1993, 1994). For example, on the basis of HERP comparisons Gold et al. (1994) conclude that "possible hazards from HA (heterocyclic amines) rank below those of most `natural pesticides' and products of cooking and food preparation; synthetic pesticide residues also rank low."

In evaluating comparisons of HERP indices, certain scientific limitations need to be considered. One is that most comparisons are made on the basis of carcinogens in a single serving, rather than on the basis of average daily exposure. After comparing on the basis of average exposures, Perera and Boffetta (1988) note that "the HERP scores of many manmade pollutants are comparable to those of naturally occurring carcinogens in the diet." A second limitation is that some agents identified by Ames et al. as natural pesticides or food carcinogens and for which HERP indices were calculated lack sufficient evidence of carcinogenicity. For example, Ames et al. (1990b) list 27 agents as carcinogenic plant chemicals; in an earlier report (1987) they identify 11 compounds as `natural pesticides' and dietary toxins. However, only 7 of the first and 5 of the second were considered by IARC to be Group 1 or 2 carcinogens, or by NTP as known to be or reasonably anticipated to be carcinogenic. A number of the compounds were classified by IARC as not classifiable as to its carcinogenicity to humans (i.e., IARC Group 3) and a few were not reviewed by IARC. Consequently, there is an uneven comparison of synthetic agents that have been formally recognized as carcinogens to naturally occurring agents with insufficient evidence. Third, the analysis is not comprehensive in that only a few selected synthetic and naturally occurring agents are compared, including some obscure exposures to natural agents (e.g., the high HERP index for a serving of comfrey root and symphytine in comfrey-pepsin tablets is compared to the low HERP index for daily intake of EDB in grains averaged over the U.S. population). Fourth, as is common to a number of assessments, the increased risks to subpopulations are not addressed, subpopulations with considerably higher exposure than the calculated average exposure (or single serving in some cases) or those with identifiable increased susceptibility. Fifth, as Wartenberg and Gallo (1990a,b) and Hoel (1990) point out, all carcinogens are implicitly assumed to act by similar mechanisms, and the approach fails to account for the non-linear regions of the dose response curve, even in known and understood cases such as vinyl chloride and AF-2 (Littlefield et al. 1980). Sixth, the fraction of untested natural and synthetic agents that would be identified as carcinogenic after adequate testing is unknown. Ames et al. (1990b) note that half of the agents they identify as natural carcinogens test positive in rodent bioassays. Of chemicals selected for carcinogenicity testing by the NTP, 68% of those chosen because they were suspected to be carcinogenic were found to be positive in at least one sex/species, in contrast to 21% of those selected primarily on the basis of exposure considerations (Fung et al. 1993). A smaller fraction was found to meet the criteria for sufficient evidence in animals by IARC. It is unclear what the finding would be for a random selection of agents from the synthetic and natural world. Finally, because the diet is a complex mixture of agents containing both carcinogenic and anticarcinogenic components, evaluation of individual ones in isolation can be misleading, particularly since some agents possess dual activity. With respect to the latter, the HERP index for caffeic acid suggests high hazard, but experimental evidence indicates the possibility for protective effects at dietary levels.

In a more recent publication by Gold and colleagues (Gold et al. 1992) the second criticism mentioned above is partially addressed in that some chemicals in foods are compared on the basis of average servings for a particular food. Summing HERP indices for the same chemical (e.g., adding d-limonene in black pepper and orange juice), and then ranking HERP indices from highest to lowest for agents they identify as natural and synthetic pesticides results in the following: caffeic acid, d-limonene, safrole, mix of hydrazines, catechol, DDT (before ban in 1972), UDMH (in 6 oz of apple juice), allyl isothiocyanate, DDE, 8-methoxypsoralen, glutamyl-p-hydrazinobenzoate, EDB (before 1984 ban), carbaryl, toxaphene, p-hydrazinobenzoate, dicofol, α-methylbenzyl alcohol, lindane, chlorobenzilate, chlorothalonil, folpet, captan. Removing those agents classified by IARC as "not classifiable as to their carcinogenicity in humans" results in the following list, with naturally occurring agents in italic: *caffeic acid, safrole, mix of hydrazines,* DDT (before ban in 1972), UDMH, DDE, *8-methoxypsoralen, glutamyl-p-hydrazinobenzoate,* EDB (before 1984 ban), toxaphene, *p-hydrazinobenzoate, α-methylbenzyl alcohol,* lindane, chlorothalonil, folpet.

Additional Comparisons

The committee made an additional attempt to compare the potential risks of naturally occurring and synthetic carcinogens in food, focusing on a selected number of substances that may be found in relatively high concentrations in the diet. These comparisons were based on an exposure potency index (EPI) defined as the ratio of dietary exposure to carcinogenic potency. Carcinogenic potency is expressed in terms of the TD_{01}, then estimated to induce an excess lifetime cancer risk of 1%. This is analogous to the HERP index used by Ames and Gold (1987), with the TD_{50} replaced by the TD_{01}. The TD_{01} is used here because it is closer to human exposure levels, yet not so low as to be highly model dependent. Because potency rankings based on the TD_{50} and TD_{01} are generally similar (Krewski et al. 1990), risk comparisons based on the EPI are expected to be similar to those based on the HERP. The TD_{01} is readily available for the series of compounds assembled by the committee in Appendix B.

Many criticisms of the comparison done by Ames and colleagues apply to the comparisons in Table 5-9 as well. Only a few of the dietary carcinogens listed in Tables 5-1 and 5-3 are considered. The committee focused on some agents for which exposures are believed to be high relative to other carcinogenic agents. Average dietary exposures are difficult to estimate, and upper end exposures even more so due to the paucity of consumption and concentration data available on which to base such estimates. Nonetheless, these crude estimates suggest that exposure to individual synthetic and natural chemicals might fall within a comparable range.

Some of the putative carcinogens in foods (excluding excess fat) are ingested in greater quantities than the others (milligrams rather than micrograms per day). These include caffeic acid, a naturally occurring compound shown to be both carcinogenic and anticarcinogenic in animal models, and BHA, a synthetic chemical; both of these are consumed at comparable levels in the human diet. While

Table 5-9 Exposure/Potency Index for Selected Naturally Occurring and Synthetic Carcinogens in the Diet[a]

Carcinogen	Exposure Potency Index	
	U.S. Population Average	High Consumers[b]
Natural		
Constitutive		
Caffeic acid		
Food	0.03-0.3	0.1-1 (average child ser 1-6 yr.)
Coffee	0.3-3	1.5-15 (upper 95 percentile consumer)
Derived		
PhIP	0.006	0.02
Urethane		
Food	<0.002	<0.005 (children)
Alcohol	0.0001-0.0003	0.0007 (average per day when consumed)
N-nitrosodi-		
methylamine	0.002-0.005	0.1
Food	0.003	0.003-0.05 (moderate wine consumption)
Beer 1980	0.00008-0.0002	
1990		
Acquired		
Aflatoxin	0.001	0.003 (90th percentile consumer)

Table 5-9 Continued

	Exposure Potency Index	
	U.S. Population	
Carcinogen	Average	High Consumers[b]

Synthetic

Pesticide residues
    DDD, DDE, and
        DDD

1954 (DDE and DDT)	0.1	
1965	0.02	
Early 1980's	0.001	1
Ethylene thiourea	0.0009; 0.003	
Unsymmetrical dimethyl hydrazine	0.014	0.1 (average intake, non-nursing infant)

Packaging migrants
    Diethylhexyl-
        phthalate

1982 report	0.07	
1991 report	0.003	0.02

Environmental
    contaminants

TCDD equivalents	0.01-0.04	0.9 (nursing infant)
Polychlorinated biphenyls	0.2	3

Intentional food
    additives
    Butylated

hydroxyanisole	0.002-0.007	0.005-0.015
Potassium bromate	--	0.004
Saccharin	0.002	0.008-0.03

Table 5-9 Continued

[a]The exposure/potency index is the ratio of dietary exposure to carcinogenic potency. Carcinogenic potency is expressed in terms of the TD_{01}, the dose causing an excess lifetime cancer risk of 1%. Intake values and references are provided in Tables 5-4 and 5-5, and TD_{01} values are provided in Appendix 5A.
[b]In calculating the exposure potency index, daily exposures for infants and children were not averaged over their lifetime.

potentially carcinogenic to humans if consumed at levels producing cancer in animal bioassays, these simple phenolic compounds are potentially anticarcinogenic at lower levels, operating through an antioxidant mechanism (see Chapter 2). The degree, therefore, that caffeic acid poses a cancer risk to humans is unclear. Although the consumption of fruits and vegetables containing caffeic acid is considered to be protective against cancer, extremely high levels of coffee consumption may pose a risk. The available scientific information does not enable us to resolve this issue.

Table 5-9 illustrates two other important points. First, some consumer subgroups might be exposed to relatively high levels of naturally occurring carcinogens, for example, high consumers of stone fruit distillates and well-done meats. When averaged out over the population, these levels may appear unimpressive, but for the individual high consumer the risk might be significant. Second, reductions in exposures to individual dietary carcinogens have been significantly reduced after the identification of these agents as carcinogens, for both synthetic agents (e.g., DDT and UDMH) and natural ones (e.g., nitrosodimethylamine and urethane). Not shown in the table are several agents for which past levels of exposure are likely to have been very high (e.g., arsenic, benzyl violet 4B, and dihydrosafrole). This suggests caution when interpreting the results of exposure calculations for dietary carcinogens.

SUMMARY AND CONCLUSIONS

Humans are exposed to a wide variety of chemical substances, naturally occurring and synthetic, in their diets, although the carcinogenic potential of most of these substances has not been evaluated. Diets high in calories and fat are associated with increased cancer risks, although the mechanisms by which these substances increase risks are not well understood. Other dietary substances known to increase cancer risk in animals and possibly in humans include the mycotoxins (e.g., aflatoxins) and the heterocyclic amines, which are formed when meat is cooked at high temperatures. Recent investigations have focused on the possibility that some naturally occurring compounds produced by plants may possess carcinogenic properties. In total, such natural toxins appear to be present in the diet in greater quantities than residues of synthetic organic pesticides. Unlike most naturally occurring dietary constituents, synthetic ones such as direct and indirect food additives and pesticide residues are highly regulated, with stringent limits placed on their allowable levels of synthetic chemicals in foods.

The risks associated with dietary carcinogens depend on the carcinogenic potency of the substance and its level of ingestion. At present, dietary epidemiologic studies have identified a small number of specific components capable of causing cancer in humans. Only a few of these agents, such as aflatoxin and arsenic compounds, occur in food and water. Exposure to most of the other known human carcinogens occurs primarily through nondietary pathways. Laboratory studies have identified a much larger number of synthetic and naturally occurring agents capable of causing cancer in experimental animals. However, prediction of human cancer risks based on laboratory results is uncertain because extrapolations must be made from high to low doses and from animals to humans. Thus, important questions remain about the relevance of findings from animal studies for predicting human cancers. In particular, rodent carcinogens, some of which may act by increasing cell proliferation only at high doses, may pose little or no risk at low doses. Although the use of the maximum tolerated dose (MTD) in rodent carcinogenicity studies has been questioned, a recent review of its use by the National Research Council (1993b) failed to identify a suitable alternative. In the future, short-term tests for DNA adduct formation, mutation, and cellular proliferation, all critical factors in carcinogenesis, may provide a stronger basis for evaluating carcinogenic risks in the absence of adequate epidemiologic data.

Estimating dietary exposures requires knowledge of food consumption patterns, which vary substantially among individuals and over time. Despite periodic nationwide surveys, food consumption data are somewhat limited, particularly for the young and the elderly. The concentrations of chemical substances with carcinogenic potential in specific foods, including both naturally occurring and synthetic pesticides, are not well characterized and can vary widely.

In addition to agents that may increase cancer risk, the human diet also includes substances that may reduce the risk of cancer. These include broad classes of foods such as fruits and vegetables, as well as specific substances such as beta-carotene and vitamin A. Because the human diet is a complex mixture of many constituents, dietary cancer risk assessment needs to take into account the potential for synergistic and antagonistic interactions among dietary components.

Methods for estimating cancer risk rely largely on epidemiologic and toxicological data. Epidemiologic studies provide direct information on cancer risks in humans but are subject to certain limitations, including inadequate exposure data and confounding due to exposure to multiple agents. Toxicological studies can be conducted under controlled conditions but provide only indirect information on human cancer risks. Several hundred chemicals have been found by the IARC and NTP to have sufficient evidence of carcinogenicity in animals.

The potency of carcinogenic agents may be quantified by the reciprocal of the TD_{50} or TD_{01}, the doses estimated to produce a 50% or 1% excess lifetime cancer risk, respectively. The Carcinogenic Potency Database, which contains TD_{50} values for about 600 rodent carcinogens, serves as a useful source of information for comparing carcinogenic potency values.

The fact that the diet is a complex mixture raises important considerations when conducting cancer risk assessments. Evidence from both epidemiologic and toxicological studies indicates that interactive effects may occur. Hence, the effect of altering the concentration of one dietary substance may influence the carcinogenic (or anticarcinogenic) activity of another. The extent of such interactions among dietary constituents is not yet well characterized.

To evaluate the relative potency of naturally occurring and synthetic carcinogens in the diet, the committee compiled data on the carcinogenic potency of about 233 chemical carcinogens, including 65 naturally occurring substances and 168 synthetics. Of those with potency values, 37 naturally occurring and 60 synthetic agents were identified in U.S. diets. The potency values were derived from bioassay data tabulated in the CPDB using an expedited estimation procedure (as described by Hoover et al. 1995, Cal/EPA 1992) or, if available, drawn from regulatory agencies that had performed a more in-depth analysis. The data set included agents identified by IARC as having sufficient evidence of carcinogenicity in humans or animals or by the NTP as known or reasonably anticipated to be human carcinogens. The committee recognized that this represented a somewhat select group of substances, but considered it instructive to analyze the relative potency on this sample.

In this analysis, carcinogenic potency was expressed in terms of the reciprocal of the TD_{01}, defined as the dose inducing an excess lifetime cancer risk of 1%. Results of the analysis indicate that the average potency of the naturally occurring carcinogens was somewhat higher than that of the synthetic carcinogens. The average of the few potencies for constitutive agents was roughly the same as for synthetic agents. Potencies for the derived, acquired, and pass-through agents were higher than the synthetic and constitutive agents, suggesting greater carcinogenic activity. However, there was wide variation in potency within the groups studied, with almost complete overlap of the potency ranges. In light of this variation, the uncertainty associated with estimates of cancer potency, and the potential problem of selective sampling, the committee concluded that these data failed to establish a clear difference between the potency of naturally occurring and synthetic carcinogens present in the human diet.

In addition to looking at potency data, characterization of risk requires a consideration of exposure. Although considerable information is available on food consumption patterns and on the concentrations of certain carcinogenic substances in foods, this information was insufficient to compare the risks posed by the naturally occurring and synthetic carcinogens considered previously. Furthermore, the committee decided that there was insufficient information on the carcinogenic potential of "natural pesticides" evolved by plants to conclude that such agents pose a greater dietary cancer risk than synthetic pesticides.

The HERP index, proposed by Ames and Gold, compares the human exposure to a rodent carcinogen with the potency in a bioassay (TD_{50}), expressed as a percentage: HERP = (human exposure/TD_{50}) x 100. Although not a direct measure of risk, larger HERP values may be viewed with greater concern than lower values. Ames and his colleagues have argued that HERP values for naturally occurring carcinogens often exceed those for synthetic carcinogens, largely because of the greater consumption of a few naturally occurring substances such as caffeic acid, which occurs in high concentrations in commonly consumed foods such as lettuce, apples, and coffee. Although Ames suggests that naturally occurring carcinogens present in the diet may pose a greater risk than synthetic dietary carcinogens, he notes that dietary exposure to both kinds is low, and should be of little concern when ingesting a balanced diet.

The observation that the HERP indices for naturally occurring carcinogens tend to exceed those for synthetic carcinogens is broadly consistent with the committee's calculation that the average potency of naturally occurring carcinogens exceeds that of synthetic carcinogens. However, the committee also notes that the analyses of HERP indices performed by Ames and colleagues are based on a select number of agents and include a number of compounds for which there is not sufficient evidence of carcinogenicity. Based on average daily consumption data, HERP indices for natural and synthetic carcinogens appear to be somewhat comparable.

Several investigators have attempted to assess the proportion of the human cancer burden attributable to different sources. In 1981, Doll and Peto estimated with some confidence that about 30% of all human cancer could be attributed to tobacco smoking. They provided as a best guess that 35% was due to dietary factors, although the precise components of diet contributing to this risk are not well understood. There also exists a high degree of uncertainty about the impact of diet on the human cancer burden, with Doll and Peto citing a plausible range of uncertainty of 10-70%. Subsequent reviews have largely supported this initial analysis.

Based on the information summarized in this chapter, the committee reached the following conclusions.

• *Diet contributes to an appreciable portion of human cancer.*
Authoritative reviews have speculated that diet plays a role in about a third of all human cancer. Although the actual figure could be somewhat higher or lower, these reviews have identified diet as a major contributor to the human cancer burden.

In most of these reviews, individual dietary constituents responsible for increased cancer risk were not identified. Nonetheless, a substantial body of evidence suggests that diets high in calories and fat appear to increase cancer risk. Human studies indicate that aflatoxin and alcoholic beverages increase the cancer risk. Animal studies have shown that a number of other chemical constituents present in food, both naturally occurring and synthetic, increase the risk of cancer.

Although the precise components of diet responsible for increased cancer risks are generally not well understood, it is felt that individual chemical constituents of the human diet, both naturally occurring and synthetic, represent generally low cancer risks. The degree to which these individual agents in aggregate pose a risk is unclear. However, excess calories and fat appear to have a substantial impact on human cancer.

• *The human diet contains both naturally occurring and synthetic agents that may affect cancer risk.*

Constituents of food present in the human diet that have been shown to increase cancer risk in animal and human studies may be naturally occurring or synthetic. The risks associated with both depend on the level of exposure and the potency of these chemicals, as well as the susceptibility of the host.

• *Excess calories and fat appear to contribute substantially to the human cancer burden.*

In animal studies, diets low in calories and fat are associated with a reduction in cancer risk. Although less conclusive, epidemiologic evidence in humans indicates that excess calories and fat play a role in the occurrence of colon, prostate, and possibly breast cancer. In terms of cancer causation, current evidence suggests that the contribution of calories and fat outweighs that of all other individual food chemicals, both naturally occurring and synthetic.

• *The potencies of known naturally occurring and synthetic carcinogens present in the human diet do not differ appreciably.*

The committee compared the potencies of 233 chemical carcinogens, 65 of which are naturally occurring and 168 are synthetic. Potency was expressed in terms of the reciprocal of the TD_{01} derived from rodent carcinogenicity studies. Although the average potency of these naturally occurring substances was greater than that of the synthetic agents, the range in potency observed within both groups was broad, with the distributions of potency spanning comparable ranges and encompassing some six orders of magnitude. Since these results are based on a select group of chemicals, it is difficult to generalize to a larger set of substances.

• *Taking calories and fat into consideration, the human cancer risk from naturally occurring substances in the diet exceeds that of synthetic dietary carcinogens. However, if calories and fat are excluded from consideration, the data now available do not permit a firm conclusion about the relative risks of naturally occurring and synthetic food chemicals. Nonetheless, the committee felt that it is plausible that naturally occurring chemicals present in food pose a greater cancer risk than synthetic chemicals.*

Cancer risk is determined by the potency of the carcinogen and the level of exposure. The mechanism by which cancer is induced can also influence risk, although these mechanisms appear similar for naturally occurring and synthetic substances. Calories and fat represent major components of the human diet and play an important role in the dietary contribution towards human cancer. Naturally occurring chemicals are present in the food supply in much larger quantities than synthetic chemicals. Although only a limited number of naturally occurring food chemicals have been tested in rodent bioassays for carcinogenic activity, the proportion of them demonstrating carcinogenic properties in such tests is comparable to the proportion of synthetic chemicals that are carcinogenic. The committee also felt that further testing of carefully selected naturally occurring food chemicals would result in the identification of additional carcinogens.

• *The great majority of individual naturally occurring and synthetic food chemicals are present in human diet at levels so low that they are unlikely to pose an appreciable cancer risk.*

Although the human diet contains both naturally occurring and synthetic carcinogens, these chemicals are generally present at very low concentrations, and are thus unlikely to pose an appreciable cancer risk. Application of pesticides to food crops is subject to stringent control. Thus, most foods contain no detectable levels of such residues and the residues that are detected are generally present at levels well below established tolerances. Similarly, with the exception of a few agents such as caffeic acid, naturally occurring carcinogens, including "natural pesticides," are also present at very low levels.

• *The human diet contains anticarcinogens that reduce cancer risk.*

The human diet contains a number of nutrients, including fibre and micronutrients such as the antioxidant vitamins A, C and E, that appear to reduce cancer risk. In addition, several nonnutritive agents, including the isoflavonoids, phenolic acids, and isothiocyanates, have been shown to demonstrate anticarcinogenic effects. Diets low in calories and fat are also associated with reduced cancer risk.

Epidemiologic studies have associated diets rich in fruits and vegetables with reduced rates of human cancer. These foods are sources of a number of constitutive chemicals with anticarcinogenic properties.

• *Carcinogens and anticarcinogens present in the diet may interact in a variety of ways, which are not fully understood.*

Fruits and vegetables contain both anticarcinogenic and carcinogenic constituents. Because such foods are associated with reduced cancer risk in humans, the anticarcinogenic properties would appear to be greater than their carcinogenic properties.

A global assessment of dietary cancer risks is more difficult. Because interactions between dietary carcinogens and anticarcinogens can occur, it is difficult to predict overall dietary risks based on an assessment of the risks for individual components. Although risk assessment methods for mixtures are available, the information on interactions among dietary constituents is limited. The large number of dietary constituents present in foods further complicates the evaluation of potential interactions.

OVERALL CONCLUSIONS

Although diet clearly contributes importantly to human cancer, the committee found it difficult to identify the specific components of diet that serve to increase or decrease cancer risk. Although excess calories and fat appear to represent the single most important component of the human diet that increases cancer risk, the epidemiological evidence in this regard is not entirely consistent. Most other dietary constituents suspected of impacting upon human cancer, both naturally occurring and synthetic, account individually for a small proportion of the diet, and may pose correspondingly low risks. Much of the available evidence on these compounds derives from studies in animals, and may or may not be indicative of a human cancer risk.

The presence of anticarcinogenic substances in many foods needs to be considered in any evaluation of dietary cancer risks. Fruits and vegetables contain antioxidant vitamins that have demonstrated anticarcinogenic properties in laboratory studies; diets rich in fruits and vegetables are in fact associated with reduced cancer risks in humans. Many commonly consumed foods such as beef steak and broccoli contain low concentrations of a number of both carcinogenic and anticarcinogenic substances.

On the basis of the information available at this time, the committee found it particularly difficult to judge whether naturally occurring or synthetic dietary components (exclusive of excess calories and fat) present the greater cancer risk to humans. Much of the information on the carcinogenic potential of these substances derives from animal tests conducted at high doses, results of which are difficult to translate directly to humans. Nonetheless, the committee found that a series of selected naturally occurring and synthetic dietary components appeared to span the same range of carcinogenic potency, and that naturally occurring and synthetic substances can cause cancer by similar mechanisms. The committee also noted that the fractions of naturally occurring and synthetic substances that are positive in animal cancer tests are comparable, and that the dietary concentrations of many naturally occurring animal carcinogens such as caffeic acid exceed those of most synthetic carcinogens present in or on food. These observations supported the committee's conclusion that natural components of the diet may prove to be of greater concern than synthetic components with respect to cancer risk, although additional evidence is required before this conclusion can be drawn with certainty.

REFERENCES

Ames, B.N., and L.S. Gold. 1990a. Chemical carcinogenesis: too many rodent carcinogens. Proc. Natl. Acad. Sci. U.S.A. 87:7772-7776.

Ames, B.N., and L.S. Gold. 1990b. Dietary carcinogens, environmental pollution, and cancer: some misconceptions. Med. Oncol. Tumor Pharmacother. 7:69-85.

Ames, B.N., and L.S. Gold. 1990c. Misconceptions on pollution and the causes of cancer. Angew. Chem. Int. Ed. Engl. 29:1197-1208.

Ames, B.N., R. Magaw, and L.S. Gold. 1987. Ranking possible carcinogenic hazards. Science 236:271-280.

Ames, B.N., M. Profet, and L.S. Gold. 1990a. Nature's chemicals and synthetic chemicals: comparative toxicology. Proc. Natl. Acad. Sci. U.S.A. 87:7782-7786.

Ames, B.N., M. Profet, and L.S. Gold. 1990b. Dietary pesticides

(99.99% all natural). Proc. Natl. Acad. Sci. U.S.A. 87:7777-7781.

Ames, B.N., M.K. Shigenaga, and T.M. Hagen. 1993a. Oxidants, antioxidants, and the degenerative diseases of aging. Proc. Natl. Acad. Sci. U.S.A. 90:7915-7922.

Ames, B.N., L.S. Gold, and W.C. Willett. 1995. The causes and prevention of cancer. JAMA, Special Issue on Cancer. Pp. 1-9

Andersen, M.E., J.J. Mills, M.L. Gargas, L. Kedderis, L.S. Birnbaum, D. Neubert, and W.F. Greenlee. 1993. Modeling receptor-mediated processes with dioxin: Implications for pharmacokinetics and risk assessment. Risk Anal. 13:25-36.

Arnold, D.L., D. Krewski, and I.C. Munro. 1983. Saccharin: A toxicological and historical perspective. Toxicology 27:179-256.

Bailar, A.J., and C.J. Portier. 1988. Effects of treatment-induced mortality and tumor induced mortality on tests for carcinogenicity. Biometrics 44:417-431.

Bailar, A.J., and C.J. Portier. 1993. An index of tumorigenic potency. Biometrics (in press).

Bartsch, H. 1991. N-Nitroso compounds and human cancer: Where do we stand? Pp. 1-10 in Relevance to Human Cancer of N-Nitroso Compounds, Tobacco Smoke and Mycotoxins, I.K. O'Neill, J. Chen, and H. Bartsch, eds. International Agency for Research on Cancer (IARC) Scientific Publications No. 105. Lyon: IARC

BATF (Bureau of Alcohol, Tobacco, and Firearms). 1987. Final cumulative information 1986-1987. Ethyl carbamate testing by all ATF laboratories.

BATF (Bureau of Alcohol, Tobacco, and Firearms). 1988. Cumulative information 1988. Ethyl carbamate testing by all ATF laboratories.

Battaglia, R., H.B. Conacher, B.D. Page. 1990. Ethyl carbamate (urethane) in alcoholic beverages and foods: A review. Food Addit. Contam. 7(4):477-496.

Benz, R.D. and H. Irausquin. 1991. Priority-based assessment of food additives database of the U.S. Food and Drug Administration center for food safety and applied nutrition. Environ. Health Perspect. 96:85-89.

Bernstein, L., L.S. Gold, B.N. Ames, M.C. Pike, and D.G. Hoel. 1985. Some tautologous aspects of the comparison of carcinogenic potency in rats and mice. Fund. Appl. Toxicol. 5:79-86.

Berry, E.M., S.H. Blondheim, H.E. Eliahou, and E. Shafrir, editors. 1987. Recent Advances in Obesity Research. London: V. John Libby. 397 pp.

Biaudet, H., T. Mavelle, and G. Debry. 1994. Mean daily intake of N-nitrosodimethylamine from foods and beverages in France in 1987-1992. Food Chem. Toxicol. 32:417-421.

Birt, D.F., H.J. Pinch, T. Barnett, A. Phan, and K. Dimitroff. 1993. Inhibition of skin tumor promotion by restriction of fat and carbohydrate calories in SENCAR mice. Cancer Res. 53:27-31.

Bogen, K.T. 1994. Cancer potencies of heterocyclic amines found in cooked foods. Food Chem. Toxicol. 32:505-515.

Bois, F.Y., L. Zeise, and T.N. Tozer. 1990. Precision and sensitivity of pharmacokinetic models for cancer risk assessment: Tetrachloroethylene in mice, rats, and humans. Toxicol. Appl. Pharm. 102:300-315.

Bois, F.Y., A. Gelman, J. Jiang, and D.R. Maszle. 1994. A toxico-kinetic analysis of tetrachloroethylene metabolism in humans. Technical Report. California Environmental Protection Agency, Office of Environmental Health Hazard Assessment, Berkeley, CA.

Bois, F.Y., G. Krowech, and L. Zeise. 1995. Modeling human inter-individual variability in metabolism and risk: The example of 4-aminobiphenyl. Risk Analysis 15(2):205-213.

Boorman, G.A., R.R. Maronpot, and S.L. Eustis. 1994. Rodent carcinogenicity bioassay: Past, present, and future. Toxicologic Pathology 22(2):105-111.

Booth, A.N., O.H. Emerson, F.T. Jones, and F. DeEds. 1957. Urinary metabolites of caffeic and chlorogenic acids. J. Biol. Chem 229:51-59.

Bowers, J., B. Brown, J. Springer, L. Tollefson, R. Lorentzen, and S. Henry. 1993. Risk assessment for aflatoxin: An evaluation based on the multistage model. Risk Anal. 13:637-642.

Bressac, B., M. Kew, J. Wands, and M. Ozturk. 1991. Selective G to T mutations of *p53* gene in hepatocellular carcinoma from Southern Africa. Nature 350:429-431.

Brown, C.C., and K.C. Chu. 1989. Additive and multiplicative models and multistage carcinogenesis theory. Risk Anal. 9:99-105.

Clinton, W.P. 1985. The chemistry of coffee. Pp. 87-92 in

Proceedings of the 11th International Scientific Colloquium on Coffee, Loma, Togo. Paris: Association Scientifique International du Café.

Cohen, S.M., and L.B. Ellwein. 1990. Cell proliferation in carcinogenesis. Science 249:1007-1011.

Cohen, S.M., D.T. Purtilo, and L.B. Ellwein. 1991. Pivotal role of increased cell proliferation in human carcinogenesis. Mod. Pathol. 4:371-382.

Crouch, E., R. Wilson, and L. Zeise. 1987. Tautology or not tautology? J. Toxicol. Environ. Health 20:1-10.

Crump, K.S. 1984. An improved procedure for low-dose carcinogenic risk assessment from animal data. J. Environ. Pathol. Toxicol. Oncol. 5:339-348.

Czok, G., W. Walter, K. Knoche, and H. Degener. 1974. Uber die Resorbierbarkeit von Chlorogensaure durch die Ratte. Zeit. fur Ernahrungswissenschaft 13:108-112.

Dennis, M.J., A. Burrell, K. Mathieson, P. Willetts, and R.C. Massey. 1994. The determination of the flour improver potassium bromate in bread by gas chromatographic and ICP-MS methods. Food Addit. Contam. 11(6):633-639.

Dewanji, A., D. Krewski, and M.J. Goddard. 1993. A Weibull model for estimation of tumorigenic potency. Biometrics 49:367-377.

DHHS (U.S. Department of Health and Human Services). 1982. Third Annual Report on Carcinogens. DHHS, Public Health Service, NTIS PB83-135855. December.

DHHS (U.S. Department of Health and Human Services). 1991. Sixth Annual Report on Carcinogens. DHHS, Public Health Service.

Doll, R. 1992. The lessons of life. Keynote address to the Nutrition and Cancer Conference. Cancer Res. (Suppl.) 52:2024s-2029s.

Doll, R., and R. Peto. 1981. The causes of cancer: Quantitative estimates of avoidable risks of cancer in the United States today. J. Natl. Cancer Inst. 66:1191-1308.

Dunn, A., A.G. Salmon, and L. Zeise. 1991. Urethane: Background. Pp. 4-9 in Risks of Carcinogenesis from Urethane Exposure, A.G. Salmon and L. Zeise, eds. CRC Press.

Elkins, E.R. 1989. Effect of commercial processing on pesticide residues in selected fruits and vegetables. J. Assoc. Off. Anal. Chem.

72(3):533-535.

Ellen, G., E. Egmond, J.W. VanLoon, E.T. Sahertian, and K. Tolsma. 1990. Dietary intakes of some essential and non-essential trace elements, nitrate, nitrite and N-nitrosoamines, by Dutch adults: Estimated via a 24-hour duplicate portion study. Food Addit. Contam. 7(2):207-221.

EPA (U.S. Environmental Protection Agency). 1986a. Guidelines for carcinogen risk assessment. Fed. Reg. 51:33992-34003

EPA (U.S. Environmental Protection Agency). 1986b. Guidelines for the Health Risk Assessment for Chemical Mixtures. Federal Register 51(185):34014-34025.

EPA (U.S. Environmental Protection Agency). 1989a. Ethylene bisdithiocarbamates; Notice of Preliminary Determination to Cancel Certain Registrations, Notice of Availability of Technical Support Document and Draft Notice of Intent to Cancel. Federal Register 54(243):52158-52185.

EPA (U.S. Environmental Protection Agency). 1989b. Preliminary Determination to Cancel Certain Daminozide Product Registrations; Availability of Technical Support Document and Draft Notice of Intent to Cancel. Federal Register 54(99):22558-22573.

EPA (U.S. Environmental Protection Agency). 1992. Ethylene bisdithiocarbamates (EBDCs); Notice of Intent to Cancel; Conclusion of Special Review. Federal Register 57:7484

Farmer, J.H., R.L. Kodell, and D.W. Gaylor. 1982. Estimation and extrapolation of tumor probabilities from a mouse bioassay with survival/sacrifice components. Risk Anal. 2:27-34.

Farrar, D., B. Allen, K. Crump, and A. Shipp. 1989. Evaluation of uncertainty in input parameters to pharmacokinetic models and the resulting uncertainty in output. Toxicol. Lett. 49:371-385.

FDA (U.S. Food and Drug Administration). 1982a. FDA compliance program report of findings. FY 79 total diet studies—adult (7305.002). Washington, DC: U.S. Department of health and Human Services, Food and Drug Administration. PB83-112722.

FDA (U.S. Food and Drug Administration). 1982b. FDA compliance program report of findings. FY 79 total diet studies—infants and toddlers (7305.002). Washington, DC: U.S. Department of health and Human Services, Food and Drug Administration. PB82-

260213.

FDA (U.S. Food and Drug Administration). 1985. Sensitivity of Method Carcinogen Policy. Congressional Federal Register 40(No. 211) §45530-45553, October 31, 1985.

FDA (U.S. Food and Drug Adminstration). 1993. Food Additives: Threshold of Regulation for Substances Used in Food-Contact Articles. Federal Register 58:52719-52729.

Finkel, A. M. 1995. Toward less misleading comparisons of uncertain risks: The example of aflatoxin and alar. Environmental Health Perspectives 103:376-385.

Finkelstein, D.M., and L.M. Ryan. 1987. Estimating carcinogenic potency from a rodent tumorigenicity experiment. Appl. Stat. 36:121-133.

Frawley, J.P. 1967. Scientific evidence and common sense as a basis for food-packaging regulations. Food Cosmet. Toxicol. 5:293-308.

Friedenreich, C.M., and T.E. Rohan. 1995. A review of physical activity and breast cancer. Epidemiology 6:311-317.

Fung, V.A., J. Huff, E.K. Weisburger, and D.G. Hoel. 1993. Predictive strategies for selecting 379 NCI/NTP chemicals evaluated for carcinogenic potential: Scientific and public health impact. Fund. Appl. Toxicol. 20:413-436.

Fürst, P., C. Fürst, and K. Wilmers. 1991. Body burden with PCDD and PCDF from food. Pp. 133-142 in Banbury Report 35: Bioloical Basis for Risk Assessment of Dioxins and Related Compounds, M.A. Gallo, R.J. Scheuplein, and C.A. van der Heijden, eds. Cold Spring Harbour Laboratory Press.

Gallo, M.A., R. Scheuplein, and C.A. van der Heijden. 1991. Banbury Report 35: Biological Basis for Risk Assessment of Dioxins and Related Compounds. Cold Spring Harbour Laboratory Press. Pp. 179-212.

Gaylor, D.W. 1989. Preliminary estimates of the virtually safe dose for tumors obtained from the maximum tolerated dose. Reg. Toxicol. Pharmacol. 9:101-108.

Gaylor, D.W., and J.J. Chen. 1986. Relative potency of chemical carcinogens in rodents. Risk Anal. 6(3):283-290.

Gaylor, D.W., and F.F. Kadlubar. 1991. Quantitative cancer risk assessment of heterocyclic amines in cooked foods. Pp. 229-236 in

Mutagens in Food: Detection and Prevention, H. Hayatsu, ed. Boca Raton, FL: CRC Press, Inc.

Gaylor, D.W., J.J. Chen, and D.M. Sheehan. 1993. Uncertainty in cancer risk estimates. Risk Anal. 13:149-154.

Gaylor, D.W., and L.S. Gold. 1995. Quick estimates of the regulatory virtually safe dose based on the maximum tolerated dose for rodent bioassays. Regul. Toxicol. Pharmacol. 22:57-63.

Gaylor, D.W., R.L. Kodell, J.J. Chen, J.A.Springer, R.J. Lorentzen, and R.J. Scheuplein. 1994. Point estimates of cancer risk at low doses. Risk Analysis 14:843-850.

Gibb, H.J., and C.W. Chen. 1986. Multistage model interpretation of additive and multiplicative carcinogenic effects. Risk Anal. 6:167-170.

Giovannucci, E., E.B. Rimm, G.A. Colditz, M.J. Stampfer, A. Ascherio, C.C. Chute, and W.C. Willett. 1993. A prospective study of dietary fat and risk of prostate cancer. J. Natl. Cancer Inst. 85:1571-1579.

Goddard, M.J., and D. Krewski. 1995. The future of mechanistic research in risk assessment: Where are we going and can we get there from here? Toxicology. 102:53-70.

Goddard, M.J., D.J. Murdoch, and D. Krewski. 1995. Temporal aspects of risk characterization. Inhalation Toxicology 7:1005-1018.

Gold, L.S., L. Bernstein and B.N. Ames. 1990. The importance of ranking possible carcinogenic hazards using HERP. Risk Anal. 10:625-33

Gold, L.S., C.B. Sawyer, R. Magaw, G.M. Backman, M. de Veciana, R. Levinson, N.K. Hooper, W. Havender, L. Bernstein, R. Peto, M.C. Pike, and B.N. Ames. 1984. A carcinogenic potency database of the standardized results of animal bioassays. Environ. Health Perspect. 58:9-319.

Gold, L.S., T.H. Slone, G.M. Backman, S. Eisenberg, M. Da Costa, M. Wong, N.B. Manley, L. Rohrback, and B.N. Ames. 1990. Third chronological supplement to the Carcinogenic Potency Database: Standardized results of animal bioassays published through December 1986 and by the National Toxicology Program through June 1987. Environ. Health Perspect. 84:215-285.

Gold, L.S., T.H. Slone, B.R. Stern, N.B. Manley, and B.N. Ames. 1992. Rodent carcinogens: Setting priorities. Science 258:261-265.

Gold, L.S., N.B. Manley, T.H. Slone, G.B. Garfinkel, L. Rohrbach, and B.N. Ames. 1993a. The fifth plot of the Carcinogenic Potency Database: Results of animal bioassays published in the general literature through 1988 and by the National Toxicology Program through 1989. Environ. Health Perspectives 100:65-135.

Gold, L.S., T.H. Slone, B.R. Stern, N.B. Manley, and B.N. Ames. 1993b. Possible carcinogenic hazards from natural and synthetic chemicals: Setting priorities in Comparative Environmental Risk Assessment, C.R. Cothern, ed. Boca Raton: Lewis Publishers.

Gold, L.S., T.H. Slone, N.B. Manley, and B.N. Ames. 1994. Heterocyclic amines formed by cooking food: Comparison of bioassay results with other chemicals in the Carcinogenic Potency Database. Cancer Letters 83:21-29.

Goldbohm, R.A., P.A. van den Brandt, P. van't veer, H.A.M. Brants, E. Dorant, F. Sturmans, and R.J.J. Hermus. 1994. A prospective cohort study on the relation between meat consumption and the risk of colon cancer. Caner Res. 54:718-723.

Goodman, M.T., L.N. Kolonel, C.N. Yoshizawa, and J.H. Hankin. 1988. The effect of dietary cholesterol and fat on the risk of lung cancer in Hawaii. Am. J. Epidemiol. 128:1241-1255.

Goodman, G., and R. Wilson. 1992. Comparison of the dependence of the TD_{50} on maximum tolerated dose for mutagens and nonmutagens. Risk Anal. 12:525-534.

Government Accounting Office (GAO). 1991. Pesticides: Food Consumption Data of Little Value to Estimate Some Exposures. GAO/RCED-91-125. U.S. General Accounting Office, Resources, Community and Economic Development Division, Washington, DC.

Harborne, J.B. 1993. Introduction to Ecological Biochemistry, 4th edition. London: Academic Press. 318pp.

Haseman, J.K., and S.K. Seilkop. 1992. An examination of the association between maximum-tolerated dose and carcinogenicity in 326 long term studies in rats and mice. Fund. Appl. Toxicology 19:207-213.

Henderson, B.E., J.T. Casagrande, M.C. Pike, T. Mack, and T. Rosario. 1983. The epidemiology of endometrial cancer in young women. Br. J. Cancer 47:749-756.

Herrmann, K. 1978. Ubersicht uber nichtessentielle inhaltsstoffe der germusearten III. Mohren, Sellerie, Pastinaken, Rote Ruben, Spinat, Salat, Endivien, Trieibzichorie, Rhabarber und Artischock. Z Lebensm Unter.-Forsch 167:262-273.

Herrmann, K. 1989. Occurrence and content of hydroxycinnamic and hydroxybenzoic acid compounds in foods. Crit. Rev. Fd. Sci. Nutri. 28(4):315-347.

Hetrick, D.M., A.M. Jarabek, and C.C. Travis. 1991. Sensitivity analysis for physiologically based pharmacokinetic models. J. Pharmacokinet. Biopharm. 19:1-20.

Higginson, J. 1988. Changing concepts in cancer prevention: Limitations and implications for future research in environmental carcinogenesis. Cancer Research 48:1381-1389.

Hoel, D. 1990. Assumptions of the HERP index. Risk Anal. 10(4):623-624.

Hoel, D.G., J.K. Haseman, M.D. Hogan, J. Huff, and E.E. McConnell. 1988. The impact of toxicity on carcinogenicity studies: Implications for risk assessment. Carcinogenesis 9:2045-2052

Hoseyni, M.S. 1992. Risk assessment for aflatoxin: III. Modeling the relative risk of hepatocellular carcinoma. Risk Anal. 12:123-128.

Howe, G.R., T. Hirohata, T.G. Hislop, J.M. Iscovich, J.-M. Yuan, K. Katsouyanni, F. Lulian, E. Marulini, B. Moda, T. Rohan, P. Tonialo, and Y. Shunghang. 1990. Dietary factors and risk of breast cancer: Combined analysis of 12 case-control studies. J. Natl. Cancer Inst. 82:561-569.

Hsu, I.C., R.A. Metcalf, T. Sun, J.A. Welsh, N.J. Wang, and C.C. Harris. 1991. Mutational hotspot in the *p53* gene in human hepatocellular carcinomas. Nature 350:427-428.

Hunter, D.J., and W.C. Willett. 1993. Diet, body size, and breast cancer. Epidemiol. Rev. 15(1):110-132.

Idle, J.R., M. Armstrong, A.V. Boddy, C. Boustead, S. Cholerton, J. Cooper, A.K. Daly, J. Ellis, W. Gregory, H. Hadidi, C. Hofer, J. Holt, J. Leathart, N. McCracken, S.C. Monkman, J.E. Painter, H. Taber, D. Walker, and M. Yule. 1992. The pharmacogenetics of chemical carcinogenesis. Pharmacogen. 2:246-258.

ILSI (International Life Sciences Institute). 1993. Approaches for Establishing A Safe Intake Level for Ingested Acetaldehyde. Washington, D.C.: ILSI North America.

Inoue, S., K. Ito, K. Yamamoto, and S. Kawanishi. 1992. Caffeic acid causes metal-dependent damage to cellular and isolated DNA through H2O2 formation. Carcinogenesis 13:1497-502.

IARC (International Agency for Research on Cancer). 1976. IARC Monographs on the Evaluation of Carcinogenic Risk of Chemicals to Man. Pp. 51-72 in Some Naturally Occurring Substances, vol. 10. Lyon, France: IARC.

IARC (International Agency for Research on Cancer). 1982. IARC Monographs on the Evaluation of Carcinogenic Risks to Humans. Volume 29: Some Industrial Chemicals and Dyestuffs. WHO, IARC. 416 pp.

IARC (International Agency for Research on Cancer). 1983. Laboratory decontamination and destruction of carcinogens in laboratory wastes: some polycyclic aromatic hydrocarbons. IARC Scientific Publications No. 49.

IARC (International Agency for Research on Cancer). 1992. Mechanisms of Carcinogenesis in Risk Identification, H. Vainio, P.N. Magee, D.B. McGregor, and A.J. McMichael editors. WHO, IARC. pp. 579-599 in IARC Scientific Publications No. 116.

IARC (International Agency for Research on Cancer). 1993. IARC Monographs on the Evaluation of Carcinogenic Risks to Humans. Lists of IARC Evaluations. WHO, IARC, Lyon. Vol. 56.

IFBC (International Food Biotechnology Council). 1990. Toxicol. Pharmacol. 12:526-528

Ito, N., M. Hirose, and S. Takahashi. 1991. Cellular proliferation and stomach carcinogenesis induced by antioxidants. Pp. 43-52 in Chemically Induced Cell Proliferation: Implications for Risk Assessment., eds. Wiley Liss.

Jackel, S.S. 1994. Update on potassium bromate. Cereal Food World 39(10):772.

Kodell, R.L., and D.W. Gaylor. 1989. On the additive and multiplicative models of relative risk. Biom. J. 31:359-370.

Kodell, R.L., D.W. Gaylor, and J.J. Chen. 1990. Carcinogenic potency correlations: Real or artifactual? J. Toxicol. Environ. Health 32:1-9.

Kodell, R.L., D. Krewski, and J.M. Zielinski. 1991. Additive and multiplicative relative risk in the two-stage clonal expansion model of carcinogenesis. Risk Anal. 11:483-490.

Kohn, M.C., and C.J. Portier. 1993. Effects of the mechanism of receptor-mediated gene expression on the shape of the dose-response curve. Risk Anal. 13(5):565-572.

Kolonel, L.N., A.M.Y. Nomura, M.W. Hinds, T. Hirohata, J.H. Hankin, and J. Lee. 1983. Role of diet in cancer incidence in Hawaii. Cancer Res. 43:2397s-2402s

Krewski, D. 1990. Measuring carcinogenic potency. Risk Analysis 10:615-617.

Krewski, D., and R.D. Thomas. 1992. Carcinogenic mixtures. Risk Anal. 12:105-113.

Krewski, D., D. Murdoch, and J.R. Withey. 1989. Recent developments in carcinogenic risk assessment (with discussion). Health Phys. 57(Supplement 1):313-325.

Krewski, D., M.J. Goddard, and J.R. Withey. 1990. Carcinogenic potency and interspecies extrapolation. Pp. 323-334 in Cancer and the Environment, Pard D: Carcinogenesis. M.L. Mendelson and R.J. Albertini, eds. New York: Wiley-Liss.

Krewski, D., M. Szyszkowicz, and H. Rosenkranz. 1990. Quantitative factors in chemical carcinogenesis: variation in carcinogenic potency. Regul. Toxicol. Pharmacol. 12:13-29.

Krewski, D., D. Gaylor, and M. Szyszkowicz. 1991. A model-free approach to low-dose extrapolation. Environ. Health Perspect. 90:279-285.

Krewski, D., M.J. Goddard, and J.M. Zielinski. 1992. Dose-response relationships in carcinogenesis. Pp. 579-599 in Mechanisms of Carcinogenesis in Risk Identification, H. Vainio, P.N. Magee, D.B. McGregor, and A.J. McMichael, eds. A.J. Lyon: IARC.

Krewski, D., D.W. Gaylor, A.P. Soms, and M. Syzszkowicz. 1993. Correlation between carcinogenic potency and the maximum tolerated dose: Implications for risk assessment. Pp. 111-171 in Issues in Risk Assessment. Washington, DC: National Academy Press.

Krewski, D., J.R. Withey, L.-F. Ku, and M.E. Andersen. 1994. Applications of physiologic pharmacokinetic modeling in carcinogenic risk assessment. Environmental Health Perspectives 102(Suppl. 11):37-50.

Krewski, D., Y. Wang, S. Bartlett, and K. Krishnan. 1995.

Uncertainty, variability, and sensitivity analysis in physiologic pharmacokinetic models. Journal of Biopharmaceutical Statistics in press.

Layton, D.W., K.T. Bogen, M.G. Knize, F.T. Hatch, V.M. Johnson, and J.S. Felton. 1995. Cancer risk of heterocyclic amines in cooked foods: An analysis and implications for research. Carcinogenesis 16(1):39-52.

Lee, I.M., R.S. Paffenbarger, Jr., and C. Hsieh. 1991. Physical activity and risk of developing colorectal cancer among college alumni. J. Natl. Cancer Inst. 83:1324-1329.

Lee, I.M., R.S. Paffenbarger, and E.C. Hseieh. 1992. Physical activity and risk of prostate cancer among college alumni. Am. J. Epidemiol. 135:169-179.

Le Marchand, L., L.N. Kolonel, L.R. Wilkens, B.C. Myers, and T. Hirohata. 1994. Animal fat consumption and prostate cancer: A prospective study in Hawaii. Epidemiology 5:276-282.

Levander, O.A. 1987. A global view of human selenium nutrition. Annu. Rev. Nutr. 7:227-250.

Littlefield, N.A., J.H. Farmer, D.W. Gaylor, and W.G. Sheldon. 1980. Effects of dose and time in a long-term, low-dose carcinogenic study. J. Environ. Pathol. Toxicol. 3:17-34.

Lutz, W.K., and J. Schlatter. 1992. Chemical carcinogens and overnutrition in diet-related cancer. Carcinogenesis 13:2211-2216.

Lyon, J.L., J.W. Gardner, and D.W. West. 1980. Cancer risk and lifestyle: Cancer among Mormons (1967-1975). Pp. 273-290 in Genetic and Environmental Factors in Experimental and Human Cancer, H.V. Gelboin, B. MacMahon, T. Matsuhara, T. Sugimura, S. Takayama, and H. Takebe, eds. Tokyo: Japanese Scientific Society Press.

Massey, R., M.J. Dennis, M. Pointer, and P.E. Key. 1990. An investigation of the levels of N-nitrosodimethylamine, apparent total N-nitroso compounds, and nitrate in beer. Food Addit. Contam. 7(5):605-615.

McCann, J., L.S. Gold, L. Horn, R. McGill, T.E. Graedel, and J. Kaldor. 1988. Statistical analysis of Salmonella test data and comparison to results of animal cancer tests. Mutat. Res. 205:183-195.

McGregor, D.B. 1992. Chemicals classified by IARC: their potency in tests for carcinogenicity in rodents and their genotoxicity and acute toxicity. Pp. 323-352 in Mechanisms of Carcinogenesis in Risk Identification. H. Vainio, P.N. Magee, D.B. McGregor, and A.J. McMichael, eds. International Agency for Research on Cancer. Lyon, France.

Metzger, B., E. Crouch, and R. Wilson. 1989. On the relationship between carcinogenicity and acute toxicity. Risk Anal. 9:169-177.

Miller, J.D. 1994. Mycotoxin Overview. Presented at the Toxicology Forum Special Meeting on Mycotoxin Health Risk, Control and Regulation. Capital Hilton, Washington DC, February 23-24.

Moolgavkar, S.H., and G. Luebeck. 1990. Two-event model for carcinogenesis: Biological, mathematical, and statistical considerations. Risk Anal. 10(2):323-341.

Moolgavkar, S.H., E.G. Luebeck, D. Krewski, and J.M. Zielinski. 1993. Radon cigarette smoke, and lung cancer: A re-analysis of the Colorado Plateau uranium miners'data. Epidemiology 4(3):204-217.

Morgan, K.J., V.J. Stults, and M.E. Zabik. 1982. Amount and dietary sources of caffeine and saccharin intake by individuals ages 5 to 18 years. Regul. Toxicol. Pharmacol. 2:296-307.

Morgan, M.G., and M. Henrion. 1990. Uncertainty: A Guide to Dealing with Uncertainty in Quantitative Risk and Policy Analysis. Cambridge: Cambridge University Press.

Munro, I.C. 1990. Safety assessment procedures for indirect food additives: an overview. Regul. Toxicol. Pharmacol. 12:2-12.

Murdoch, D.J., D. Krewski, and J. Wargo. 1992. Cancer risk assessment with intermittent exposure. Risk Analysis 12:569-577.

National Institute on Alcohol Abuse and Alcoholism. 1988. Alcohol Epidemiologic Data System. Surveillance Report #10. Apparent per capita alcohol consumption: National, state, and regional trends, 1977-1986. U.S. Department of Health and Human Services.

NRC (National Research Council). 1978. Saccharin: Technical Assessment of Risks and Benefits. Washington, DC: National Academy Press.

NRC (National Research Council). 1979a. Use and Intake of Food and Color Additives. Washington, DC: National Academy Press.

NRC (National Research Council). 1979b. The 1977 Survey of

Industry on the Use of Food Additives. Washington, DC: National Academy Press.

NRC (National Research Council). 1981. The Health Effectsof Nitrate, Nitrite, and N-Nitroso Compounds. National Academy of Sciences. Washington, DC: National Academy Press.

NRC (National Research Council). 1982. Diet, Nutrition and Cancer. Washington, DC: National Academy Press.

NRC (National Research Council). 1987. Pharmacokinetics in Risk Assessment. Pp. 441-468 in Drinking Water and Health, Volume 8. Washington, DC: National Academy Press.

NRC (National Research Council). 1988. Complex Mixtures: Methods for In Vivo Toxicity Testing. Washington, DC: National Academy Press.

NRC (National Research Council). 1989b. Drinking Water and Health. Vol. 9. Selected Issues in Risk Assessment. Washington, DC: National Academy Press.

NRC (National Research Council). 1989a. Diet and Health: Implications for Reducing Chronic Disease Risk. Food and Nutrition Board, Committee on Diet and Health. Washington, DC.: National Academy Press.

NRC (National Research Council). 1993b. Issues in Risk Assessement: Use of the Maximum Tolerated Dose in Animal Bioassays for Carcinogenicity. Washington, DC: National Academy Press.

NRC (National Research Council). 1993a. Pesticides in the Diets of Infants and Children. Washington, DC: National Academy Press.

NRC (National Research Council). 1994. Science and Judgment in Risk Assessment. Washington, DC: National Academy Press.

National Toxicology Program (NTP). 1995. DRAFT NTP Technical Report on the Effect of Dietary Restriction on Toxicology and Carcinogenesis Studies in F344/N Rats and B6C3F1 Mice. NTIP Technical Report Series No. 460. NIH Publication No. 95-3376. U.S. Department of Health and Human Services, Public Health Service, National Institutes of Health, Research Triangle Park, NC.

Nomura, A., and L.N. Kolonel. 1991. Prostate cancer: A current perspective. Epidemiol. Rev. 13:200-227.

Pariza, M.W., and R.K. Boutwell. 1987. Historical perspective:

Calories and energy expenditure in carcinogenesis. Amer. J. Clin. Nutrit. 45(Suppl):151-156.

Parodi, S., M. Taningher, P. Boero, and L. Santi. 1982. Quantitative correlations amongst alkaline DNA fragmentation, DNA covalent binding, mutagenicity in the Ames test and carcinogenicity, for 21 compounds. Mutat. Res. 93:1-24.

Pennington, J.A., B.E. Young, and D.B. Wilson. 1989. Nutritional elements in U.S. diets: Results from the Total Diet Study, 1982 to 1986. J. Am. Diet Assoc. 89:639-644.

Perera, F., and P. Boffetta. 1988. Perspectives on comparing risks of environmental carcinogens. JNCI 80:1282-1293.

Peters, R.K., D.H. Garabrant, M.C. Yu, and T.M. Mack. 1989. A case-control study of occupational and dietary factors in colorectal cancer in young men by subsite. Cancer Res. 49:5459-5468.

Peto, R., M.C. Pike, N.E. Day, R.G. Gray, P.N. Lee, S. Parish, J. Peto, S. Richards, and J. Wharendorf. 1980. Guidelines for simple, sensitive significance tests for carcinogenic effects in long term animal experiments. Pp. 311-426 in IARC Monographs on the Evaluation of the Carcinogenic Risk of Chemicals to Humans: Supplement of Long-Term and Short-Term Screening Assays for Carcinogens: A Critical Appraisal. International Agency for Research on Cancer. Lyon, France.

Peto, R., M. Pike, L. Bernstein, L.S. Gold, and B. Ames. 1984a. The TD_{50}: A proposed general convention for the numerical description of the carcinogenic potency of chemicals in chronic exposure animal experiments. Environ. Health Perspect. 58:1-9

Peto, R., R. Gray, P. Brantom., and P. Grasso. 1984b. Nitrosamine carcinogenesis in 5120 rodents: Chronic administration of sixteen different concentrations of NDEA, NDMA, NPYR, and NPIP in the water of 4400 inbred rats with parallel studies on NDEA alone of the effect of age of starting (8, 6, or 20 weeks) and of species (rats, mice hamsters). Pp. 617-665 in N-Nitroso Compounds: Occurrence, Biological Effects and Relevance to Human Cancer, I.K. O'Neill, R.G. Borstell, C.T. Miller, J. Long, and H. Bartsch, eds. IARC Scientific Publications No. 57. Lyon France: IARC.

Piegorsch, W.W., and D.G. Hoel. 1988. Exploring relationships between mutagenic and carcinogenic potencies. Mutat. Res. 196:161-

175

Pignatelli, B., Malaveille, C. Chen, A. Hautefeuille, P. Thuillier, N. Muñoz, B. Moulinier, F. Berger, H. DeMontclos, H. Oshima, R. Lambert, and H. Bartsch. 1991. N-Nitroso compounds, genotoxins and their precursors in gastric juice from humans with and without precancerous lesions of the stomach. In Relevance to Human Cancer of N-Nitroso Compounds, Tobacco Smoke and Mycotoxins, I.K. O'Neill, J. Chen, H. Bartsch, eds. International Agency for Research on Cancer (IARC) Scientific Publication No. 105. Lyon: IARC.

Pohland, A.E. 1994. Worldwide Occurrence of Fumonisins. Proceedings of Toxicology Forum Special Meeting on Mycotoxin Health Risk, Control, and Regulation, Feb. 23-24, 1994. Washington, DC: Toxicology Forum.

Portier, C.J., and D.G. Hoel. 1987. Issues concerning the estimation of TD_{50}. Risk Anal. 7:437-449.

Portier, C.J., and N.L. Kaplan. 1989. Variability of safe dose estimates when using complicated models of the carcinogenic process. A case study: Methylene chloride. Fund. Appl. Toxicol. 13:533-544.

Potter, J.D., M.L. Slattery, R.M. Bostick, and S.M. Gapstur. 1993. Colon cancer: A review of the epidemiology. Epidemiol. Rev. 15(2):499-545.

Prentice, R.L., and L. Sheppard. 1990. Dietary fat and cancer: Consistency of the epidemiologic data, and disease prevention that may follow from a practical reduction in fat consumption. Cancer Causes and Control 1:81.

Preussmann, R. 1984. Occurrence nad exposure to N-nitroso compounds and precursors. Pp. N-Nitroso Compounds: Occurrence, Biological Effects and Relevance to Human Cancer, I.K. O'Neill, R.C. von Borstel, C.T. Miller, J. Long, and H. Bartsch, eds. International Agency for Research on Cancer (IARC) Scientific Publication No. 57. Lyon: IARC.

Ranum, P. 1992. Potassium bromate in bread baking. Creal Food World (37(3):253-258.

Reith, J.P., and T.B. Starr. 1989. Experimental desing constraints on carcinogenic potency estimates. J. Toxicol. Environ. Health 27:287-296.

Reitz, R.H., P.G. Watanabe, M.J. McKenna, J.F. Quast, and P.J.

Gehring. 1980. Effects of vinylidene chloride on DNA synthesis and DNA repair in the rat and mouse: A comparative study with dimethylnitrosamine. Toxicol. Appl. Pharmacol. 52:357-370.

Reitz, R.H., A.L. Mendrala, R.A. Corley, J.F. Quast, M.L. Gargas, M.E. Andersen, D.A. Staats, and R.B. Connolly. 1990. Estimating the risk of liver cancer associated with human exposures to chloroform using physiologically-based pharmacokinetic modeling. Toxicol. Appl. Pharmacol. 105:443-459.

Risch, B., and K. Herrmann. 1988. Hydroxyzimtsäure-Verbindungen in citrus-früchten. Z Lebensm Unters.-Forsch 187:530-534.

Risch, H.A., M. Jain, L. Marrett, and G.R. Howe. 1994. Dietary fat intake and risk of epithelial ovarian cancer. J. Natl. Cancer Inst. 86:1409-1415.

Roe, F.J.C. 1988. How do hormones cause cancer? Pp. in Theories of Carcinogenesis. O. H. Iversen, ed. New York: Hemisphere Publishing Corporation.

Rose, D.P., A.P. Boyar, and E.L. Wynder. 1986. International comparisons of mortality rates for cancer of the breast, ovary, prostate, and colon, and per capita food consumption. Cancer. 58:2363.

Rosenkranz, H.S. 1992. Structure-activity relationships for carcinogens with different modes of action. Pp. 271-277 in Mechanisms of Carcinogenesis in Risk Identification, H. Vainio, P.N. Magee, D.B. McGregor, and A.J. McMichael, eds. International Agency for Research on Cancer Scientific Publications No. 116, Lyon.

Rulis, A.M. 1986. De minimis risk and the threshold of regulation. Pp. 29-37 in Food Protection Technology, C.W. Felix, ed. Chelsea, MI: Lewis Publishers.

Rulis, A.M. 1989. Establishing a threshold of regulation. Pp. 271-278 in Risk Assessment in Setting National Priorities, J.J. Bonin, and D.E. Stevenson, eds. New York: Plenum.

Rulis, A.M. 1992. Threshold of regulation: Options for handling minimal risk situations. Pp. 132-139 in Food Safety Assessment. ACS Sympos. Series 484.

Sawyer, C., R. Peto, L. Bernstein, and M. Pike. 1984. Calculation of carcinogenic potency from long-term animal experiments. Biometrics 40:27-40.

Scanlan, R.A. 1983. Formation and occurrence of nitrosamines in food. Cancer Research 43:2435-2440.

Scanlan, R.A., and J.F. Barbour. 1991. N-Nitrosodimethylamine content of US and Canadian beer. In Relevance to Human Cancer of N-Nitroso Compounds, Tobacco Smoke and Mycotoxins, I.K. O'Neill, J. Chen, and H. Bartsch, eds. International Agency for Research on Cancer (IARC) Scientific Publication No. 105. Lyon: IARC.

Scheuplein, R.J. 1990. Perspectives on toxicological risk—an example: Food-borne carcinogenic risk. Pp. 351-371 in Progress in Predictive Toxicology. D.B. Clayson, I.C. Munro, P. Shubik, and J.A. Swenberg, eds. Elsevier Science Publ., B.V.

Schrauzer, G.N., and D.A. White. 1978. Selenium in human nutrition: Dietary intakes and effects of supplementation. Bioinorg. Chem. 8:303-318.

Schubert, A., M. M. Holden, and W.R. Wolf. 1987. Selenium content of a core group of foods based on a critical evaluation of published analytical data. J. Am. Diet Assoc. 87:285-299.

Shibamoto, T., and L.F. Bjeldanes. 1993. Introduction to Food Toxicology. New York: Academic Press.

Simonich, S.L., and R.A. Hites. 1994. Importance of vegetation in removing polycyclic aromatic hydrocarbons from the atmosphere. Nature 370:49-51.

Springer, J. 1994. Risk Assessment: FDA's most recent risk assessment. Presented at the Toxicology Forum Special Meeting on Mycotoxin Health Risk, Control and Regulation. Capital Hilton, Washington DC, February 23-24.

Steinmetz, K.A., and J.D. Potter. 1991. Vegetables, fruit, and cancer. I. Epidemiology (Review). Cancer Causes Control 5:325-357

Stich, H.F. 1991. The beneficial and hazardous effects of simple phenolic compounds. Mutation Research 259:307-324.

Stich, H.F. 1992. Teas and tea components as inhibitors of carcinogen formation in model systems and man. Preventive Medicine 21:377-84.

Stolz, D.R., B. Stavric, R. Stapley, R. Klaassen, R. Bendall, and D. Krewski. 1984. Mutagenicity screening of foods. II. Results with fruits and vegetables. Environ. Mut. 6:343-354

Sugimura, T. 1985. Carcinogenicity of mutagenic heterocyclic amines formed during the cooking process. Mut. Res. 150:33-41.

Sugimura, T. 1986. Studies on environmental chemical carcinogenesis in Japan. Science 233:312-318.

Sweet, D.V., ed. 1987. Registry of Toxic Effects of Chemical Substances (RTECS). 1986 Edition. National Center for Occupational Safety and Health. Washington, D.C.

Takayama, S., Y. Nakatsure, M. Masuda, H. Ohgaki, S. Sato, and T. Sugimura. 1984. Demonstration of carcinogenicity in F344 rats of 2-amino-3-methylimidazo[4,5-f]quinoline from broiled sardine, fried beef and beef extract. Gann 75:467-570.

Tanaka ,T., W.S. Barnes, G.M. Williams, and J.H. Weisburger. 1985. Multipotential carcinogenicity of the fried food mutagen 2-1mino-3-methylimidazo[4,5-f]quinoline in rats. Jpn. J. Cancer Res. 76:570-576.

Tanaka ,T., T. Kojima, T. Kawamor, A. Wang, M. Suzui, K. Okamoto, and H. Mori. 1993. Inhibition of 4-nitroquinoline-1-oxide-induced rat tongue carcinogenesis by the naturally occurring plant phenolics caffeic, ellagic, chlorogenic and ferulic acids. Carcinogenesis 14:1321-5.

Technical Assessment Systems. 1995a. Exposure®. Detailed Distributional Dietary Exposure Analysis. Washington, D.C.: Technical Assessment Systems, Inc.

Technical Assessment Systems. 1995b. TASDIET®. International Diet Research System. Washington, D.C.: Technical Assessment Systems, Inc.

Tennant, R.W., M.R. Elwell, J.W. Spalding, and R.A. Griesemer. 1991. Evidence that toxic injury is not always associated with induction of chemical carcinogenesis. Molecular Carcinogenesis 4:420-440.

Toda, S., M. Kumura, and M. Ohnishi. 1991. Effects of phenolcarboxylic acids on superoxide anion and lipid peroxidation induced by superoxide anion. Planta Medica 57:8-10.

Travis, C.C., and R.K. White. 1988. Interspecies scaling of carcinogenic potency. Risk Analysis 8:119-125.

Travis, C.C., S.A. Richter Pack, A.W. Saulsbury, and M.W. Yambert. 1990a. Prediction of carcinogenic potency from toxicology data.

Mutat. Res. 241:21-36.

Travis, C.C., A.W. Saulsbury, and S.A. Richter Pack. 1990b. Prediction of cancer potency using a battery of mutation and toxicity data. Mutagenesis 5:213-219.

Travis, C.C., L.A. Wang, and M.J. Waehner. 1991. Quantitative correlation of carcinogenic potency with four different classes of short-term test data. Mutagenesis 6:353-360.

Tricker, A.R., B. Pfundstein, E. Theobald, R. Preussmann, and B. Spiegelhalder. 1991. Mean daily intake of volatile N-nitrosoamines from foods and beverages in West Germany in 1989-1990. Food Chem. Toxicol. 29:729-732.

Turnbull, G.J., P.N. Lee, and F.J.C. Roe. 1985. Relationship of body weight to longevity and to risk of development of nephropathy and neoplasia in Sprague-Dawley rats. Food Chem. Toxicol. 23:355-362.

Turturro, A., P.H. Duffy, and R.W. Hart. 1993. Modulation of toxicity by diet and dietary macronutrient restriction. Mutation Research 295:151-164.

USDA (U.S. Department of Agriculture). 1987. Nationwide Food Consumption Survey. Continuing Survey of Food Intake of Individuals. Women 19-50 years and their children 1-5 years, 4 days, 1985. Report No. 85-4. Nutrition Monitoring Division, Human Nutrition Information Service. Hyattsville, MD

USDA (U.S. Department of Agriculture). 1992. Nutrient Database for Standard Reference. Release 10 Tape. Human Nutrition Information Service. Hyattsville, MD

Vainio, H., M. Sorsa, and A.J. McMichael. 1990. Complex Mixtures and Cancer Risk. IARC Sci. Publ. No. 104. International Agency for Research on Cancer. Lyon, France

Van Ryzin, J. 1980. Quantitative risk assessment. J. Occup. Med. 22(5):321-326.

Van't Veer, P., F.J. Kok, H.A.M. Brants, T. Ockhuizen, F. Sturmans, and R.J.J. Hermus. 1990. Dietary fat and the risk of breast cancer. Int. J. Epidemiol. 19:12-18.

Watanabe, K., F.Y. Bois, and L. Zeise. 1992. Interspecies extrapolation: A reexamination of acute toxicity data. Risk Analysis 12(2):301-310.

Wartenberg, D., and M.A. Gallo. 1990a. The fallacy of ranking possible carcinogenic hazards using the TD50. Risk Analysis 10(4):609-613.

Wartenberg, D., and M.A. Gallo. 1990b. A response to comments. Risk Analysis 10(4):629-633.

Wattenberg, L.W., J.B. Coccia, and L.K.T. Lam. 1980. Inhibitory effects of phenolic compounds on benzo(a)pyrene-induced neoplasia. Cancer Res. 40:2820-2823.

Wegstaff, J. 1991. Dietary exposure to furocoumarins. Regulatory Toxicology and Pharmacology 14:261-272.

Weinberg, R.A. 1989. Oncogenes, antioncogenes and the molecular bases of multistep carcinogenesis. Cancer Res. 49:3713-3721.

Welsch, C.W. 1992. Cancer Research. 52(Suppl. 7):20405.

Welsch, C.W., J.L. House, B.L. Herr, S.J. Eliasberg, and M.A. Welsch. 1990. Enhancement of mammary carcinogenesis by high levels of dietary fat: A phenomenon dependent on ad libitum feeding. JNCI 82:1615-1620.

Welsh, E.A., J.M. Holden, W.R. Wolf, et al. 1981. Selenium in self-selected diets of Maryland residents. J. Am. Diet Assoc. 79:277-285.

West, D.W., M.L. Slattery, L.M. Robison, K.L. Schuman, M.H. Ford, A.W. Mahoney, J.L. Lyon, and A.W. Sorensen. 1989. Dietary intake and colon cancer: Sex- and anatomic site-specific associations. Amer. J. Epidemiol. 130:883-894.

Whittemore, A.S., A.H. Wu-Williams, M. Lee, et al. 1990. Diet, physical activity, and colorectal cancer among Chinese in North America and China. J. Natl. Cancer Inst. 82:915-926.

WHO (World Health Organization. 1979. DDT and Its Derivatives. Environmental Health Criteria 9. Geneva: WHO.

WHO (World Health Organization. 1988. PCBs, PCDDs and PCDFs in Breast Milk: Assessment of Health Risks. Environmental Health Series 29. Europe, Copenhagen: WHO, Regional Office.

WHO (World Health Organization. 1991. Lindane. Environmental Health Criteria 124. Geneva: WHO International Programme on Chemical Safety.

WHO (World Health Organization. 1993. Polychlorinated Biphenyls and Terphenyls (Second Edition). Environmental Health Criteria 140. Geneva: WHO, International Programme on Chemical Safety.

Willett, W.C., M.J. Stampfer, G.A. Colditz, B.A. Rosner, and F.E.

Speizer. 1990. Relation of meat, fat, and fiber intake to the risk of colon cancer in a prospective study among women. N. Engl. J. Med. 323:1664-1672.

Winter, M., and K. Herrmann. 1986. Esters and glucosides of hydroxycinnamic acids in vegetables. J. Agri. Food Chem. 34:616-620.

Wu-Williams, A.H., L. Zeise, and D. Thomas. 1992. Risk assessment for aflatoxin B1: A modeling approach. Risk Anal. 12:559-567.

Yeh, F.-S. M.-C. Yu, C.-C. Mo, S. Luo, M.J. ong, and B.E. Henderson. 1989. Hepatitis B virus, aflatoxins, and hepatocellular carcinoma in southern Guangxi, China. Cancer Res. 49:2506-2509.

Youngman, L.D., J.Y. Park, and B.N. Ames. 1992. Protein oxidation associated with aging is reduced by dietary restriction of protein or calories. Proc. Natl. Acad. Sci. U.S.A. 89:9112-9116.

Zeise, L., R. Wilson, E.A.C. Crouch, and M. Fiering. 1982. Use of toxicity to estimate carcinogenic potency. In Health and Environmental Effects Document: Non-Regulatory and Cost Effective Control of Carcinogenic Hazard. Report to the Department of Energy, Health and Assessment Division, Office of Energy Research. Energy and Environmental Policy Center, Harvard University, Cambridge, September.

Zeise, L., R. Wilson, and E.A.C. Crouch. 1984. Use of acute toxicity to estimate carcinogenic risk. Risk Anal. 4(3):187-199.

Zeise, L., E.A.C. Crouch, and R. Wilson. 1986. A possible relationship between toxicity and carcinogenicity. J. Am. Coll. Toxicol. 5:137-151

Zeise, L. 1989. Issues in State risk assessment. Pp. 135-144 in Proceedings—Pesticides and Other Toxics: Assessing Their Risks, J.E. White, ed. University of California at Riverside.

Zhou, Y.C., and R.L. Zheng. 1991. Phenolic compounds and as analog as superoxide anion scavengers and antioxidants. Biochem. Pharmacol. 42:1177-1179.

Zimmerli, B., and J. Schlatter. 1991. Ethyl carbamate: Analytical methodology, occurrence, formation, biological activity and risk assessment. Mutation Research 259:325-350.

6

Conclusions, Recommendations, and Future Directions

As indicated in the original statement of task to this committee, the purpose of this report is to examine the occurrence, toxicologic data, mechanisms of action, and potential role of natural carcinogens in the causation of cancer, including relative risk comparisons with synthetic carcinogens, and a consideration of anticarcinogens. The committee was also asked to develop a strategy for selecting additional natural substances for toxicological testing.

This subject is immense because by far the major source of exposure to naturally occurring chemicals is the diet, and the concern that dietary factors might play a major role in human cancer causation. Therefore, this committee addressed its charge by focusing its attention on naturally occurring and synthetic dietary chemicals with carcinogenic potential. This report does not consider non-cancer effects or broader aspects of environmental exposure, such as air, water (other than drinking water), or occupational hazards; nor are the carcinogenic effects of radiation or physical agents covered in this report. Some of the latter aspects have been covered in previous NRC reports.

The committee was also asked to assess the impact of naturally occurring chemicals on the initiation, promotion, and progression of tumors. In this report, these stages of carcinogenesis were considered from a mechanistic point of view, but most carcinogenicity data on the compounds reviewed do not provide precise information on the specific stage or stages of the multistage process at which these compounds act. Because the terms "initiator," "promoter," and "progressor" are especially difficult to apply to specific agents, particularly as they pertain to human carcinogenesis, the committee chose to use the more contemporary classification of agents as genotoxic and nongenotoxic. Although the committee recognized the importance of the legal and regulatory aspects of the subject of naturally occurring dietary carcinogens, it was felt that these aspects were beyond the purview of its task. A strengthening of the scientific base of the subject of naturally occurring carcinogens will provide a better foundation for regulatory policy and actions.

The purpose of this chapter is to review the committee's major conclusions and recommendations. Several specific principles emerged from the deliberations, including 1) that the great majority of individual naturally occurring and synthetic chemicals in the diet are present at levels below a significant biologic effect, so low that they are unlikely to pose an appreciable cancer risk and 2) that the macronutrients and excess total calories present the greatest dietary cancer risk in the United States. Nevertheless, it was apparent that the existing database and methods are insufficient to identify the precise roles of individual naturally occurring dietary chemicals in human cancer causation and prevention. Therefore, this chapter concludes with a set of proposals for future directions of research, including fundamental mechanistic studies and development of more sophisticated methods that can be applied in laboratory assays and in human populations. Advances in these areas of research will be greatly enhanced by taking advantage of powerful new concepts and methods in analytical and structural chemistry, cellular biology, and molecular genetics.

CONCLUSIONS

Several broad perspectives emerged from the committee's deliberations. First, the committee concluded that based upon existing exposure data the great majority of individual naturally occurring and synthetic chemicals in the diet appear to be present at levels below which any significant biologic effect is likely, and so low that they are unlikely to pose an appreciable cancer risk. The NRC report *Diet and Health* (NRC 1989) concluded that macronutrients and excess calories are likely the greatest contributors to dietary cancer risk in the United States. It is not clear the degree to which, in aggregate, naturally occurring and synthetic chemicals present an appreciable risk. It is apparent that existing concentration and exposure data and current cancer risk assessment methods are insufficient to definitively address the aggregate roles of naturally occurring or synthetic dietary chemicals in human cancer causation and prevention.

The committee's other major conclusions are listed below. They address the complexity and variability of the human diet, cancer risk from the diet, mechanisms and properties of synthetic vs. naturally occurring carcinogens, the role of anticarcinogens, and models for identifying dietary carcinogens and anticarcinogens.

Complexity of the Diet

• The human diet is a highly complex and variable mixture of naturally occurring and synthetic chemicals. Of these, the naturally occurring far exceed the synthetic in number and quantity. The naturally occurring chemicals include macronutrients (fat, carbohydrate, and protein), micronutrients (vitamins and trace metals), and non-nutrient constituents. Only a small number of specific carcinogens and anticarcinogens have been identified in the human diet (e.g., aflatoxins have been identified in the human diet, however it seems unlikely that important carcinogens are yet to be identified). In part, this may reflect the limited number of studies performed.

• Human epidemiologic data indicate that diet contributes to an appreciable portion of cancer, but the precise components of diet responsible for increased cancer risk are generally not well understood.

Carcinogenicity and Anticarcinogenicity

• Current epidemiologic evidence suggests the importance of protective factors in the diet, such as those present in fruits and vegetables.

• Current evidence suggests that the contribution of excess macronutrients and excess calories to cancer causation in the United States outweighs that of individual food microchemicals, natural and synthetic. This is not necessarily the case in other parts of the world.

• Epidemiologic data indicate that alcoholic beverages (specifically ethanol, the macronutrient found in alcoholic beverages) consumed in excess are associated with increased risk for specific types of cancer.

• Given the greater abundance of naturally occurring substances in the diet, the total exposure to naturally occurring carcinogens (in addition to excess calories and fat) exceeds the exposure to synthetic carcinogens. The committee reviewed data, including those generated by the Department of Agriculture and the Department of Health and Human Services through the Nationwide Food Consumption Surveys, the National Health and Nutrition Examination Surveys, and other related databases, regarding dietary exposure. However, data are insufficient to determine whether the dietary cancer risks from naturally occurring substances exceeds that for synthetic substances (e.g., databases do not include concentration data on many of the potential carcinogenic constituents found in foods). Indeed, at the present time quantitative statements cannot be made about cancer risks for humans from specific dietary chemicals, either naturally occurring or synthetic.

• Current regulatory practices have applied far greater stringency to the regulation of synthetic chemicals in the diet than to naturally occurring chemicals. The committee reviewed IARC, NTP, and other data to ascertain the status of carcinogenicity testing of naturally occurring versus synthetic chemicals. Only a very small fraction of naturally occurring chemicals has been tested for carcinogenicity. Naturally occurring dietary chemicals known to be potent carcinogens in rodents include agents derived through food preparation, such as certain heterocyclic amines generated during cooking, and the nitrosamines and agents acquired during food storage, such as aflatoxins and some other fungal toxins.

• The human diet also contains anticarcinogens that can reduce cancer risk. For example, the committee evaluated relevant literature on antioxidant micronutrients, including vitamins A, C, E, folic acid, and selenium, and their suggested contributions to cancer prevention. Human diets that have a high content of fruits and vegetables are associated with a reduced risk of cancer, but the specific constituents responsible for this protective effect and their mechanisms of action are not known with certainty. The vitamin and mineral content of fruits and vegetables may be important factors in this relationship. In addition, fruits and vegetables are dietary sources of many non-nutritive constituents, such as isoflavonoids, isothiocyanates and other sulfur-containing compounds, some of which have inhibited the carcinogenic process in experimental animal studies. Foods high in fiber content are associated with a decreased risk of colon cancer in humans, but it is not yet clear that fiber per se is the component responsible for this protective effect.

• Carcinogens and anticarcinogens present in the diet can interact in a variety of ways that are not fully understood. This makes it difficult to predict overall dietary risks based on an assessment of the risks from individual components based on uncertainties associated with rodent to human extrapolation and high-dose to low-dose extrapolation. It is likely that there is also considerable inter-individual variation in susceptibility to specific chemicals or mixtures due to either inherited or acquired factors.

Synthetic Versus Naturally Occurring Carcinogens

• Overall, the basic mechanisms involved in the entire process of carcinogenesis—from exposure of the organism to expression of tumors—are qualitatively similar, if not identical, for synthetic and naturally occurring carcinogens. The committee concluded that there is no notable biologic difference(s) between synthetic and naturally occurring carcinogens. To assess relative potency, the committee compiled and analyzed data on over 200 carcinogens—65 of which were naturally occurring. The data set included agents identified by IARC as having sufficient evidence of carcinogenicity in humans or animals, or by the NTP as known or reasonably anticipated to be human carcinogens. Based in part on this limited sample, the committee concluded that there is no clear difference between the potency of naturally occurring and synthetic carcinogens that may be present in the human diet. In general, both types of chemicals have similar mechanisms of action, similar positivity rates in rodent bioassay tests for carcinogenicity, and encompass similar ranges of carcinogenic potencies. Consequently, naturally occurring and synthetic chemicals can be evaluated by the same epidemiologic or experimental methods and procedures.

• Although there are differences between specific groups of synthetic and naturally occurring chemicals with respect to properties such as lipophilicity, degree of conjugation, resistance to metabolism, and persistence in the body and environment, it is unlikely that information on these properties, if available, will enable predictions to be made of the degree of carcinogenicity of a naturally occurring or synthetic chemical in the diet. Both categories of chemicals—naturally occurring and synthetic—are large and diverse. Predictions based on chemical or physical properties are problematic, due to the likely overlap of values between the categories.

Models for Identifying Carcinogens and Anticarcinogens

• The committee evaluated the current methods for assessing carcinogenicity, and concluded that current strategies for identifying and evaluating potential carcinogens and anticarcinogens are essentially the same. They can be grouped into epidemiologic studies, in vivo experimental animal models, and in vitro systems. The committee recognized the value and limitations of these tests, specifically for identifying dietary carcinogens and anticarcinogens.

• In its assessment of traditional epidemiologic approaches to identifying dietary carcinogens and anticarcinogens, the committee concluded that these can be beneficially expanded by incorporating into research designs biochemical, immunologic, and molecular assays that utilize human tissues and biologic fluids. Furthermore, incorporating the identification of biologic markers into these approaches may provide early indicators of human carcinogenicity— long before the development of tumors.

• The committee analyzed the applicability of rodent bioassays— specifically the long-term bioassays conducted by the National Toxicology Program—for identifying dietary carcinogens and anti-carcinogens. The committee concluded that, despite their limitations, rodent models (involving high dose exposures) have served as useful screening tests for identifying chemicals as potential human carcinogens and anticarcinogens. Concerns about the use of data generated from these models for predicting the potential carcinogenicity and anticarcinogenicity of chemicals in our food are due to the fact that they do not mimic human exposure conditions, i.e., we are exposed to an enormous complex of chemicals, many at exceedingly low quantities, in our diet.

RECOMMENDATIONS

The committee's recommendations, derived from the conclusions just presented, are listed below. The committee was charged to examine the risk from naturally occurring versus synthetic components of the diet on human cancer. Numerous and extensive gaps in the current knowledge base became apparent. These gaps are so large—and resources are so limited—that careful prioritization of further research efforts is essential. The following recommendations emphasize the need for expanded epidemiologic studies, more human exposure data, improved and enhanced testing methods, more detailed data on dietary components, and further mechanistic studies, if these gaps are to be filled. Research might prove feeble, however, when the complexity and variability of diets and food composition, as well as human behavior, are considered.

Epidemiologic Studies and Human Exposure

• *Improved methods are needed to enable the incorporation of relevant cellular and molecular markers of exposure, susceptibility, and preneoplastic effects (DNA damage, etc.) into epidemiologic studies.*

While existing markers are useful, additional molecular markers of exposure and susceptibility need to be developed, and their relevance and predictivity to the carcinogenic process evaluated. These markers should then be incorporated into traditional epidemiologic studies. In particular, methods are needed to identify high- and low-risk populations. Biologic markers for both genotoxic and nongenotoxic agents need to be developed and validated.

• *Additional data on the concentrations and human exposures to naturally occurring and synthetic chemicals in foods are needed.*

In order to determine the exposures to specific dietary chemicals, it is necessary to know the concentration of a specific chemical in individual food commodities as well as the consumption of those food commodities. At present, the concentrations are known for relatively few chemicals. In addition, more information is needed on the factors that modify these concentrations.

Current methods for assessing food consumption based on recall or food diaries have limitations; they may entail a substantial degree of error and lack of reproducibility. Furthermore, the sample sizes of existing food consumption surveys are limited, particularly when subpopulations such as infants and children or the elderly are considered. In order to minimize the resources needed to acquire these data, consideration should be given to building on other large population-based studies, such as the Women's Health Initiative Study currently supported by the National Institutes of Health.

Testing

• *Improved bioassay screening methods are needed to test for carcinogens and anticarcinogens in our diet.*

The rodent bioassay currently used in screening chemicals for potential carcinogenicity or anticarcinogenicity has major problems and uncertainties, especially in providing quantitative estimates of dietary cancer risk to humans or the magnitude of protection by anticarcinogens. These uncertainties relate to the variability of the composition and caloric content of the human diet and the bioassay's inability to mimic this range of variability. In addition, human exposure levels to individual naturally occurring or synthetic chemicals are far lower than experimental test conditions. (The committee recognized that of the NTP bioassays netting positive results, only 6% were from levels exclusively at the maximum tolerated dose.) Uncertainties also result from variation in responses among species. The factors causing these and other uncertainties should be further evaluated and minimized wherever possible. New methods are needed for assessing complex mixtures such as those present in food. Because some chemicals may produce or prevent cancer in animals by mechanisms not relevant to humans, or do so only at high doses, information on the mechanisms of action of chemical carcinogens and anticarcinogens is crucial to improving the science of human risk assessment.

• *Further testing of naturally occurring chemicals present in the food supply for carcinogenic and anticarcinogenic potential should be conducted on a prioritized basis.*

At present, only a limited number of naturally occurring substances present in the human diet have been subjected to testing for carcinogenic and anticarcinogenic potential. Selected additional substances should be subjected to appropriate testing in order to develop a more comprehensive database on which to base comparisons of the potential cancer risks or protective effects of naturally occurring and synthetic chemicals in the diet. Because resources for toxicological testing are limited and because there is a vast number of naturally occurring dietary chemicals, further testing of appropriately selected naturally occurring food chemicals requires the establishment of selection criteria. For potential carcinogens, priority should be assigned to those suspected naturally occurring non-nutritive chemicals that occur at relatively high concentrations in commonly consumed foods, and/or those whose consumption is associated with diets or life styles known to be deleterious. Research should only be conducted when there is substantial evidence that an important problem exists and when there is a reasonable expectation of a meaningful result. Unless a suspected carcinogen or anticarcinogen occurs at high and measurable levels in a diet, its risk to humans cannot be predicted using present methods (experimental animal studies or human epidemiologic investigations).

Additional criteria should be based on our knowledge of known carcinogens and anticarcinogens. For example, naturally occurring chemicals could also be accorded a higher priority for testing if they 1) fall in the same chemical class as known chemical carcinogens or anticarcinogens, 2) contain chemical groups also found in known chemical carcinogens or anticarcinogens, 3) are likely, based on structural comparisons with known chemical carcinogens or anticarcinogens, to form reactive intermediates, in vivo, 4) are known to be mutagenic and/or to bind to DNA, 5) share biologic effects similar to those of known nongenotoxic carcinogens, or 6) are likely, based on structural comparisons with known chemicals, to be unusually stable (i.e., long lasting) in vivo.

High priority for identifying potential anticarcinogens might be given additional consideration, in view of the fact that they do offer the possibility of new approaches to cancer control and prevention.

· *To help fill the data gaps on the cancer risk of dietary constituents, improved short-term screening tests for carcinogenic and anticarcinogenic activity should be developed, especially for detecting nongenotoxic effects that are relevant to carcinogenesis.*

Existing short-term screening tests, usually employing cell culture systems, often provide useful information, but new methods need to be developed and validated. Emphasis should be placed on developing systems that use human genes, enzymes, cells, or tissues. Since most of the present short-term tests detect DNA reactive compounds, new methods are needed for screening chemicals for nongenotoxic endpoints such as cell proliferation, hormonal effects, receptor mediated events, and effects on cell-cell interactions, gene expression, differentiation, and apoptosis (programmed cell death). Great promise exists for the use of transgenic mice.

Dietary Factors

· *The risk of cancer from excess calories and fat should be further delineated vis-à-vis naturally occurring and synthetic dietary chemicals.*

There is considerable evidence that excessive calorie (energy) intake (i.e., in excess of body needs and including fat) is associated with increased cancer risk for several sites. In rodents, and especially in humans, mammary cancer is associated both with excess calories and with high proportion of calories as fat. The mechanism(s) responsible for this effect have not been clearly identified. Possible mechanisms that have been implicated include: increased cell proliferation, decreased cell death, changes in hormonal status, and alterations in the activity of enzymes which metabolize endogenous and environmental agents, and increased oxidative stress. Further studies are needed to elucidate the precise mechanisms and to better define what is optimal or excess caloric intake. Dietary fat has also been associated with increased risk of some forms of cancer, but it is not clear if this is related to the high caloric contribution of fat, to specific constituents in foods high in saturated fats (such as specific fatty acids or other lipid oxidation products), or heterocyclic amines produced in cooking. These relationships and the underlying mechanisms need further study and clarification.

· *The specific chemicals that provide the protective effects of vegetables and fruits should be identified and their protective mechanisms delineated.*

The consumption of diets rich in fruits and vegetables is associated with reduced incidence of several forms of human cancer. The specific factors accounting for this relationship are not known with certainty and require further investigation. A number of vitamins, minerals and non-nutritive components of fruits and vegetables have been identified which may contribute to the protective properties of these foods. Further research is needed on the independent and interactive effects of these compounds and on the identification of additional protective components. At present, a sound recommendation for cancer prevention is to increase fruit and vegetable intake. Concerning specific plant derived chemicals, we do not have adequate information to recommend supplementation beyond the recommended daily requirements for particular vitamins or other nutrients.

FUTURE DIRECTIONS

It is apparent from the above list of recommendations that new research approaches are required to elucidate the precise roles of naturally occurring and synthetic dietary chemicals in human cancer causation and prevention. These needs merge with those related to the broader issue of the roles that chemicals in the general environment may play in cancer causation and prevention. The following section provides a broad outline of options available for future directions of research in this area.

Resources

The conclusions and recommendations of this report indicate that a better understanding is needed of the role of specific dietary naturally occurring and synthetic chemicals in cancer causation and prevention. This is an extremely complex task. Progress in this area will require expertise and extensive further research in several disciplines, including food chemistry, analytical chemistry, toxicology, nutrition, carcinogenesis, biochemistry, molecular biology, and epidemiology. It would be highly desirable, therefore, to develop multi-disciplinary teams to conduct research in this broad area and to develop new resources. One approach would be to develop specific programs committed to this field of research. It is also apparent from this report that answers to these questions will not come simply by further analyzing the existing database, since it is often fragmentary and inconclusive. In addition, because of the vast number of chemicals present in a typical diet, new concepts and methods must be developed to address this problem, and extensive research is required so that results obtained in various model systems can be extrapolated with greater validity to human populations. It is essential, therefore, that additional intellectual and physical resources be developed to meet these needs.

Fundamental Mechanistic Studies

A major limitation in this field that we do not understand the precise mechanisms that underlie the multistage process of carcino-genesis and how chemicals in the diet are able to alter this process. Recent advances in the cellular biology and molecular genetics of cancer are beginning to provide insight into the details. These findings indicate that the carcinogenic process is often associated with activation of dominant-acting cellular oncogenes and/or the inactivation of recessive tumor suppressor genes that normally influence growth. Evidence also indicates that the carcinogenic process is associated with abnormalities in cyclin and cyclin-related genes that control the cell cycle and proliferation and inhibit the processes of apoptosis and differentiation. Advances are also being made in identifying abnormalities in genes responsible for tumor invasion and metastasis, i.e., genes that control cell-cell interac-tions, cell locomotion, extracellular proteases, and angiogenesis. In addition, genetically-based variations in susceptibility to cancer are being identified in human populations.

Progress is also being made in identifying the ways in which various chemicals interact with critical cellular targets either to increase or decrease the process of carcinogenesis. Most of the progress relates to chemicals that act by binding directly to DNA (genotoxic agents), including mechanisms involved in metabolic activation or deactivation of these chemicals and the protective role of DNA repair. In addition, the roles of endogenous processes of DNA damage, including oxidative damage, deamination, depurina-tion, and the formation of exocyclic adducts, are being identified.

Furthermore, research is studying the interaction of chemicals with cellular components other than DNA that might be involved in carcinogenesis or its prevention. In this group are the interac-tions of chemicals with cellular receptors, membranes, protein kin-ases, and transcription factors, as well as alterations in the metabo-lism of endogenous hormones and growth factors. Also being iden-tified are alterations in pathways of signal transduction, the cascade of cytoplasmic events involving numerous protein kinases that eventually trigger alterations in gene expression in the nucleus by affecting the function of specific transcription factors. Elucidation of the specific pathways altered by various chemicals, particularly those that do not interact directly with DNA, should provide not only insight into the carcinogenic process but also knowledge necessary for extrapolating from results obtained at high doses in rodents or in cell culture systems to the human situation, which usually involves low dose exposures.

As discussed in Chapter 4, a number of dietary intervention studies are in progress or are being developed, as well as chemoprevention studies that employ micronutrients or related compounds. It would be desirable to incorporate specific analytic assays and biologic markers into these studies to provide mechanistic insights and more sensitive indicators of response. More detailed information on the actual exposure to the substances being evaluated and on cellular responsiveness to various stimuli would also be useful.

Epidemiology

The advantages and limitations of various types of epidemiologic studies, including ecologic, case-control, cohort, intervention, and molecular epidemiology studies are discussed in Chapter 4. Since results from these studies have suggested that a major fraction of human cancer is due to dietary factors, it is appropriate to extend this approach to identify with greater certainty the specific factors and types of cancer involved and populations affected.

Molecular epidemiology holds considerable promise in this regard. As discussed in detail in Chapter 4, laboratory procedures are now available for measuring a variety of biologic markers related to exposure and susceptibility in samples obtained from relatively large populations. These include markers that are related predominantly to DNA-altering chemicals. The markers provide information on the following: 1) genetic and acquired host susceptibility,

2) metabolism and tissue levels of carcinogens, 3) levels of covalent adducts formed between carcinogens and DNA or other macromolecules, and 4) early cellular responses to carcinogen exposure. Future progress in this field requires improvements in the sensitivity, specificity, reproducibility, and predictive value of the assays for such biologic markers. The procedures for collecting specimens must be minimally invasive.

In addition, there is a critical need to develop markers related to cell proliferation, apoptosis, receptors, protein kinases, and altered gene expression, since, as mentioned above, certain carcinogens might exert their effects through these mechanisms.

To assess exposure, previous epidemiologic studies on diet, nutrition, and cancer relied largely on dietary recall methods and, in some instances, on the levels of various nutrients in blood, tissues, and urine. These approaches have proved useful in identifying both potential risk factors and protective factors for cancer. Biologic markers that better reflect long-term intakes are needed, since currently used assays of nutrient levels in blood and urine generally reflect only recent consumption patterns (NRC 1993a). Such markers could be particularly helpful in further assessing the role of dietary fat in cancer causation. In addition, since dietary recall is subject to considerable error, methods are needed that will improve the accuracy of these assessments or correct for errors when they are non-differential (e.g., Rosner and Willett 1988).

To further explore the hypothesis that excessive caloric intake *per se* may be a major risk factor for human cancer, biologic markers that assess specific effects of excess or limited caloric intake need to be developed. These might include assays related to carcinogen metabolism, oxidative damage, signal transduction and gene expression, cell proliferation, and apoptosis.

Biologic markers related to oxidative damage may prove to be of considerable importance, since several antioxidants in the diet (e.g., vitamin C, vitamin E, certain carotenoids) have been implicated as protective factors. Such markers may include 1) urinary levels of oxidized DNA bases, 2) analyses of DNA samples for strand breaks or oxidized bases (thymine glycol, 8-hydroxyguanine, etc.), 3) blood and tissue levels of malondialdehyde, an oxidation product of lipids, and 4) markers of enzymes that detoxify activated forms of oxygen, such as catalase and superoxide dismutase (Cerutti and Trump 1991, Pryor 1993, Teebor et al. 1988).

Aside from histopathology, there are few markers for detecting preneoplastic lesions (e.g., colonic adenomatous polyps). The further development of such markers would make cohort and intervention studies more feasible and enhance the assessment of various hypotheses related to diet and cancer, since such markers could greatly shorten the required interval for follow-up and also improve intervention strategies.

A number of intervention studies based on dietary modification or the use of chemopreventive agents (vitamin A and related retinoids, beta-carotene, vitamins E and C, calcium etc.) are in progress or are being developed (see Chapter 4). It would be desirable to incorporate some of the above biologic markers into these studies, in order to refine the assessment of biologic responses in individuals and to provide mechanistic insights.

Rodent and In Vitro Assays

Rodent bioassays, short-term tests in rodents, and in vitro assays, including recently developed cellular and molecular biology methods, are summarized in Chapter 4. The committee agreed that although many of these assays provide useful information, it is important to stress that they serve only as screening tests (NRC 1993b). Better extrapolation of the results obtained to the human situation requires new approaches, particularly those that provide insights into the underlying mechanisms. Experimental animals are being developed, and numerous other potentially useful models are being developed. These may provide better screening tests and also provide mechanistic insight.

The current standard NTP rodent bioassay employs only one

type of diet, although other fairly extensive studies have been conducted on the effects of dietary factors on carcinogenesis in rodents (see Chapters 2 and 4). Further studies in which dietary constituents, particularly caloric intake and fat content, are varied, either alone or in combination with other factors, are needed. These studies should also have a mechanistic approach, should incorporate some of the types of biologic markers mentioned above, and should test specific and novel hypotheses. A recent approach, interesting although fraught with difficulties, is to feed rodents a homogenate of an actual daily human Western-type diet, to assess the total effects of the human diet on cancer induction, when testing alone or in combination with specific natural or synthetic chemicals (Rozen et al. 1996).

The above considerations also apply to the use of rodent carcinogenicity assays to detect naturally occurring and synthetic dietary chemicals that inhibit tumor formation, i.e., anticarcinogens. A major difficulty with current protocols is that they require large doses of potent carcinogens, which frequently necessitates the use of high doses of anticarcinogens. Assays more realistically approximating human exposure to dietary chemicals are necessary.

It is of critical importance to obtain greater insight into interactions among multiple chemicals, since food is a highly complex mixture of agents that can increase or decrease the risk of carcinogenesis. The study of complex mixtures has been limited, largely because examining such interactions is difficult and expensive (NRC 1988). Several complex interactions between agents in the human diet (and other types of agents) have been identified, e.g., the interaction of aflatoxin and hepatitis B and C viruses, in the causation of liver cancer; nitrosamines and the bacterium *Helicobacter pylori* in the causation of stomach cancer; cigarette smoke and asbestos in the causation of lung cancer; and others. Nevertheless, more complexities exist in the diet, and these need to be evaluated. In particular, the interaction between carcinogenic and anticarcinogenic components of the diet needs to be better delineated, including interactions affecting metabolism and other types of cellular responses to chemicals. As described in previous chapters of this report, several components of the diet have been identified that can increase or decrease the risk of developing cancer in experimental animal or in vitro assays. Determining with greater certainty which of these components are significant contributors to cancer risk in humans is necessary so that an optimum diet can be recommended to the American public (NRC 1982). Obviously, intensive research is required on this subject.

A critical parameter in carcinogenesis is the number of cell divisions in a target tissue. This number can be increased by a variety of mechanisms that either increase cell births or decrease cell deaths. Greater understanding of these mechanisms is needed, as are better assays, especially in humans, for quantitating cell division, apoptosis, differentiation and other processes known to affect carcinogenesis. Assays for these processes are needed that do not require that human tissue be removed to assess the effects of various dietary factors. Quantitative assays in rodent tissues are being developed, but more sensitive and specific assays are needed.

The use of human tissues and cell systems for studies on carcinogenesis, including mechanistic studies, is strongly encouraged. Powerful new tools have been provided by the advent of epithelial human cell lines and the ability to genetically engineer derivatives of these cells that display increased or decreased expression of specific genes (for example, genes that encode drug metabolizing enzymes and genes that alter oxidative stress). In addition, the development of specific strains of transgenic mice or of mice in which specific genes have been inactivated also provide new approaches to carcinogen testing and mechanistic studies. It is hoped that these new approaches will provide greater insight into the carcinogenic process in both rodents and humans, as well as provide a more rational approach to our understanding of chemical interactions in carcinogenesis and anticarcinogenesis and of their relevance to humans.

Analytic Methods in Structure-Activity Analyses

Rapid advances are being made in analytical methods and in methods for elucidating the complex structure of natural products. These methods should be applied to the analysis of various human dietary constituents. Advances in this general area, coupled with powerful computer-based methods for cataloging and analyzing chemical structures and activities, should also accelerate progress in the field of structure-activity analyses to predict carcinogenicity. To date, these methods have been applied largely to carcinogens that are genotoxic. It is essential to expand this approach to nongenotoxic carcinogens and also it to the detection and development of anticarcinogenic substances.

Engineering a More Optimal Diet

Processing has long been used to remove or reduce unwanted constituents, and to introduce, increase, or restore desirable constituents, including essential nutrients. As we identify those naturally occurring constituents that either enhance or inhibit human cancer, and define the conditions and concentrations that govern their actions, we can expect processing to play a large role in increasing the protective potential of diet, as it has previously played a role in improving nutritional quality.

Over many centuries plants, and to a lesser degree animals, have been optimized as human food sources by selection and breeding for such desirable characteristics as safety, size, color, flavor, yield, and resistance to disease. During this century, scientists have been able to use the principles of Mendelian genetics to expedite this process. With the exception of flavor and toxic constituents in foods, the chemical compounds responsible for the improved characteristics have not been well characterized, nor has such information usually been required.

The recent advances in genetic engineering and biotechnology (see Chapter 2) should facilitate further improvements in the quality of the food supply with respect to cancer prevention. Specifically, as naturally occurring dietary chemicals that either enhance or inhibit human cancer risk are identified, these chemicals will be candidates for appropriate modification through food biotechnology. However, in contrast to earlier approaches, this new technology requires much greater knowledge of the specific compounds involved, together with knowledge of their biosynthesis in the source organism. Depending on the compound involved, such information may or may not now be available in the biochemical literature, although it can be acquired through technology now or soon to be available.

CLOSING REMARKS

At the present time, cancers are the second leading cause of mortality in the United States, resulting in over 500,000 deaths per year. Unless current trends are reversed, cancer will be the major cause of death in the early part of the 21st century. Conventional wisdom states that dietary factors play an important role in the causation of a major fraction of these cancers. Although synthetic chemicals present in the diet cannot be ignored as potential carcinogenic risks, it seems likely that it is the naturally occurring compounds in our diet, together with excess fat and total calories, that have the greatest effect on cancer causation and prevention. This subject is, therefore, of major relevance to public health protection and disease prevention. However, the assessment by this committee indicates several inadequacies in 1) the specific naturally occurring chemicals (or mixtures) that are involved in cancer causation; 2) the mechanisms by which they act; 3) which types of cancer they affect; and 4) the magnitude of these effects. New research approaches, at both the fundamental and applied levels, are urgently required to address this important problem.

Coupled with the requirement for research efforts in these areas is the need to better characterize the chemical composition of our diet and its variations in the American population. Advances in analytic and survey techniques should facilitate this endeavor.

Finally, as specific naturally occurring dietary chemicals are identified that either enhance or inhibit cancer risks in humans, it will be possible to better formulate specific dietary guidelines for the American public. It may also be possible to utilize this information to modify the composition of our food sources, through food processing, breeding methods, and genetic engineering and other advances in biotechnology, so as to optimize the quality of the diet with respect to cancer prevention. Above all, a major effort will be needed to educate the American public regarding appropriate life style modifications if we are to achieve these goals.

REFERENCES

Cerutti, P.A., and B.F. Trump. 1991. Inflammation and oxidative stress in carcinogenesis. Cancer Cells 3:1-7.

NRC (National Research Council). 1982. Diet, Nutrition and Cancer. Washingtion, DC: National Academy Press.

NRC (National Research Council). 1988. Complex Mixtures: Methods for In Vivo Toxicity Testing. Washingtion, DC: National Academy Press.

NRC (National Research Council). 1989. Diet and Health: Implications for Reducing Chronic Disease Risk. Food and Nutrition Board, Committee on Diet and Health. Washington, DC: National Academy Press.

NRC (National Research Council). 1993a. Pesticides in the Diets of Infants and Children. Washington, DC: National Academy Press.

NRC (National Research Council). 1993b. Issues in Risk Assessment. Washington, DC: National Academy Press.

Pryor, W.A., 1993. Measurment of oxidative stress in humans. Cancer Epidemiology, Biomarkers and Prevention 2:289-292.

Rozen, P., V. Liberman. F. Lubin, S. Angel, R. Owen, N. Trostler, T. Skolnik, and D. Kritchevsky. 1996. A new dietary model to study colorectal carcinogenesis: Experimental design, food preparation and experimental findings. Nutrition and Cancer. in press.

Rosner, B., and W.C. Willett. 1988. Interval estimates for correlation coefficients corrected for within-person variation: Implications for study design and hypothesis testing. Am. J. Epidemiol. 127:377-386.

Teebor, G.W., R.J. Boorstein, and J. Cadet. 1988. The repairability of oxidative free radical mediated damage to DNA: A review. International J. Radiat. Res. 54:131-150.

Weinstein, I.B., R.M. Santella, and F. Perera. 1995. Molecular Biology and Epidemiology of Cancer. Pp. 83-110 in Cancer Prevention and Control, P. Greenwald, B.S. Kramer, and D.L. Weed, ed. New York: Marcel Dekker, Inc.

Appendix A

Selected Substances in Food Subjected to Some Degree of Carcinogenicity Testing in Animals and for Which Some Positive Results Have Been Reported

Substance	Nature of Supporting Evidence	Extent of Natural Occurrence in Foods	References
From Higher Plants			
Allyl isothiocyanate	Bladder papillomas in male rats; negative in mice and female rats; clastogenic, mutagenic	Raw cabbage, 0.04-2.7 ppm; horseradish, 2,000 ppm; black mustard seed, 10,000 ppm	NTP, 1982; Ishidate et al., 1988; McGregor et al., 1988
Anthraquinone, 1-hydroxy	Cecum, colon, and liver tumors in male rats		Mori et al., 1990
Asarone, α- and β- (oil of calamus)	Malignant tumors in the duodenal region" in male and female rats	Asarum and acorns spp (sweet flag) ≈20,000 ppm	Taylor et al., 1967

359

Substance	Nature of Supporting Evidence[a]	Extent of Natural Occurrence in Foods[b]	References[c]
Benzaldehyde	Forestomach tumors in male and female mice	Found in over 40 foods; fruits and vegetables, 0.2-1 ppm; white bread, 5.0-10 pm; wines, 0.01-1.0 ppm; cocoa, coffee, tea, 2.0 ppm; shellfish, 0.01 ppm	NTP, 1990a
Caffeine	Increased multiplicity but not incidence of spontaneous mammary gland tumors in female mice	Tea, coffee, maté, guaraná, cola nuts; 0.5 to 5.0% of the plant product	Welsch et al., 1988
Capsaicin	Duodenal adenocarcinoma in male and female mice (significant only when all treated groups combined); not mutagenic	In pungent (hot) red peppers (q.v.); <0.1 to 1.0% of dry fruit	Toth et al., 1984 (as reported by Watts, 1985)
Capsicum annuum; (hot) peppers	Liver tumors in rats	Widely used spice, especially in warmer climates	Hoch-Ligeti, 1950
Chrysazin	Colon tumors in male rats		Mori et al., 1985

Ecdysone, alpha	Liver tumors in male and female Egyptian toads	Insects and crustaceans, spinach, plants, relationship to food	El-Mofty et al., 1987
Estragole	Liver tumors in female mice; forms DNA adducts	Apple, bilberry <0.03 ppm; basil and oregano ≈100 ppm; tarragon ≈1%; anise and star anise ≈5.0%	Miller et al., 1983; Randerath et al., 1985
Ethyl acrylate	Negative in 2 strains of male and female rats; forestomach tumors in male mice, male and female rats	Dill ≈1.0 ppm; pineapple, 0.8 ppm; raspberry; durian	Miller et al., 1985; NTP, 1986
Eugenol	Data equivocal for liver tumors in female and male mice.	Oranges, cherries and many fruits ≈0.02 ppm; tomato, carrot ≈0.2 ppm, wines, liquors ≈0.1 ppm; cottage cheese, fish ≈3.0 ppm; anise ≈0.2%; cloves ≈10%	NTP, 1983

Substance	Nature of Supporting Evidence[a]	Extent of Natural Occurrence in Foods[b]	References[c]
Furfural	In male rats 2/50 at high dose only showed cholangio-carcinomas; none in females. In male mice, increased incidence of adenomas and carcinomas in high dose group; in females, increased incidence of adenomas at high dose	Cocoa, coffee, 55-255 ppm; wine, tr-10 ppm; whiskies, cider, sherry, wines, 1-30+ ppm, sauerkraut, tomato, cinnamon, cloves, wheaten bread, 1-14 ppm; many fruits, tr.-1 ppm	NTP, 1990
Gossypol	Neck myxosarcomas in female mice	Cottonseed meal, limit of .045% (U.S.) and .06% (P.A.G.) free gossypol	Dhaliwal et al, 1987
D-Limonene	Kidney tumors in male rats	Citrus juices ≈200 ppm; citrus oils 50-90%; other fruits and vegetables 1-30 ppm; coffee, tea ≈1 ppm; spices, trace -5%	NTP, 1990b
Piper nigrum, (black and white) pepper	Lung, liver, and skin tumors in male and female mice; liver tumors in male and female Egyptian toads	Widely used spice	Concon et al., 1979; El-Mofty et al., 1988; El-Mofty et al., 1991

Phytic acid	Kidney tumors in male and female rats	Oil seed, legumes, cereal grains	Hiasa et al., 1992
Ptaquiloside	Ileal, mammary, and bladder tumors in female rats	Bracken fern ("fiddle-heads")	Hirono et al., 1984; Hirono et al., 1987
Quercetin	Intestinal and bladder tumors in male and female "albino" rats; kidney tumors in male F344/N rats; liver tumors in female F344 rats; mutagenic	Ubiquitous in food plants, esp. in rinds of plant fruits	Pamukcu et al., 1980; Dunnick and Hailey, 1992; NTP, 1992
Safrole	Liver tumors in 3 strains male and female mice; liver tumors in 2 strains male rats, 1 strain female rats; clastogenic, forms DNA adducts	Cocoa, nutmeg, mace, black pepper, $\approx 0.2\%$	Lipsky et al., 1981; Innes et al., 1969; Vesselinovitch et al., 1979; Wislocki et al., 1977; Borchert et al., 1973; Boberg et al., 1983; Miller et al., 1983; Ishidate et al., 1988; Randerath et al., 1985
Sesamol	Forestomach tumors in male rats and male and female mice	Sesame seeds and oil	Hirose et al., 1990; Tamano et al., 1992
Shikimic acid	Leukemia in male and female mice; glandular stomach tumors in male mice	Important biosynthetic precursor in most plants	Evans and Osman, 1974

Substance	Nature of Supporting Evidence[a]	Extent of Natural Occurrence in Foods[b]	References[c]
8-methoxypsoralen (Xanthotoxin)	Kidney and Zymbal's gland tumors in male rats; mutagenic, clastogenic		NTP, 1989
Xylitol	Bladder tumors in mice; adrenal gland tumors in rats	Carrots, lettuce, onions, raspberries, and spinach	Anonymous, 1977

In addition to the list above, the committee is aware of other data on carcinogenic effects of benzene, cycasin, methoxyazoxymethylacetate, and styrene. See Appendix B.

From Edible Fungi

Substance	Nature of Supporting Evidence[a]	Extent of Natural Occurrence in Foods[b]	References[c]
Acetaldehyde methylformyl-hydrazone	Lung, forestomach, clitoral tumors in female mice; preputial, lung tumors in male mice	Several species of edible mushrooms, especially of the genus *Gyromitra*	Toth et al., 1981
Glutamyl *p*-hydrazino-benzoic acid	Subcutaneous tumors in male mice	Edible mushrooms (*Agaricus bisporus*) and several *Gyromitra* species	Toth, 1986

p-Hydrazino-benzoic acid	Aorta and large artery tumors in male and female mice	McManus et al., 1987

From Fungal Contaminants of Food

In addition to aflatoxin B_1, the committee is aware of other data on carcinogenic effects for aflatoxin B_2, aflatoxin G_1, aflatoxin G_2, *Fusarium moniliforme* toxins, *Penicillium islandicum* toxins (e.g., islanditoxin), T-2 toxin, ochratoxins, and sterigmatocystin. See Chapter 2 and Appendix B.

Carcinogens Formed During Traditional Preparation and Processing

Benz[a]anthracene	Benign liver and lung tumors in mice	Coconut oil, 0.5-13.7 ng/g; broiled meat, 0.2-1.1 ng/g; broiled fish, 0.6-2.9 ng/g; smoked fish, 0.2-189 ng/g; ham, 1.3-12 ng/g; cereal, 0.4-6.8 ng/g; lettuce, 6.1-15.4 ng/g; tomatoes 0.3 ng/g; spinach, 16.1 ng/g; roasted coffee, 0.5-42.7 ng/g; tea, 2.9-36 ng/g; whisky, 0.04-0.08 ng/g	Klein, 1963

Substance	Nature of Supporting Evidence[a]	Extent of Natural Occurrence in Foods[b]	References[c]
Benzo[a]pyrene	Forestomach tumors in mice; mammary tumors in female rats	Margarine, 0.9-36 ng/g; coconut oil, 0.3-8.2 ng/g; broiled meat, 0.17-50 ng/g; broiled fish, 0.2-0.9 ng/g; smoked fish, 1-78 ng/g; ham, <0.5-14.6 ng/g; bacon, 0.16-0.25 ng/g; cereal, 0.19-4.13 ng/g; potatoes, 0.09 ng/g; flour, 0.73; bread, 0.23; toasted bread, 0.39-0.56; lettuce, 2.8-12.8; tomatoes, 0.2-0.22; spinach, 7.4; fruits, 0.5-30; roasted coffee, 0.3-15.8; tea, 3.9-21.3; whisky, 0.04	Neal and Rigdon, 1967; McCormick, 1981
Catechol	Glandular stomach tumors in male and female rats		Hirose et al., 1990
Dibenz[a,h]anthracene	Forestomach and lung tumors in mice		Larinow and Soboleva, 1938; Lorenz and Stewart, 1948; Snell and Stewart, 1962, 1963

In addition to the list above, the committee is aware of other data on carcinogenic effects of 7H-Dibenzo[c,g]-carbazole, Dibenzo[a,h]-pyrene, Dibenzo[a,il]-pyrene, Me-A-alpha-C(2-Amino-3-methyl-9H-pyrido-[2,3-b]indole), and 5-methylchyrysene. N-Nitroso-N-demethylamine is discussed in Chapter 2, and the committee also is aware of other data on carcinogenic effects on N-Nitroso-N-dibutylamine, N-Nitroso-diethylamine, N-Nitroso-methylethylamine, N-Nitroso-nornicotine, N-Nitroso-piperidine, and N-Nitroso-pyrrolidine. See Appendix B.

IQ(2-Amino-3-methylimidazo[4,5-f]quinoline)	Lung, liver, and forestomach tumors in male and female mice; mammary gland, Zymbal gland, and liver tumors in female rats; liver, Zymbal gland, colon, and small intestine tumors in male and female rats; liver tumors in male and female monkeys	Fried ground beef, 0.5-20 ng/g; broiled beef, 0.19 ng/g; sun-dried, broiled sardines, 20 ng/g; broiled salmon, 0.3-1.8 ng/g; fried fish, 0.16 ng/g; fried egg, 0.1 ng/g	Ohgaki et al, 1984, 1986; Tanaka et al, 1985; Takayama et al, 1984; Adamson et al, 1990, 1991
MeIQ	Liver tumors in female mice; forestomach tumors in male and female mice; Zymbal gland, oral cavity, and colon tumors in male and female rats; mammary gland tumors in female rats; skin tumors in male rats	Fried fish, 0.03 ng/g; grilled, sun-dried sardines, 20-72 ng/g; broiled sardines, 16.6 ng/g	Ohgaki et al, 1986; Kato et al, 1989

Substance	Nature of Supporting Evidence[a]	Extent of Natural Occurrence in Foods[b]	References[c]
MeIQx	Liver tumors in male and female mice; lung tumors in female mice; lymphoma and leukemia in male mice; liver and Zymbal gland tumors in male and female rats; clitoral gland tumors in female rats; skin tumors in male rats.	Fried ground beef, 0.45-12.3 ng/g; broiled beef, 2.11 ng/g; fried fish, 6.44 ng/g; broiled mutton, 1.01 ng/g; broiled salmon, 1.4-5 ng/g; dried, smoked mackerel, 0.8 ng/g; broiled chicken, 2.33 ng/g; canned roasted eel, 1.1 ng/g	Ohgaki et al., 1987, Kato et al., 1988
PhIP2-Amino-1-methyl-6-phenylimidazo[4,5-]pyridine	Lymphoma in male and female mice, colon tumors in male rats, mammary gland tumors in female rats, and colon tumors in female rats	Broiled chicken 38.1 ng/g, broiled 42.5 ng/g, fried fish 69.2 ng/g, fried ground beef 15 ng/g	Felton et al 1986, Esumi et al 1989, Ito et al 1991, Wakabayashi et al 1992

In addition to PhIP, the committee is aware of other data on carcinogenic effects of A-alpha-C (2-Amino-9H-pyrido[2,3-b]indole), Glu-P-1 (2-Amino-6-methyldipyrido[1,2-a:3',2'-d]-imidazole, Glu-P-2 (2-Aminodipyrido[1,2-a:3',2'-d]-imidazole, Trp-P-1 (Tryptophan-P-1), and Trp-P-2 (Tryptophan-P-2).

REFERENCES

Adamson, R.H., U.P. Thorgeirsson, E.G. Snyderwine, S.S. Thorgeirsson, J. Reeves, D.W. Dalgard, S. Takayama, and T. Sugimura. 1990. Carcinogenicity of 2-amino-3-methylimidazo(4,5-f)quinoline in nonhuman primates: Induction of tumors in three macaques. Jpn. J. Cancer Res. 81(1):10-14.

Adamson, R.H., E.G. Snyderwine, U.P. Thorgeirsson, H.A.J. Schut, R.J. Turesky, S.S. Thorgeirsson, S. Takayama, and T. Sugimura. 1991. Metabolic processing and carcinogenicity of heterocyclic amines in nonhuman prmiates. Xenobiotics and Cancer 289-301.

Anonymous. 1977. Saccharin Fails Ames Test, Xylitol Passes. Chem Eng News 55(50): 8.

Boberg, E.W., E.C. Miller, J.A. Miller, A. Poland, and A. Liem. 1983. Strong evidence from studies with brachymorphic mice and pentachlorophenol that 1'suffooxysafrole is the major ultimate electrophilic and carcinogenic metabolite of 1'hydroxysafrole in mouse liver. Cancer Res. 43(11)P5163-P5173.

Borchert, P., J.A. Miller, E.C. Miller, T.K. Shires. 1973. 1'-Hydroxysafrole, a proximate carcinogenic metabolite of safrole in the rat and mouse. Cancer Res. 33(3):P590-P600.

Concon, J.M., D.S. Newburg, and T.W. Swerczek. 1979. Black pepper (Piper nigrum): Evidence of carcinogenicity. Nutr. Cancer 1:22-26.

Dhaliwal, M.K., J.O. Norman, S. Pathak, and D.L. Busbee. 1987. Cytogenetic analysis of a gossypol-induced murine myxosarcoma. J. Natl. Cancer Inst. 78(6):1203-1209.

Dunnick, J.K., and J.R. Hailey. 1992. Toxicity and carcinogenicity studies of quercetin, a natural component of foods. Fundam. Appl. Toxicol. 19(3):P423-P431.

El-Mofty, M., I. Sadek, A. Soliman, A. Mohamad, and S. Sakre. 1987. Alpha-ecdysone, a new bracken fern factor responsible for neoplasm induction in the Egyptian toad (Bufo regularis). Nutr. Cancer 9(2-3):103-107.

El-Mofty, M.M., A.A. Soliman, A.F. Abdel-Gawad, S.A. Sakr, and M.H. Shwaireb. 1988. Carcinogenicity testing of black pepper (Piper nigrum) using Egyptian toad (Bufo regularis) as a quick biological test animal. Oncology 45(3):P247-P252.

El-Mofty, M.M., V.V. Khudoley, and M.H. Shwaireb. 1991. Carcinogenic effect of force-feeding an extract of black pepper (Piper nigrum) in Egyptian toads (Bufo regularis). Oncology 48(4):347-350.

Esumi, H., H. Ohgaki, E. Kohzen, S. Takayama, and T. Sugimura. 1989. Induction of lymphoma in CDF₁ mice by the food mutagen, 2-amino-1-methyl-6-phenylimidazo[4,5-*b*]pyridine. Jpn. J. Cancer Res. 80, 1176-1178.

Evans, I.A., and M.A. Osman. 1974. Carcinogenicity of bracken and shikimic acid. Nature 250(464)P348-P349.

Felton, J.S., M.G. Knize, N.H. Shen, P.R. Lewis, B.D. Andresen, J. Happe, and F.T. Hatch. 1986. The isolation and identification of a new mutagen from fried ground beef: 2-amino-1-methyl-6-phenylimidazo[4,5-*b*]pyridine (PhIP). Carcinogenesis (7):1081-1086.

Hiasa, Y., Y. Kitahori, J. Morimoto, N. Konishi, S. Nakaoka, and H. Nishioka. 1992. Carcinogenicity study in rats of phytic acid "Daiichi", a natural food additive. Food Chem Toxicol. 30:117-25.

Hirono, I., S. Aiso, T. Yamaji, H. Mori, K. Yamada, H. Niwa, M. Ojika, K. Wakamatsu, H. Kigoshi, and K. Niiyama. 1984. Carcinogenicity in rats of ptaquiloside isolated from bracken. Gann 75:833-6.

Hirono, I. 1987. Naturally occurring carcinogens of plant origin: toxicology, pathology, and biochemistry. Bioactive Molecules, volume 2.

Hirose, M., S. Fukushima, T. Shirai, and R. Hasegawa. 1990. Stomach carcinogenicity of caffeic acid, sesamol and catechol in rats and mice. Jpn. J. Cancer Res. 81:207-12.

Hoch-Ligeti, C. 1950. Production of liver tumours by dietary means; Effect of feeding chillies (Capsicum frutescens and annuum) to rats. Fifth Intl Cancer Congress, Paris. 606-611.

Innes, J.R.M., B.M. Ulland, M.G. Valerio, L. Petrucelli, L. Fishbein, E.R. Hart, A.J. Pallotta, R.R. Bates, H.L. Falk, J.J. Gart, M. Klein, I. Mitchell, and J. Peters. 1969. Bioassay of pesticides and industrial chemicals for tumorigenicity in mice: A preliminary note. J. Natl. Cancer Inst. 42(6):1101-1114.

Ishidate, M. Jr., M.C. Harnois, and T. Sofuni. 1988. A comparative anaylsis of data on the clastogenicity of 951 chemical substances tested in mammalian cell cultures. Mutat. Res. 195(2):151-213.

Kato, T., H. Ohgaki, H. Hasegawa, S. Sato, S. Takayama, and T. Sugimura. 1988. Carcinogenicity in rats of a mutagenic compound, 2-amino-3,8-dimethylimidazo[4,5-*f*]quinoxaline. Carcinogenesis 9:71-73.

Kato, T., H. Migita, H. Ohgaki, S. Sato, S. Takayama, and T. Sugimura. 1989. Induction of tumors in the Zymbal gland, oral cavity, colon, skin and mammary gland of F344 rats by a mutagenic comound 2-amino-3,4-dimethylimidazo[4,5-*f*]quinoline. Carcinogenesis 10:601-603.

Klein M. 1963. Susceptibility of strain B6AF/J hybrid infant mice to tumorigenesis with 1,2-benzanthracene, deosycholic acid and 3-methylcholanthracene. Cancer Res 23:1701-1707.

Larinow, L.T., and N.G. Soboleva. 1938. Gastric tumors experimentally produced in mice by means of benzopyrene and dibenzanthracene. Vestn Rentgenol Radiol 20:276.

Lipsky, M.M., D.E. Hinton, J.E. Klaunig, and B.F. Trump. 1981. Biology of hepatocellular neoplasia in the mouse. I. Histogenesis of safrole-induced hepatocellular carcinoma. J. Natl. Cancer Inst. 67:365-76.

Lipsky, M.M., D.E. Hinton, J.E. Klaunig, P.J. Goldblatt, and B.F. Trump. 1981a. Biology of hepatocellular neoplasia in the mouse. II. Sequential enzyme histochemical analysis of BALB/c mouse liver during safrole-induced carcinogenesis. J. Natl. Cancer Inst. 67:377-92.

Lipsky, M.M., D.E. Hinton, J.E. Klaunig, and B.F. Trump. 1981b. Biology of hepatocellular neoplasia in the mouse. III. Electron microscopy of safrole-induced hepatocellular adenomas and hepatocellular carcinomas. J. Natl. Cancer Inst. 67:393-405.

Lorenz, E. and H.L. Steward. 1948. Tumors of alimentary tract in mice fed carcinogenic hydrocarbons in mineral oil emulsions. JNCI 9:173.

McCormick, D.L., F.J. Burns, and R.E. Albert. 1981. Inhibition of benz[a]pyrene-induced mammary carcinogenesis by retinyl acetate. J. Natl. Cancer Inst. 66(3):P559-P564.

McGregor, D.B., A. Brown, P. Cattanach, and I. Edwards. 1988. Responses of the L5178Y tk+/tk- mouse lymphoma cell forward mutation assay: III. 72 coded chemicals. Environ Mol Mutagen

12(1):85-154.

McManus, B.M., B. Toth, and K.D. Patil. 1987. Aortic rupture and aortic smooth muscle tumors in mice. Induction by p-hydrazinobenzoic acid hydrochloride of the cultivated mushroom Agaricus bisporus. Lab Invest 57(1):78-85.

Miller, E.C., A.B. Swanson, D.H. Phillips, T.L. Fletcher, A. Liem, and J.A. Miller. 1983. Structure-activity studies of the carcinogenicities in the mouse and rat of some naturally occurring and synthetic alkenylbenzene derivatives related to safrole and estragole. Cancer Res. 43(3):1124-1134.

Miller, T.A., and V.L. Salgado. 1985. The Pyrethroid insecticides. pp.43-97.

Mori, H., N. Yoshimi, H. Iwata, Y. Mori, A. Hara, T. Tanaka, and K. Kawai. 1990. Carcinogenicity of naturally occurring 1-hydroxyanthraquinone in rats: Induction of large bowel, liver and stomach neoplasms. Carcinogenesis 11(5):799-802.

Mori, H., S. Sugie, K. Niwa, M. Takahashi, and K. Kawai. 1985. Induction of intestinal tumours in rats by chrysazin. Br J. Cancer 52(5):781-3.

NTP (National Toxicology Program). 1982. NTP Technical Report on the Carcinogenesis Bioassay of Allyl Isothiocyanate in F344/N Rats and B6C3F$_1$ Mice. NTP Technical Report TR-81-36. Research Triangle Park, North Carolina and Bethesda, Maryland: National Toxicology Program.

NTP (National Toxicology Program). 1983. NTP Technical Report on the Carcinogenesis Studies of Eugenol in F344/N Rats and B6C3F$_1$ Mice. NTP Technical Report TR 223. Research Traingle Park, N.C.: National Toxicology Program.

NTP (National Toxicology Program). 1986b. NTP Technical Report on the Carcinogenesis Studies of Ethyl Acrylate in F344/N Rats and B6C3F$_1$ Mice. NTP Technical Report TR 259. Research Triangle Park, N.C.: National Toxicology Program.

NTP (National Toxicology Program). 1989. NTP Technical Report on Toxicology and Carcinogenesis Studies of 8-Methoxypsoralen in F344/N Rats. NTP Technical Report TR 359. Research Triangle Park, N.C.: National Toxicology Program.

NTP (National Toxicology Program). 1990. NTP Technical Report on

Toxicology and Carcinogenesis Studies of Furfural in F344/N Rats and B6C3F₁ Mice. NTP Technical Report TR 382. Research Triangle Park, N.C.: National Toxicology Program.

NTP (National Toxicology Program). 1990a. NTP Technical Report on Toxicology and Carcinogenesis Studies of Benzaldehyde in F344/N Rats and B6C3F₁ Mice. NTP Technical Report TR 378. Research Triangle Park, N.C.: National Toxicology Program.

NTP (National Toxicology Program). 1990b. NTP Technical Report on the Toxicology and Carcinogenesis Studies of d-Limonene in F344/N Rats and B6C3F₁ Mice. NTP Technical Report TR 347. Research Triangle Park, N.C.: National Toxicology Program.

NTP (National Toxicology Program). 1992. NTP Technical Report on the Toxicology and Carcinogenesis Studies of Quercetin in F344/N Rats. NTP Technical Report TR 409. Research Triangle Park, N.C.: National Toxicology Program.

Neal, J., and R.H. Rigdon. 1967. Gastric tumors in mice fed bezo(a)pyrene: A quantitative study. Tex. Rep. Biol. Med. 25(4):P553-P557.

Ohgaki, H., K. Kusama, N. Matsukura, K. Morino, H. Hasegawa, S. Sato, S. Takayama, and T. Sugimura. 1984. Carcinogenicity in mice of mutagenic compound, 2-amino-3-methylimidazo-(4,5-f)-quinoline, from broiled sardine, cooked beef and beef extracts. Carcinogenesis 5(7):921-924.

Ohgaki, H., H. Hasegawa, M. Suenaga, T. Kato, S. Sato, S. Takayama, and T. Sugimura. 1986. Induction of hepatocellular carcinoma and highly metastatic squamous cell carcinomas in the forestomach of mice by feeding 2-amino-3,4-dimethylimidazo[4,5-f]quinoline. Carcinogenesis 7(11):P1889-P1893.

Ohgaki, H., H. Hasegawa, M. Suenaga, S. Sato, S. Yakayama, and T. Sugimura. 1987. Carcinogenicity in mice of a mutagenic compound, 2-amino-3,8-dimethylimidazo[4,5-f]quinoxaline (MeIQx) from cooked foods. Carcinogenesis 8:665-668.

Pamukcu, A.M., S. Yalciner, J.F. Hatcher, and G.T. Bryan. 1980. Quercitin, a rat intestinal and bladder carcinogen present in bracken fern (Pteridium aquilinum). Cancer Res. 40:3468-3472.

Randerath, K., E. Randerath, H.P. Agrawal, R.C. Gupta, M.E. Schurdak, and M.V. Reddy. 1985. Postlabeling methods for carcinogen-DNA adduct analysis. Environ. Health Perspect. 62:P57-P65.

Snell, K.C. and H.L. Stewart. 1962. Pulmonary adenomatosis induced in DBA/2 mice by oral administration of debenz[a,h]anthracene. JNCI 28:1043.

Snell, K.C. and H.L. Stewart. 1963. Induction of pulmonary adenomatoses in DBA/2 mice by the oral administration of dibenz[a,h]anthracene. Acta Un Int Cancer 19:692-694.

Takayama, S., Y. Nakatsuru, M. Masuda, H. Ohgaki, S. Sato, and T. Sugimura. 1984. Demonstration of carcinogenicity in F-344 rats of 2 amino-3-methylimidazo-4 5-f quinoline from broiled sardine fried beef and beef extract. Gann 75(6):467-470.

Tamano, S., M. Hirose, H. Tanaka, E. Asakawa, K. Ogawa, and N. Ito. 1992. Forestomach neoplasm induction in F344/DuCrj rats and B6C3F1 mice exposed to sesamol. Jpn. J. Cancer Res. 83(12):P1279-P1285.

Tanaka, T., W.S. Barnes, G.M. Williams, and J.H. Weisburger. 1985. Multipotential carcinogenicity of the fried food mutagen 2 amino-3-methylimidazo-4 5-f-quinoline in rats. Jpn. J. Cancer Res. (Gann) 76(7):570-576.

Taylor, J.M., W.I. Jones, E.C. Hagan, M.A. Gross, D.A. Davis, and E.L. Cook. 1967. Toxicity of Oil of Calamus (Jammu Variety). Tox and App Pharm 10:405.

Toth, B, E. Rogan, and B. Walker. 1984. Tumorogenicity and mutagenicity studies with capsaicin of hot peppers. Anticancer Res. 4(3):117-9.

Toth, B., J.W. Smith, and K.D. Patil. 1981. Cancer induction in mice with acetaldehyde methylformylhydrazone of the false morel mushroom. J. Natl. Cancer Inst. 67(4):P881-P887.

Toth, B. 1986. Carcinogenesis by N2-[gamma-L(+)-glutamyl]-4-carboxyphenylhydrazine of Agaricus bisporus in mice. Anticancer Res. 6(5):917-20.

Wakabayashi, K., M. Nagao, H. Esumi, and T. Sugimura. 1992. Food-derived mutagens and carcinogens. Cancer Res. 52 (Suppl.):2092s-2098s.

Welsch, C.W., J.V. DeHoog, and D.H. O'Connor. 1988. Influence of caffeine consumption on carcinomatous and normal mammary gland development in mice. Cancer Res. 48(8):2078-82.

Wislocki, P.G., E.C. Miller, J.A. Miller, E.C. McCoy, and H.S. Rosenkranz. 1977. Carcinogenic and mutagenic activities of safrole, 1'-hydroxysafrole, and some known or possible metabolites. Cancer Res. 37(6):1883-1891.

Vesselinovitch, S.D., K.V. Rao, and N. Mihailovich. 1979. Transplacental and lactational carcinogenesis by safrole. Cancer Res. 39:4378-4380.

Appendix B

Agents with Potential Carcinogenic Activity and Their Occurrence in the Diet

This appendix is a compilation of all agents classified by IARC as known (1), probable (2A), or possible (2B) human carcinogens, or by the NTP as known or reasonably anticipated to be carcinogenic to humans. The appendix is subdivided into four tables in terms of dietary occurrence as follows:

- Table B-1: Agents That Might Be Encountered in U.S. Diets
- Table B-2: Agents Formerly Encountered in U.S. Diets
- Table B-3: Agents Rarely or Accidentally Encountered in U.S. Diets
- Table B-4: Agents Unlikely to Have Ever Been Present in U.S. Diets

CAVEATS AND DISCLAIMERS

The classification of these agents as potential carcinogens is based on epidemiological data in only 20% of the cases. In most cases, the classification is based on findings in high-dose animal experiments, usually conducted in more than one species. The IARC 2B classification typically signifies sufficient evidence of carcinogenicity from animal studies. Limited evidence in animals, without other highly suggestive data from human or mechanistic studies would not result in a 2B rating. The committee relied on IARC and NTP classifications of potential carcinogens as a means of obtaining a large set of agents of potential concern that have been systematically and rigorously evaluated by the same criteria.

The carcinogenic risk posed by a substance is a function of its exposure and potency, which in some cases can differ dramatically for different routes of exposure. Listings in this table should not be interpreted as indicating that the actual risk to humans is significant. In some cases, it is possible that there is no risk under the conditions of human exposure. Definitive conclusions regarding human risk are difficult to reach, as discussed in Chapter 5. The primary purpose of this table is to provide a collection of substances that form the basis for the risk comparisons made in Chapter 5.

For the majority of agents listed, the IARC monographs, FDA tabulations, NRC reports, and assistance from several groups provided enough information to unequivocally assign agents to one of the four tables. In a few cases, the assignment of agents to a given table was difficult (e.g., agents with past exposures, several dyes, drugs, and chemical intermediates). For example, before passage of the first Food and Drug Act of 1906, many unevaluated substances, many of them harmful, found their way into the food supply. Table B-2 (Agents Formerly Encountered in U.S. Diets), therefore, covers only the period since 1906. Even today, occurrences of exposure to trace levels of chemical intermediates and dyes used in food packaging are difficult to establish. A food packaging component often can be regarded as an indirect additive. A component is virtually never used in all types of packaging. Constituents that are used in the manufacture of food packaging components are generally present, if at all, as unwanted impurities, typically at very low levels. Also, veterinarians have considerable latitude in prescribing drugs in treating livestock and poultry. Thus, parallel problems are encountered with drug residues and with pesticide residues as well. The number of all these is large, and establishing exposure with any accuracy to a quantitatively minor substance in our complex food supply entails major problems of surveillance, sampling, and analysis.

Inadvertent accidental exposures can be difficult to anticipate or recognize. The PBB contamination of animal feed and resulting human exposure in Michigan is an obvious case that the committee noted. However, other cases suggest that our assessment of such exposures may be too limited, and thus the list in Table B-3 might well be inappropriately short. These include the use of phenobarbital to increase the metabolic elimination of chlordane in cattle feeding on contaminated pineapple leaves, illegal use of anabolic steroids in European meat production (Daeseleire, 1992), and related precautionary notes of Truhaut et al. (1985).

TD_{01} ESTIMATION

As indicated by the TD_{01} values listed, the carcinogenic activity of these substances spans at least eight orders of magnitude, and human exposures perhaps even a wider range, starting in some cases at infinitesimal levels. Thus, although TD_{01} values and related risk numbers present the appearance of accuracy, it is inappropriate in general to treat the results as providing for actual predicions of health risks.

TD_{01} values are derived from cancer potency or unit risk values available from U.S. EPA or Cal/EPA, using the approximation

$$TD_{01} = 0.01 \cdot q_{human}$$

where q_{human} is an upper bound estimate of the slope of the cancer dose-response curve in humans. In general, an upper confidence limit on the value q_{human} estimates was obtained by fitting the multistage model to dose-response data from animal cancer bioassays, thereby providing a lower confidence limit on the TD_{01}. This procedure included corrections for differences in pharmacokinetics at high and low doses, study length, and animal body size. Time-dependent forms of the multistage model were used for cases of poor survival in some study groups, provided sufficient data were available. In a few cases, the estimate of potency was derived directly from human data. For a large number of agents, potency was derived by systematically applying the data selection criteria of regulatory agents to the Canrcinogenic Potency Database (CPDB) of Gold and colleagues. These criteria have been described by Hoover et al. (1995) and Cal/EPA (1992) and are highlighted below:

- Data sets showing statistically significant dose-related increases in cancer incidence were used, unless the CPDB indicated that the authors considered the results unrelated to exposure to the carcinogen.
- Data sets were excluded from consideration if the end point was specified as all tumor bearing animals or combined unrelated tumors.
- When several studies were available, the highest quality study was selected. The quality of the study was judged on the basis of such factors as the numbers of animals, dose selection, duration, etc.
- Where there were multiple studies of similar quality conducted in the most sensitive species, the geometric mean of potencies derived from these studies was calculated. When both sexes of the same species/strain were tested under the same laboratory conditions, and no other adequate studies were available for that species, the data set for the more sensitive sex was selected.
- Potency was derived from data sets for malignant tumors, combined malignant and benign tumors, or tumors that would have likely progressed to malignancy.

In a few cases, the committee derived cancer potency values directly from bioassay data using the data selection criteria and techniques described above.

Table B-I. Agents[a] That Might Be Encountered in U.S. Diets

Agent	IARC Classification[b]	Occurrence[c]	TD01[d] (mg/kg·d)
A-alpha-C (2-Amino-9H-pyrido[2,3-b]indole)	2B	N: Derived (cooking)	2.50E-02
Acetaldehyde	2B	N: Constitutive, derived and added. Also S (synthesized for food additive use)	Carcinogenicity by oral route uncertain
Acrylamide	2A	S: Tap water; constituent of food packaging	2.22E-03
Acrylonitrile	2A	S: constituent of food packaging; pesticide	1.00E-02
Aflatoxins	1	N: Acquired (mycotoxin)	
Aflatoxin B1	1	N: Acquired (mycotoxin)	2.17E-04
Aflatoxin M1	2B	N: Acquired (mycotoxin)	
Alcoholic beverages	1	N and S	
p-Aminoazobenzene	2B	S: food color trace impurity	
4-Aminobiphenyl	1	S: food color impurity	4.76E-04
Amitrole	2B	S: pesticide	1.06E-02
Androgenic (anabolic) steroids	2A	N: Constitutive S: veterinary product and food residue	
Aramite	2B	S: pesticide	3.33E-01
Arsenic	1	N: Pass-through. Also, indirect additive from tap water and previously through pesticidal use	1.89E-03

Agent	IARC Classification[b]	Occurrence[c]	TD01[d] (mg/kg-d)
Asbestos	1	N: Added through tap water.	Carcinogenicity by oral route uncertain
Atrazine	2B	S: pesticide	
Benz(a)anthracene	2A	N: Derived (cooking)	5.00E-04
Benzene	1	N: Constitutive; derived (cooking); added (food packaging constituent, tap water)	1.00E-01
Benzidine	1	S: trace food color impurity	2.00E-05
Benzo(b)fluoranthene	2B	N: Derived (cooking); pass-through	5.56E-04
Benzo(j)fluoranthene	2B	N: Derived (cooking); pass-through	1.30E-03
Benzo(k)fluoranthene	2B	N: Derived (cooking); pass-through	
Benzo[a]pyrene	2A	N: Derived (cooking); pass-through	8.33E-04
Beryllium and beryllium compounds	2A	N: Pass-through and added (tap water)	
Betel quid with tobacco	1	N: Direct	
Bracken fern	2B	N: Direct; a food	
Bromodichloromethane	2B	S: In tap water; N: Present in marine microalgae (non-food occurrence)	7.69E-02
1,3-Butadiene	2A	S: Food packaging constituent	5.56E-03
Butylated hydroxyanisole	2B	S: Direct and indirect food additive	5.00E+01
Cadmium and cadmium compounds	1	N: Pass-through and added (tap water)	Carcinogenicity by oral route uncertain

Agent	Classification	Notes	Value
Caffeic acid	2B	N: Constitutive	5.88E-01
Captafol	2A	S: pesticide	6.67E-02
Carbon tetrachloride	2B	S: Pesticide; tap water contaminant	5.56E-02
Chlordane	2B	S: pesticide	7.69E-03
Chlordecone (Kepone)	2B	S: pesticide	6.25E-04
Chlorinated paraffins (Ave. chain length C12; approx. 60% chlorine by weight)	2B	S: General industrial use	1.12E-01
α-Chlorinated toluenes	2B	S:pesticides	3.23E-01
Chloroform	2B	S: insecticide; tap water contaminant	7.14E-02
3-Chloro-2-methylpropene		S: plastics and pesticides intermediate	
Chlorophenols	2B	S: general industrial use	
2,4,6-Trichlorophenol	2B	S: pesticide	1.43E-01
p-Chloro-o-toluidine and its strong acid salts	2A	S: pesticide	3.70E-02
Chromium (VI) compounds	1	N: Pass-through and added (tap water)	2.44E-01
Citrus Red No. 2	2B	S: orange skin colorant	
Cobalt and cobalt compounds	2B	N: Constitutive (essential in B12); pass through. Also indirect additive	
Coffee (urinary bladder)	2B	N: Traditional food beverage	
p-Cresidine	2B	S: food color intermediate	6.67E-02

Agent	IARC Classification[b]	Occurrence[c]	TDO1[d] (mg/kg-d)
Danthron (Chrysazin; 1,8-Dihydroxyanthraquinone)	2B	N: plant constituent drug; S: Synthesized for use as drug	1.32E-01
DDD		S: persistent lipophilic pesticide	2.94E-02
DDE		S: Metabolite of DDT	2.94E-02
DDT	2B	S: persistent lipophilic pesticide	2.94E-02
2,4-Diaminotoluene	2B	S: food packaging constituent	2.50E-03
Dibenz(a,h)acridine	2B	N: Derived (cooking)	
Dibenz(a,j)acridine	2B	N: Derived (cooking)	
Dibenz(a,h)anthracene	2A	N: Derived (cooking); pass through (plant uptake fuel combustion byproducts)	2.44E-03
7H-Dibenzo(c,g)carbazole	2B	N: Derived	1.32E-05
Dibenzo(a,e)pyrene	2B	N: Derived	
Dibenzo(a,h)pyrene	2B	N: Derived	3.23E-05
Dibenzo(a,i)pyrene	2B	N: Derived	3.45E-05
Dibenzo(a,l)pyrene	2B	N: Derived and added (tap water)	
1,2-Dibromo-3-chloropropane	2B	S: pesticide; persistent in groundwater	1.43E-03
p-Dichlorobenzene	2B	S: indirect additive (pesticide and other)	2.50E-01
1,2-Dichloroethane (Ethylene dichloride)	2B	S: pesticide fumigant; general industrial use	1.43E-01
Dichloromethane	2B	S: used in food processing; fumigant	7.14E-01

384

Agent	Classification	Use/source	Value
1,3-Dichloropropene	2B	S: soil fumigant	2.33E-01
Dichlorvos (DDVP)	2B	S: insecticide	3.45E-02
Di(2-ethylhexyl)phthalate	2B	S: plasticizer	1.19E+00
Diethylstilbesterol	1	S: growth promoter in cattle production	2.86E-05
Diethyl sulfate	2A	S: general industrial use	1.03E-02
Dimethylformamide	2B	S: food packaging constituent	
Dimethyl sulfate	2A	S: indirect food additive	7.69E-04
1,6-Dinitropyrene	2B	S: Diesel combustion; assume uptake by food plants	2.22E-04
1,8-Dinitropyrene	2B	S: Diesel combustion; assume uptake by food plants	1.32E-04
1,4-Dioxane	2B	S: food packaging constituent	3.70E-01
Epichlorohydrin	2A	S: food packaging constituent	1.25E-01
Estrogen, non-steroidal	1		
Estrogen, steroidal	1	N: Constitutive and added (drug residues) S: synthetic growth promoters	
Estradiol 17ß (and esters)	2B	N: Constitutive and added (drug residues)	2.56E-04
Estrone (and estrone benzoate)	(Steroidal estrogens, group 1; estrone - sufficient in animals)	N: Constitutive	

Agent	IARC Classification[b]	Occurrence[c]	TD01[d] (mg/kg-d)
Ethinyl estradiol	(Steroidal estrogens, group 1; ethinyl estradiol - sufficient in animals)	S: Added (meat residues)	
Ethyl acrylate	2B	N: Constitutive; S: Food packaging constituent; added flavoring ingredient	
Ethylene oxide	1	S: fumigant	3.23E-02
Ethylene thiourea	2B	S: pesticidal breakdown product	2.22E-01
Formaldehyde	2A	N: Derived and added (preservative in defoaming agent; in food packaging).	Carcinogenicity by oral route uncertain
Glu-P-1 (2-Amino-6-methyldipyrido[1,2-a:3',2'-d]-imidazole	2B	N: Derived (cooking)	2.08E-03
Glu-P-2 (2-Aminodipyrido[1,2-a:3',2'-d]-imidazole)	2B	N: Derived (cooking)	7.14E-03
Glycidaldehyde	2B	N: Derived	
Heptachlor	2B	S: pesticidal contaminant, in food chain	2.22E-03
Hexachlorobenzene	2B	S: pesticidal contaminant, in food chain	5.56E-03
Hexachlorocyclohexanes (HCH)	2B	S: pesticidal contaminant, in food chain	
alpha isomer	2B	S: pesticidal contaminant, in food chain	3.70E-03
beta isomer	3	S: pesticidal contaminant, in food chain	6.67E-03

386

gamma isomer	3	S: pesticidal contaminant, in food chain	9.09E-03
technical grade	2B	S: pesticidal contaminant, in food chain	2.50E-03
Hot mate (Ilex paraguariensis)	2A	N: Added	
Indeno(1,2,3-cd)pyrene	2B	N: Pass-through; derived	
Isoprene	2B	N: Constitutive	
IQ (2-Amino-3-methylimidazo[4,5-f]quinoline)	2A	N: Derived (cooking)	7.14E-03
Lead and lead compounds, inorganic	2B	N: Pass-through	
Me-A-alpha-C (2-Amino-3-methyl-9H-pyrido-[2,3-b]indole)	2B	N: Derived (cooking)	8.33E-03
Medroxyprogesterone acetate	2B	S	
MeIQ	2B	N: Derived (cooking)	4.76E-03
MeIQx	2B	N: Derived (cooking)	2.94E-03
Mestranol	(Steroidal estrogens, group 1; mestranol - sufficient in animals)	S: Estrogen steroid used in meat production	
5-Methoxypsoralen (in the presence of UVA)	2A	N: Constitutive	
8-Methoxypsoralen (xanthotoxin) plus UV radiation	1	N: Constitutive (excluding UV radiation)	

Agent	IARC Classification[b]	Occurrence[c]	TD01[d] (mg/kg-d)
5-Methylchrysene	2B	N: Pass-through (assume food plant uptake)	7.69E-05
Methylmercury compounds	2B	N: Derived	
N-Methyl-N'-nitro-N-nitrosoguanidine	2A	N: Derived	1.20E-03
Mirex	2B	S: pesticidal contaminant, in food chain	5.56E-04
5-(Morpholinomethyl)-3-[(5-nitrofurfurylidene-amino]-2-oxalolidione	2B	S: veterinary drug	2.56E-03
Nickel, metallic	2B	N: Pass-through	
Nickel compounds	1	N: Pass-through	
Nitrilotriacetic acid, and its salts	2B	S: Industrial use	1.89E+00
Nitrilotriacetic acid, trisodium salt monohydrate	(2B)	S: Industrial use	1.00E+00
6-Nitrochrysene	2B	S: byproduct of fuel combustion; assume uptake by food plants	2.50E-05
Nitrofen (technical grade)	2B	S: herbicide	1.22E-01
2-Nitrofluorene	2B	S: byproduct of diesel fuel combustion Assume deposition on food plants	1.28E-03
2-Nitropropane	2B	S: used in adhesives which contact food	3.70E-01

Chemical	Group	Notes	Value
1-Nitropyrene	2B	N: incomplete combustion detected in grilled chicken; S: in diesel and gasoline exhaust particulates	9.09E-03
4-Nitropyrene	2B	S: byproduct of fuel combustion; assume deposition on food plants	4.00E-04
N-Nitroso-N-dibutylamine	2B	N: Derived	9.09E-04
N-Nitrosodiethylamine	2A	N: Derived	2.78E-04
N-Nitrosodimethylamine	2A	N: Derived (also constitutive in plant not consumed in US)	6.25E-04
N-Nitrosodi-N-propylamine	2B	N: Derived; also S (pesticidal impurity)	1.43E-03
N-Nitrosomethylethylamine	2B	N: Derived	4.55E-04
N-Nitrosopiperidine	2B	N: Derived	1.06E-03
N-Nitrosopyrrolidine	2B	N: Derived	4.76E-03
N-Nitrososarcosine	2B	N: Derived	7.14E-02
Ochratoxin A	2B	N: Acquired (mycotoxin)	4.76E-04
Pentachlorophenol	2B	S: wood perservative and herbicide, in food chain	5.56E-01
Phenyl glycidyl ether	2B	S: Food-packaging constituent	7.14E-02
o-Phenylphenate, sodium	2B	S: fungicide	3.33E+00
PhIP (2-Amino-1-methyl-6-phenylimidazo[4,5-b]pyridine	2B	N: Derived (cooking)	2.00E-03
Pickled vegetables (traditional in China)	1	N and S	

Agent	IARC Classification[b]	Occurrence[c]	TD01[d] (mg/kg-d)
Polychlorinated biphenyls	2A	S: General industrial use, in food chain	1.30E-03
Polychlorinated biphenyls (> 60% chlorine by weight)	2A	S: General industrial use, in food chain	2.00E-03
Potassium bromate	2B	S: Flour bromination; low residue	2.04E-02
Progestins	2B	N: Constitutive S: synthetic hormones	
Progestrone		N: Constitutive and added (drug residues)	
Propylene oxide	2A	S: food product and package sterilant; used in food starch production	4.17E-02
Propylthiouracil	2B	S	1.00E-02
Radon and its decay products	1	N: Added through tap water	
Saccharin	2B	S: Non-nutritive sweetening agent; was used as preservative	7.69E+01
Safrole	2B	N: Constitutive and added	4.55E-02
Salted fish (Chinese style)	1	N: Direct; a food	
Silica, crystalline	2A	N: Added	Carcinogenicity by oral route uncertain
Sodium *o*-phenylphenate	2B	S: Fungicide and antibacterial agent	
Sterigmatocystin	2B	N: Acquired (mycotoxin)	2.86E-04
Styrene	2B	N: Constitutive and added; (S: food-packaging constituent)	
Styrene oxide	2A	S: food-packaging constituent	6.25E-02

			TD_{01}[d]
Sulfallate		S: herbicide	5.26E-02
Testosterone	2B (Androgenic steroid, group 2A; testosterone sufficient in animals)	N: constitutive and added (drug residue)	
Tetrachlorodibenzo-p-dioxin	2B	S: Widespread environmental contaminant in food chain	7.69E-08
Tetrachloroethylene	2B	S: General industrial use; contaminant of food and water	1.96E-01
Toluene diisocyanate	2B	S: Food-packaging constituent	2.56E-01
Toxaphene (polychlorinated camphenes)	2B	S: Pesticidal contaminant of food and water	8.33E-03
Toxins derived from *Fusarium moniliforme*	2B	N: Acquired (mycotoxin)	
Trp-P-1 (Tryptophan-P-1)	2B	N: Derived	3.85E-04
Trp-P-2 (Tryptophan-P-2)	2B	N: Derived	3.13E-03
Urethane (Ethyl carbamate)	2B	N: Derived	1.00E-02
Vinyl chloride	1	S: Food-packaging constituent	3.70E-03

[a] Agents identified by IARC as known (1), probable (2A), or possible (2B) human carcinogens or by the NTP as known or reasonably anticipated to be carcinogens (NTP K or NTP R, if the agent has not been classified as 1, 2A, or 2B by IARC).

[b] For definition of terms and overall evaluations, see Preamble, pp.28-29 (IARC 1993).

[c] Where possible, synthetic agents (S) are distinguished from naturally occurring (N) (as defined in Chapter 1). Naturally occurring agents are subclassified into constitutive, derived, acquired, or added (as defined in Chapters 1 and 2).

[d] TD_{01} is the chronic dose in mg/kg/day causing a 1% increase in tumors in experimental animals.

Table B-2. Agents[a] Previously but No Longer Encountered in U.S. Diets

Agent	IARC Classification[b]	Occurrence[c]	TD01[d] (mg/kg-d)
Benzyl violet 4B	2B	S:Was direct food color additive	5.00E-01
Carbon black extracts	2B	S: Use of food colorant 'channel black' disapproved in 1976. Note IARC listing of extracts, not carbon black	
Chloramphenicol	2A	N: Antibiotic, in soil. S: Synthetically produced antibiotic; meat residues.	
Chlorphenoxy herbicides	2B	S: All uses in food production cancelled by 1974.	
Diethylstilbesterol	1	S: growth promoter in cattle production	2.86E-05
Dihydrosafrole	2B	S: was food flavorant (35 years ago)	2.27E-01
4-Dimethylaminoazo-benzene	2B	S: Was food colorant in U.S. prior to 1918	2.17E-03
1,1-Dimethylhydrazine (UDMH)	2B	S: agricultural chemical breakdown product	3.57E-03
Ethylene dibromide	2A	S: was widely used fumigant. Currently a groundwater contaminant in a few locations	4.00E-02

393

Agent	IARC Classification[b]	Occurrence[c]	TD01[d] (mg/kg-d)
Methylthiouracil	2B	S: Was growth promoter in meat production (swine and sheep)	2.50E-02
N-[4-(5-Nitro-2-furyl)-2-thiazolyl]acetamide	2B	S: used in veterinary applications	6.67E-03
Oil Orange SS	2B	S: General food colorant until 1956	
Ponceau 3R	2B	S: Food color delisted in 1961	6.25E-01
Thiourea	2B	N: Indirect additive (was citrus fungicide, chemical intermediate for pesticide production); is constitutive for nonfood plants.	1.39E-01

[a] Agents identified by IARC as known (1), probable (2A), or possible (2B) human carcinogens or by the NTP as known or reasonably anticipated to be carcinogens (NTP K or NTP R, if the agent has not been classified as 1, 2A, or 2B by IARC).

[b] For definition of terms and overall evaluations, see Preamble, pp.28-29 (IARC 1993).

[c] Where possible, synthetic agents (S) are distinguished from naturally occurring (N) (as defined in Chapter 1). Naturally occurring agents are subclassified into constitutive, derived, acquired, or added (as defined in Chapters 1 and 2).

[d] The TD_{01} is the chronic dose in mg/kg/day causing a 1% increase in tumors in experimental animals. Values derived from epidemiologic data are indicated in bold face.

Table B-3. Agents[a] Rarely or Accidentally Encountered in U.S. Diets

Agent	IARC Classification[b]	Occurrence[c]	TD01[d] (mg/kg-d)
Acetamide	2B	N: Derived (constitutive in a non-food plant)	1.43E-01
Antimony trioxide	2B	N: metallic compound; uses include as glassware constituent	
Auramine	2B	S: may have been food dye in some countries	1.14E-02
p-Chloroaniline	2B	S: intermediate; pesticide degradant	
Cycasin	2B	N: Constitutive	
Danthron (Chrysazin; 1,8-Dihydroxyanthraquinone)	2B	N: plant constituent drug; S: synthesized for use as drug.	1.32E-01
Glasswool	2B	S: Use in food processing	
Hexamethylphosphor-amide	2B	S: General industrial use	1.61E-04
Methylazoxymethanol acetate	2B	N: Constitutive (of cycasin)	
4,4'-Methylenedianiline	2B	S: Indirect food additive through use as curing agent in resins used to coat large containers in alcoholic beverage production	6.25E-03
4,4'-Methylenedianiline dihydrochloride	(2B)	S: See cell above	8.33E-03

Agent	IARC Classification[b]	Occurrence[c]	TD01[d] (mg/kg·d)
N-Nitrosodiethanolamine	2B	S: Impurity in herbicide atrazine; contaminant in cutting fluids and some cosmetics	3.57E-03
N-Nitrosomethyl-vinylamine	2B	N: Derived	6.25E-05
N-Nitroso-N-methylurethane	2B	N: Derived	9.09E-05
Polybrominated biphenyls	2B	S: was flame retardant; now minimal and localized food chain contaminant	3.33E-04
Ponceau MX	2B	S: Was drug and cosmetic color in US; used as a food colorant elsewhere	2.22E+00
beta-Propiolactone	2B	S: Industrial use	7.14E-04
Reserpine	3	N: Indirectly added veterinary drug	9.09E-04
o-Toluidine	2B	S: Chemical intermediate (e.g., pesticides, dyes) ; N: constitutive	5.56E-02
o-Toluidine hydrochloride	(2B)	S	7.69E-02

[a] Agents identified by IARC as known (1), probable (2A), or possible (2B) human carcinogens or by the NTP as known or reasonably anticipated to be carcinogens (NTP K or NTP R, if the agent has not been classified as 1, 2A, or 2B by IARC).
[b] For definition of terms and overall evaluations, see Preamble, pp.28-29 (IARC 1993).
[c] Where possible, synthetic agents (S) are distinguished from naturally occurring (N) (as defined in Chapter 1). Naturally occurring agents are subclassified into constitutive, derived, acquired, or added (as defined in Chapters 1 and 2).
[d] The TD_{01} is the chronic dose in mg/kg/day causing a 1% increase in tumors in experimental animals.

Table B-4. Agents[a] Unlikely Ever to Have Been Present in U.S. Diets

Agent	IARC Classification[b]	Occurrence[c]	TD01[d] (mg/kg-d)
2-Acetylaminofluorene	(NTP R)	S: was intended for pesticidal use but never marketed	2.63E-03
Adriamycin	2A	N: Antibiotic; also S (synthesized for use)	
AF-2 (2-(2-furyl)-3(5-nitro-2-furyl)acrylamide]	2B	S: Food additive previously in Japan	4.17E-02
2-Aminoanthraquinone	3 (NTP R)	S: dye and pharmaceutical intermediate	3.03E-01
o-Aminoazotoluene	2B	S: dye	2.63E-03
1-Amino-2-methylanthraquinone	3 (NTP R)	S: dye intermediate	6.67E-02
2-Amino-5-(5-nitro-2-furyl)-1,3,4-thiadiazole	2B	S: drug	6.25E-04
o-Anisidine	2B	S: dye intermediate; water pollutant	7.14E-02
o-Anisidine hydrochloride	(2B)	S: dye intermediate	9.09E-02
Azaserine	2B	N: mycotoxin. S (synthesized) drug.	9.09E-04
Azacytidine	2A	N: antibiotic (drug)	
Azathioprine	1	S: drug	5.56E-03
Benzidine based dyes	2A	S: dyes	
Benzotrichloride	2B	S: Dye and herbicide intermediate	7.69E-04

Agent	IARC Classification[b]	Occurrence[c]	TD01[d] (mg/kg-d)
Bischloroethyl nitrosourea (BCNU)	2A	S: drug	2.17E-04
Bis(chloromethyl)ether	1	S: chemical intermediate	
Bischloromethyl methyl ether	1	S: chemical intermediate	
Bleomycins	2B	N: antibiotic; drug	
beta-Butyrolactone	2B	S: chemical intermediate	1.00E-02
Carrageenan, degraded	2B	S: Produced synthetically from seaweed.	
Ceramic fibres	2B	S: used in thermal insulation	
Chlorambucil	1	S: drug	2.27E-05
Chlorendic acid	2B	S: chemical intermediate	1.10E-01
Chlornaphazine	1	S: drug	
1-(2-Chloroethyl)-3-cyclohexyl-1-nitrosourea	2A	S: drug	
1-(2-Chloroethyl)-3-(4-methylcyclohexyl)-1-nitrosourea	1	S: drug	
Chloromethyl methyl ether (technical grade)	1	S: chemical intermediate	4.17E-03
4-Chloro-o-phenylenediamine	2B	S: dye intermediate	6.25E-01
Chlorozotocin	2A	S: drug	4.17E-05
C.I. Acid Red 114	2B	S: dye	
C.I. Basic Red 9 monohydrochloride	(NTP R)	S: dye	4.00E-02

Compound	Classification	Use/Notes	Value
C.I. Direct Blue 15	2B	S: dye	
Cisplatin	2A	S: drug	
Coal-tars	1	S: used in various pharmaceutical, cosmetic, and biocidal preparations	
Cupferron	(NTP R)	S: chemical reagent	4.55E-02
Cyclophosphamide (anhydrous)	1	S: drug	1.64E-02
Cyclophosphamide (hydrated)	1	S: drug	1.75E-02
Cyclosporin (Ciclosporin)	1	N: antibiotic. Drug.	
Dacarbazine	2B	S: drug	2.04E-04
Danthron (Chrysazin; 1,8-Dihydroxyanthraquinone)	2B	N: plant constituent drug. S: Synthesized for use as drug.	1.32E-01
Daunomycin	2B	N: antibiotic. drug.	
N,N'-Diacetylbenzidine	2B	S: dye intermediate	
2,4-Diaminoanisole	2B	S: dye intermediate	4.35E-01
2,4-Diaminoanisole sulfate	(2B)	S: dye intermediate	7.69E-01
4,4'-Diaminodiphenyl ether (4,4'-Oxydianiline)	2B	S: chemical intermediate	7.14E-02
3,3'-Dichlorobenzidine	2B	S: dye intermediate; curing agent	8.33E-03
3,3'-Dichlorobenzidine dihydrochloride	(2B)	S: dye intermediate; curing agent	
3,3'-Dichloro-4,4'-diaminodiphenyl ether	2B	S: may not be commercially used	
Diepoxybutane	2B	S: chemical intermediate, curing agent	
1,2-Diethylhydrazine	2B	S: an experimental rocket fuel	

Agent	IARC Classification[b]	Occurrence[c]	TD01[d] (mg/kg·d)
Diglycidyl resorcinol ether (DGRE)	2B	S: used as or in epoxy resins	5.88E-03
Diisopropyl sulfate	2B	S: chemical intermediate	
3,3'-Dimethoxybenzidine (o-Dianisidine)	2B	S: dye and chemical intermediate	2.04E-03
3,3'-Dimethoxybenzidine dihydrochloride	(2B)	S: dye and chemical intermediate	2.70E-03
trans-2-[(Dimethylamino)-methylimino]-5-[2-(5-nitro-2-furyl)vinyl]-1,3,4-oxadiazole	2B	S: possibly used in pharmaceutical	2.27E-02
2,6-Dimethylaniline (2,6-Xylidine)	2B	N: present in tobacco leaves; S: chemical intermediate	1.75E+00
3,3'-Dimethylbenzidine (o-Tolidine)	2B	S: dye intermediate	1.33E-04
3,3'-Dimethylbenzidine dihydrochloride	(2B)	S: dye intermediate	1.79E-04
Dimethylcarbamoyl chloride	2A	S: pesticide intermediate	7.69E-04
1,2-Dimethylhydrazine	2B	S: experimental rocket fuel	1.82E-05
Dimethylvinylchloride	(NTP R)	S: chemical intermediate	2.22E-01
Direct Black 38 (technical grade)	2A	S: dye	1.35E-03
Direct Blue 6 (technical grade)	2A	S: dye	1.35E-03
Direct Brown 95 (technical grade)	2A	S: dye	1.49E-03
Erionite	1	N: Natural zeolite	
Ethyl methanesulfonate	2B	S: No evidence of commercial use	

Chemical	Classification	Use	Value
Formaldehyde	2A	N: pyrolysis product S: many industrial uses	5.56E-01
2-(2-Formylhydrazino)-4-(5-nitro-2-furyl)thiazole	2B	S: No evidence of commercial use	4.35E-03
Griseofulvin	2B	N: antibiotic. S/N (acquired): occasional veterinary drug	7.14E-01
HC Blue 1	2B	S: in hair dyes	1.96E-01
Hydrazine	2B	S: rocket fuel	5.88E-04
Hydrazine sulfate	2B	S: used in metal refining	3.33E-03
Hydrazobenzene (1,2-Diphenylhydrazine)	3 (NTP - R)	S: colorant of waxes, resins, soaps, fats	1.15E-02
Iron dextran complex	2B	S: drug	
Lasiocarpine	2B	N: Acquired (contamination of cereal grains in Asia)	1.28E-03
Lead acetate	2B	S: general industrial uses. Was used in medicine and hair dyes	3.57E-02
Lead phosphate	2B	S: limited industrial use	
Lead subacetate	2B	S: analytical reagent. Astringent in lotions.	2.63E-01
Magenta (containing CI Basic Red 9)	2B	S: dye	
Melphalan	1	S: cancer drug	7.69E-05
Merphalan	2B	S: cancer drug	
2-Methylaziridine (Propyleneimine)	2B	S: chemical and pharmaceutical intermediate	3.85E-04

Agent	IARC Classification[b]	Occurrence[c]	TD01[d] (mg/kg-d)
4,4'-Methylene bis(2-chloroaniline)	2A	S: curing agent for polyurethane prepolymers	6.67E-03
4,4'-Methylene bis(N,N-dimethyl)benzeneamine	3 (NTP - R)	S: dye intermediate; antioxidant in grease and oil	2.17E-01
4,4'-Methylene bis(2-methylaniline)	2B	S: dye intermediate	1.09E-02
Methyl methanesulfonate	2B	S: commercial use unknown	1.01E-01
2-Methyl-1-nitroanthraquinone (of uncertain purity)	2B	S: dye intermediate	2.33E-03
Metronidazole	2B	S: human drug; some veterinary use.	5.00E-02
Michler's ketone	(NTP R)	S: dye intermediate	1.16E-02
Mitomycin C	2B	N: antibiotic	1.22E-06
Monocrotaline	2B	N: Constitutive in bush teas; not believed consumed in US	1.00E-03
MOPP and other combined chemotherapy including alkylating agents	1	S: cancer drug	
Mustard gas (sulfur mustard)	1	S: cancer drug	
Myleran (1,4-butanediol dimethylsulfonate)	1	S: cancer drug	
Nafenopin	2B	S: experimental drug	

402

2-Naphthylamine (beta-Naphthylamine)	1	N: pyrolysis product (will clarify). S: dye intermediate	5.56E-03
Niridazole	2B	S: drug	
5-Nitroacenaphthene	2B	S: dye intermediate not commercially used in US	7.69E-02
1-[(5-Nitrofurfurylidene)-amino]-2-imidazolidinone	2B	S: antibacterial agent, reported used to treat urinary tract infections	5.56E-03
Nitrogen mustard	2A	S: vesicant in chemical warfare. potential cancer drug.	
Nitrogen mustard hydrochloride	(NTP - R)	S: antineoplastic and immunosuppressant in human and veterinary medicine	
Nitrogen mustard N-oxide	2B	S: cancer drug and chemical sterilant	
N-Nitroso-N-ethylurea	2A	S: No known commercial use. Environmental occurrence unknown	3.70E-04
3-(N-Nitrosomethyl-amino)propionitrile	2B	N: Derived	
4-(N-Nitrosomethylamino)-1-(3-pyridyl)-1-butanone (NNK)	2B	N: Derived	
N-Nitroso-N-methylurea	2A	S: No known commercial use. Environmental occurrence unknown	8.33E-05
N-Nitrosomorpholine	2B	S: No evidence of commercial use. Impurity in methylene chloride and chloroform	1.49E-03
N'-Nitrosonornicotine	2B	N: Derived	7.14E-03

Agent	IARC Classification[b]	Occurrence[c]	TD01[d] (mg/kg-d)
Noresthisterone	2B	S: human drug	
Oxymethalone	(NTP R)	S: human drug	
Panfuran S (containing dihdroxymethyl-furatrizine)	2B	S: human drug	
Phenacetin	2A	S: human and veterinary analgesic and antipyretic	4.55E+00
Phenazopyridine	2B	S: human drug	5.88E-02
Phenazopyridine hydrochloride	2B	S: human drug	6.67E-02
Phenobarbital	2B	S: human and veterinary sedative and anticonvulsant	2.17E-02
Phenoxybenzamine	2B	S: human drug	3.23E-03
Phenoxybenzamine hydrochloride	2B	S: human drug	3.70E-03
Phenytoin	2B	human and veterinary anticonvulsant	
Procarbazine	(2A)	S: cancer drug	7.14E-04
Procarbazine hydrochloride	2A	S: cancer drug	8.33E-04
1,3-Propane sultone	2B	S: chemical intermediate	4.17E-03
Rockwool	2B	S: thermal and acoustic insulant	
Selenium sulfide	3 (NTP R)	S: topical drug in human and veterinary medicine	
Slagwool	2B	S: thermal and acoustic insulant	

Agent	Classification	Use	Value
Solar radiation	1	N	
Streptozotocin	2B	N: antibiotic	9.09E-05
Talc containing asbestiform fibres	1	N	
Tetranitromethane	(NTP R)	S: diesel and rocket fuel additive	7.69E-04
Thioacetamide	2B	S: previously used with mercury as mordant	1.64E-03
4,4'-Thiodianiline	2B	S: dye intermediate	6.67E-04
Thorium dioxide	(NTP K)	N: limited commercial use. was radio-opaque for x-ray imaging.	
Treosulfan	1	S: cancer drug	
Trichlormethine (Trimustine hydrochloride)	2B	S: cancer drug	
Tris(1-aziridinyl)phosphine sulfide (Thiotepa)	1	S: cancer drug	8.33E-04
Tris(2,3-dibromopropyl)phosphate	2A	S: flame retardant	4.35E-03
Trypan blue	2B	S: biological stain	
Ultraviolet radiation A	2A	N	
Ultraviolet radiation B	2A	N	
Ultraviolet radiation C	2A	N	
Uracil mustard	2B	S: cancer, immunosuppressive, antiviral and antibacterial drug	
Vinyl bromide	2A	S: general industrial use	1.85E-02

Agent	IARC Classification[b]	Occurrence[c]	TD01[d] (mg/kg·d)
4-Vinylcyclohexene	2B	S: Byproduct of chemical production processes	
4-Vinylcyclohexene diepoxide	2B	S: General industrial use	

[a] Agents identified by IARC as known (1), probable (2A), or possible (2B) human carcinogens or by the NTP as known or reasonably anticipated to be carcinogens (NTP K or NTP R, if the agent has not been classified as 1, 2A, or 2B by IARC).

[b] For definition of terms and overall evaluations, see Preamble, pp.28-29 (IARC 1993).

[c] Where possible, synthetic agents (S) are distinguished from naturally occurring (N) (as defined in Chapter 1). Naturally occurring agents are subclassified into constitutive, derived, acquired, or added (as defined in Chapters 1 and 2).

[d] The TD_{01} is the chronic dose in mg/kg/day causing a 1% increase in tumors in experimental animals.

Appendix C

Chemical Compounds Occurring in Dietary Plants that Have Been Reported to Inhibit Carcinogenesis in Vivo[a]

Class	Compound Name	Inducer	Species (Route[b])
Amino acid	Cysteine	1,2-Dimethylhydrazine	Mouse (po)
	(DL)-Tryptophan	Benzidine	Mouse (po)
Arylheptanoid	Curcumin	Methylazoxymethanol	Mouse (po)
		N-Methyl-N'nitroso-urea	Rat (po)
		Benzo(a)pyrene	Rat (po)
		TPA	Mouse (ext)
		TPA	Mouse (ip)
		20-Methylcholanthrene	Mouse (sc)
		DMBA + Croton oil	Mouse (ext)

Class	Compound Name	Inducer	Species (Route[b])
Benzenoid	Gingerol	Azoxymethane	Rat (po)
Carotenoid	Canthaxanthin	Benzo(a)pyrene DMBA	Mouse (po) rat (po)
Carotenoid	β-Carotenal, 8-Apo	Benzo(a)pyrene	Mouse (po)
	α-Carotene	Spontaneous liver CA	Mouse (po)
	β-Carotene	Benzo(a)pyrene N-methyl-N'-nitroso-urea DMN-OAC DMBA	Mouse (ext) Rat Hamster (po) Mouse (ext)
	Fucoxanthin	N-Ethyl-N'-Nitro-N-nitroso-guanidine	Mouse (po)
Coumarin	Aesculetin	DMBA	Rat (po)

408

	Compound		Model
	Coumarin	Benzo(a)pyrene	Mouse (po)
	Umbelliferone	Benzo(a)pyrene	Mouse (po)
Cyclitol	Myoinositol		Mouse (po)
	Phytic acid[c]	DMBA	Rabbit (po)
Diterpene	Cafestol	DMBA	Hamster (po)
	Cafestol Palmitate	DMBA	Rat (po)
	Kahweol	DMBA	Hamster (po)
Flavonoid	Amorphinospirone	TPA	Mouse (ext)
	Apigenin	DMBA/TPA	Mouse (ext)
	Myricetin	DMBA + Benzo(a)pyrene + TPA	Mouse

409

Class	Compound Name	Inducer	Species (Route[b])
	Quercetin[c]	Azoxymethanol	Mouse (po)
		DMBA	Rat (po)
		Teleocidin	Mouse (ext)
		Benzo(a)pyrene	Mouse (ext)
		Benzo(a)pyrene	Mouse (ip)
		Benzo(a)pyrene diol epoxide	Mouse (ip)
	Robinetin	Benzo(a)pyrene	Mouse (ext)
		Benzo(a)pyrene	Mouse (ip)
		Benzo(a)pyrene diol	Mouse (ip)
	Rutin	Azoxymethanol	Mouse (po)
Indole Alkaloid	Indole-3-carbinol	4-Nitroquinoline-1-oxide	Rat (po)
		Diethylnitrosamine + N-methylnitrosourea + N,N-dibutyl-nitrosamine	Rat (po)
		Spontaneous mammary tumors	Mouse (po)
Isoflavonoid	Biochanin A	Benzo(a)pyrone	Mouse (ip)

Lactone	α-Angelicalactone	Benzo(a)pyrene	Mouse (po)
Lignan	Sesamin	DMBA	Rat (po)
Monoterpene	Carveol	DMBA	Rat (po)
	Limonene[c]	DMBA	Rat (po)
		4-(Methylnitrosamino)-1-(3-pyridyl)-1-butanone	Rat (po)
		Same	Rat (ip)
		N-Ethyl-N-Hydroxy-nitrosamine	Rat (po)
	(-) Menthol	DMBA	Rat (po)
	para-Mentha-2-8-dien-1-ol	Benzo(a)pyrene	Mouse (po)

411

Class	Compound Name	Inducer	Species (Route)[b]
Organic acid	Fumaric acid	N-Methyl-N'-nitroso-urea	Hamster (po)
		N-Methyl-N-benzylnitroso-amine	Rat (po)
		N-Ethyl-N-nitrosurea	Rat (po)
		3'-Methyl-4-(Dimethyl-amino)azobenzene	Rat (po)
Phenolic acid	Gallic acid		Mouse (po)
	Protocatechuic acid	Azoxymethane	Rat (po)
Phenylpropanoid	Caffeic acid	4-Nitroquinoline-1-oxide	Rat (po)
		Benzo(a)pyrene	mouse (po)
	Chlorogenic acid	4-Nitroquinoline-1-oxide	Rat (po)
	Cinnamic acid, *ortho*-hydroxy	Benzo(a)pyrene	Mouse (po)
	Eugenol[c]	DMBA	Mouse (ext)

	Ferulic acid	4-Nitroquinoline-1-oxide	Rat (po)
		Benzo(a)pyrene	Mouse (po)
	Myristicin	Benzo(a)pyrene	Mouse (po)
	Myristicin, dihydro	Benzo(a)pyrene	Mouse (po)
Sesquiterpene	Nerolidol	Azoxymethane	Rat (po)
Sterol	Sitosterol	MNU	Rat (po)
Sulfur compound	Diallyldisulfide	DMBA or TPA	Mouse (ext)

413

Class	Compound Name	Inducer	Species (Route[b])
	Diallysulfide	Nitrosomethylbenzylamine	Rat (po)
		DMBA	Hamster (po)
		DMBA	Rat (po)
		DMBA or TPA	Mouse (ext)
		MNNG	Rat (po)
		1,2-Dimethylhydrazine	Mouse (po)
		Diethylnitrosamine	Pig (po)
		+ N-methylnitrosourea	
		+N,N-dibutylnitrosamine	
		N-Nitrosodiethylamine	Rat (ip)
		4-(Methylnitrosoamino)-1 butanone	Rat (ip)
		N-Nitrosodimethylamine	Rat (ip)
	Benzyl isothiocyanate	Diethylnitrosamine	Rat (po)
		Diethylnitrosamine	Mouse (po)
		Benzo(a)pyrene	Mouse (po)
		NNK	Mouse (po)
		4-(Methylnitrosamino)-1-(3-pyridyl)-1-butanone	Mouse (po)

Isothiocyanate, Phenethyl	4-(Methylnitrosamino)-1-(3-pyridyl)-1-butanone	Mouse (po)
	N-Nitrosomethylbenzyl-amine	Rat (po)
	Same	Mouse (po)
	NNK	Mouse (po)
Sinigrin	4-Nitroquinoline-1-oxide	Rat (po)
Ellagic acid	4-(methylnitrosamino)-1-(3-Pyridyl)-1-butanone	Mouse (po)
	4-Nitroquinoline-1-oxide	Rat (po)
	N-Nitrosobenzmethylamine	Rat (po)
	Azoxymethane	Rat (po)
	DMBA	Rat (po)
	Benzo(a)pyrene	Mouse (ext)
	Benzo(a)pyrene	Mouse (ip)
	Benzo(a)pyrene diol epoxide	Mouse (ext)
	Benzo(a)pyrene diol epoxide	Mouse (ip)
	3-Methylcholanthrene	Mouse (po)
Tannin		

Class	Compound Name	Inducer	Species (Route)[b]
	(-)-Epigallocatechin-3-gallate		Rodents
		X-ray	Mouse (po)
		Spontaneous liver tumors	Mouse (po)
		N-Ethyl-N'Nitro-N-nitrosoguanidine	Mouse (po)
		Nitrosamine-4-(methyl-nitrosamino)-1-(3-pyridyl)-1-butanone	Mouse (po)
	Tannic acid	DMBA + benzo(a)pyrene + TPA	Mouse
		Benzo(a)pyrene	Mouse (po)
Triterpene	Glycyrrhetinic acid	Teleocidin	Mouse (ext)
		Azoxymethane	Rat (po)
		Methylazoxymethane	Mouse (po)
		DMBA	Mouse (po)
		DMBA or TPA	Mouse (ext)
	Limonin	DMBA	Hamster (ext)

	Oleanolic acid	Azoxymethane	Rat (po)
		DMBA	Mouse (ext)
		TPA	Mouse (ext)
	Ursolic acid	DMBA	Mouse (ext)
		TPA	Mouse (ext)
Triterpene glycoside	Glycyrrhizin	DMBA	Mouse (po)
Xanthine Alkaloid	Caffeine[c]	Estradiol + progesterone	Mouse (po)
		Diethylstilbestrol	rat (ip)

[a]Data obtained from the NAPRALERT database of natural products. On-line access is available through the Scientific and Technical Network (STN) of Chemical Abstract Services. Data presented are intended to be illustrative but may not be complete.

[b]The following abbreviations are used to indicate route:

ext: external
po: oral, in diet or drinking water, sometimes gastric administration
ip: intraperitoneal
sc: subcutaneous

[c]Plant species containing this compound are listed in Appendix A.